Nursing Management of the Neurosurgical Patient

AN INTERPROFESSIONAL APPROACH

Nursing Management of the Neurosurgical Patient

AN INTERPROFESSIONAL APPROACH

NEWTON MEI, MD
Assistant Professor of Medicine
Assistant Director and Director of Education
Farber Hospitalist Service
Division of the Department of Neurological Surgery
Departments of Medicine and Neurological Surgery
Thomas Jefferson University
Philadelphia, Pennsylvania

LAUREN MALINOWSKI-FALK, MSN, BA, CRNP, AGACNP-BC
Nurse Practitioner
Farber Hospitalist Service
Division of the Department of Neurological Surgery
Departments of Medicine and Neurological Surgery
Thomas Jefferson University
Philadelphia, Pennsylvania

ALLISON M. LANG, MSN, CRNP, AGACNP-BC
Nurse Practitioner
Farber Hospitalist Service
Division of the Department of Neurological Surgery
Departments of Medicine and Neurological Surgery
Thomas Jefferson University
Philadelphia, Pennsylvania

JESSE EDWARDS, MD, FHM
Assistant Professor of Medicine
Farber Hospitalist Service
Division of the Department of Neurological Surgery
Departments of Medicine and Neurological Surgery
Thomas Jefferson University
Philadelphia, Pennsylvania

RENÉ DANIEL, MD, PhD, FACP, FHM
Associate Professor of Medicine and Neurological Surgery
Director, Farber Hospitalist Service
Division of the Department of Neurological Surgery
Departments of Medicine and Neurological Surgery
Thomas Jefferson University
Philadelphia, Pennsylvania

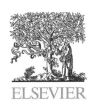

ELSEVIER

Elsevier
3251 Riverport Lane
St. Louis, Missouri 63043

NURSING MANAGEMENT OF THE NEUROSURGICAL PATIENT:
AN INTERPROFESSIONAL APPROACH   ISBN: 9780-323-93447-3

Executive Content Strategist: Lee Henderson
Content Development Specialist: Nicole Congleton
Publishing Services Manager: Deepthi Unni
Senior Project Manager: Manchu Mohan
Book Designer: Ryan Cook

Cover design by Russell Falk. Cover image from iStock.

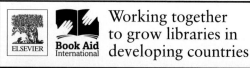

Printed in India
Last digit is the print number: 9   8   7   6   5   4   3   2   1

*To my mother, Winnie Tam Mei: My achievements and success
would not have been possible without you
To my beloved family and friends: Thank you for your unwavering
support and invigorating inspiration*

NM

*For my uncle Robert "Mario" Levito, who did not let his glioblastoma
stop him from dancing through life*

LMF

*To my father, Rick, and late mother, Rosie, who taught me to persevere.
I'll never forget the "5 Ps," Dad.*

AML

For Belén and the Mardlin family

JE

*To the unsung heroes of the Jefferson nursing staff,
who take care of neurosurgical patients with the highest degree of professionalism and
sacrifice*

RD

CONTRIBUTORS

Hadi Abou-Rass, BS, DO
Physician
Thomas Jefferson University
Philadelphia, Pennsylvania

Naomi Owusu Acheampong, MSN, CRNP
Neurology
Thomas Jefferson University
Philadelphia, Pennsylvania

Michael P. Baldassari, BA, MD
Resident Physician
Department of Neurosurgery
Thomas Jefferson University
Philadelphia, Pennsylvania

Johanna Beck, MD
Child & Adolescent Psychiatry Fellow
Psychiatry
Thomas Jefferson University
Philadelphia, Pennsylvania

Rebecca Belfonti, MSN, CRNP, AGACNP-BC, PCCN
Certified Registered Nurse Practitioner
Interventional Radiology
Thomas Jefferson University
Philadelphia, Pennsylvania

Carol Blyzniuk, BSN, RN
Department of Neurosurgery
Thomas Jefferson University
Philadelphia, Pennsylvania

Matthew Brown, MD
Assistant Professor
Department of Neurosurgery
Jefferson Health
Philadelphia, Pennsylvania

René Daniel, MD, PhD, FACP, FHM
Associate Professor of Medicine and
    Neurological Surgery
Director, Farber Hospitalist Service
Division of the Department of Neurological
    Surgery
Departments of Medicine and Neurological
    Surgery
Thomas Jefferson University
Philadelphia, Pennsylvania

Teresita Devera, MSN, RN, APN-BC
Nurse Practitioner
Functional Neurosurgery
Thomas Jefferson University
Philadelphia, Pennsylvania

Donyell Doram, BS, MD
Internal Medicine Attending
Neuroscience
Thomas Jefferson University
Philadelphia, Pennsylvania

Jesse Edwards, MD, FHM
Assistant Professor of Medicine
Farber Hospitalist Service
Division of the Department of Neurological
    Surgery
Departments of Medicine and Neurological
    Surgery
Thomas Jefferson University
Philadelphia, Pennsylvania

Christopher J. Farrell, MD
Associate Professor of Neurological Surgery
Neurological Surgery
Thomas Jefferson University
Philadelphia, Pennsylvania

Shannon Feldman, MSN, CRNP, AGACNP-BC
Acute Care Nurse Practitioner
Department of Neurosurgery
Thomas Jefferson University
Philadelphia, Pennsylvania

Renae Fisher, MD
Department of Rehabilitation Medicine
Thomas Jefferson University
Philadelphia, Pennsylvania

Monét A. Gambrel, BSN, RN
Registered Nurse
Department of Neurosurgery
Thomas Jefferson University
Philadelphia, Pennsylvania

Bharath Ganesh, MD, FACP
Clinical Instructor
Medicine and Neurological Surgery
Thomas Jefferson University
Philadelphia, Pennsylvania

Eric Gladstone, DO
Hospitalist
Departments of Hospital Medicine and
    Neurosurgery
Thomas Jefferson University
Philadelphia, Pennsylvania

Shelly Gupta, MD
Clinical Instructor
Department of Neurosurgery and Medicine
Thomas Jefferson University
Philadelphia, Pennsylvania

Kristin Gustafson, DO
Associate Professor
Rehabilitation Medicine
Sidney Kimmel Medical College
Thomas Jefferson University
Philadelphia, Pennsylvania

Ellina Hattar, MD
Resident Physician
Department of Neurosurgery
Thomas Jefferson University
Philadelphia, Pennsylvania

Kevin Hines, MD
Neurological Surgery
Thomas Jefferson University
Philadelphia, Pennsylvania

**Diane Ferrara Hoffman, MSN, RN, CRNP,
ACNP-BC, RNFA**
Nurse Practitioner, RN First Assistant
Department of Neurosurgery
Thomas Jefferson University
Philadelphia, Pennsylvania

Rebecca T. Hsu, BS, MD
Resident
Department of Neurology
Thomas Jefferson University
Philadelphia, Pennsylvania

Kelly Hufford, PT, DPT
Physical Therapist
Department of Rehabilitation Medicine
Thomas Jefferson University
Philadelphia, Pennsylvania;
Physical Therapist
Department of Rehabilitation Medicine
Main Line Health
Malvern, Pennsylvania

Liam P. Hughes, MD
Resident
Department of Neurosurgery
Johns Hopkins University
Baltimore, Maryland

Khadija Israel, MSW, LMSW
Silver School of Social Work
New York University
New York, New York

Rebecca Jonas, MD
Department of Neurological Surgery
Thomas Jefferson University
Philadelphia, Pennsylvania

Elise Lambertson, MSN, CRNP
Department of Neurology
Thomas Jefferson University
Philadelphia, Pennsylvania

Allison M. Lang, MSN, CRNP, AGACNP-BC
Nurse Practitioner
Farber Hospitalist Service
Division of the Department of Neurological
    Surgery
Departments of Medicine and Neurological
    Surgery
Thomas Jefferson University
Philadelphia, Pennsylvania

Anthony Joseph Macchiavelli, MD, SFHM, FACP
Clinical Assistant Professor of Vascular Medicine
Surgery
Jefferson Health
Philadelphia, Pennsylvania

Swathi Maddula, MD
Clinical Instructor
Hospital Medicine
Thomas Jefferson University
Philadelphia, Pennsylvania

**Lauren Malinowski-Falk, MSN, BA, CRNP,
AGACNP-BC**
Nurse Practitioner
Farber Hospitalist Service
Division of the Department of Neurological
    Surgery
Departments of Medicine and Neurological
    Surgery
Thomas Jefferson University
Philadelphia, Pennsylvania

Laura Esquivel Martinez, PhD Candidate, LMSW
Silver School of Social Work
New York University
New York, New York;
Social Worker
Outpatient Care Managment
Mount Sinai
New York, New York

Newton Mei, MD
Assistant Professor of Medicine
Assistant Director and Director of Education
Farber Hospitalist Service
Division of the Department of Neurological
    Surgery
Departments of Medicine and Neurological
    Surgery
Thomas Jefferson University
Philadelphia, Pennsylvania

Nikolaos Mouchtouris, MD
Department of Neurosurgery
Thomas Jefferson University
Philadelphia, Pennsylvania

Mina Na, DO
Spinal Cord Injury Medicine Fellow
Physical Medicine and Rehabilitation
Thomas Jefferson University
Philadelphia, Pennsylvania

Aniket Natekar, MD, MSc
Department of Neurology
Ohio Health
Columbus, Ohio

Dina G. Orapallo, MSN, AGACNP-BC
Vascular Medicine
Thomas Jefferson University
Philadelphia, Pennsylvania

Grace Pae, MSN, CRNP
Department of Medicine
Thomas Jefferson University
Philadelphia, Pennsylvania

Crystal Pak, BSN, MSN, CRNP
Department of Neurosurgery
Thomas Jefferson University
Philadelphia, Pennsylvania

Alexandra Pisani, BSN, RN, SCRN
Registered Nurse
Thomas Jefferson University
Philadelphia, Pennsylvania

Malissa Pynes, MD
Department of Neurology
Thomas Jefferson University
Philadelphia, Pennsylvania

Lauren Alice Robinson, MSN, AGACNP-BC, CCRN
Advanced Practice Provider
Surgical Critical Care Services
Penn Medicine;
Endocrinology Advanced Practice Provider
Endocrinology, Diabetes, and Metabolic Diseases
Jefferson University Physicians
Philadelphia, Pennsylvania

Madeline Schuler, BSN, RN, SCRN
Registered Nurse
Nursing
Thomas Jefferson University
Philadelphia, Pennsylvania

Ashwini Sharan, MD
Professor of Neurosurgery and Neurology
Department of Neurosurgery
Sidney Kimmel Medical College
Thomas Jefferson University
Philadelphia, Pennsylvania

Laura Sweeney, MSN, CRNP, FNP, AGACNP, CNRN
Nurse Practitioner
Department of Neurosurgery
Thomas Jefferson University
Philadelphia, Pennsylvania

Victor S. Wang, MD
Resident Physician
Department of Neurology
Thomas Jefferson University
Philadelphia, Pennsylvania

Heather Lynn Yenser, MSN
Nurse Practitioner
Vascular Medicine
Thomas Jefferson University
Philadelphia, Pennsylvania

Jinah Yoo, MSN, AGPCNP-BC, CWOCN
Nurse Practitioner
Department of Urology
Thomas Jefferson University
Philadelphia, Pennsylvania

Yichao Ethan Zhao, MD, MSc
Neurohospitalist
Internal Medicine
Thomas Jefferson University
Philadelphia, Pennsylvania

David Hernán Aguirre-Padilla, MD, PhD(c)
Assistant Professor; Stereotactic & Functional
    Neurosurgeon; Director, Neuromodulation
    and Functional Neurosurgery Program
Faculty of Medicine, Department of
    Neurosurgery—Center Campus
University of Chile;
San-Borja Arriarán Clinical Hospital
Santiago de Chile, Chile

Jennifer Coyle, MSN, RN, SCRN
Clinical Practice Leader
Jefferson Health
Philadelphia, Pennsylvania

Jessica Dawe, MD, FRCPC
Neurologist
Valley Regional Hospital
Kentville, Nova Scotia, Canada

Parneet Grewal, MD
Physician
Medical University of South Carolina
Charleston, South Carolina

Stephanie Hittle, MSN, RN, AGACNP-BC
Nurse Practitioner
Erlanger Health System
Chattanooga, Tennessee

Michael Karsy, MD, PhD, MSc
Neurosurgeon
Assistant Professor, Neurosurgery
Global Neurosciences Institute
Drexel University College of Medicine
Philadelphia, Pennsylvania

Olivia McSpedon, MSN, RN
Nurse Educator, ASU/INICU
Jefferson Hospital for Neuroscience
Philadelphia, Pennsylvania

Elanagan Nagarajan, MD
Assistant Professor of Neurology
UT College of Medicine, Chattanooga
Erlanger Health System
Chattanooga, Tennessee

Lucas Rodrigues de Souza, MD, MSc
Neurosurgeon
Hospital das Clínicas da Universidade
    Federal de Minas Gerais
CEO/Medical director
Instituto Mineiro de Neurocirurgia e
    Acupuntura
Belo Horizonte, MG, Brazil

Ellen Smith, MSN, RN-BC, PCCN-K
Clinical Practice Leader
Thomas Jefferson University Hospital
Philadelphia, Pennsylvania

PREFACE

Neurosurgical patients have complex medical, surgical, and psychosocial needs. Interdisciplinary management is essential for the successful care of neurosurgical patients—with nurses at the forefront. This handbook provides a framework of care for these patients. Anyone who provides care and helps manage neurosurgical patients will find the information in this book practical, straightforward, easy to understand, and easy to apply in practice.

This handbook is divided into six sections and comprises 33 chapters. This format aims to capture the journey of a neurosurgical patient, starting with preoperative care, followed by surgery and inpatient postoperative management of common medical issues and complications, and concluding with discharge to rehabilitation units. Diagrams, flowcharts, and illustrations are included throughout each chapter to help readers understand the care and treatment of each condition. Furthermore, each chapter ends with a clinical vignette and questions to demonstrate how the key points of each chapter apply to clinical scenarios.

- **Section 1** outlines the components of a thorough neurologic exam and the medical assessment necessary for surgery to proceed. As stressed in the handbook, establishing a baseline neurologic examination and ensuring medical optimization preoperatively can help the care team prevent and detect complications that may arise during the patient's hospitalization.
- **Sections 2 and 3** discuss neurologic ailments and common surgical procedures for the brain and spine. Topics for the brain include strokes, tumors, brain bleeds, headaches, and encephalitis. Topics for the spine include spinal cord injuries, elective spinal cord surgeries, cord compression, spinal infections, and spinal cord stimulators.
- **Section 4** discusses management of the common medical complications that occur in hospitalized neurosurgical patients. These topics include diabetes, acute kidney injury, venous thromboembolism, airway management, anemia, thrombocytopenia, constipation, ileus, nutrition, wound care, and postoperative fever.
- **Section 5** covers techniques to achieve adequate pain management in neurosurgical patients with complex, often multifaceted needs. This section also explains the role of a social worker in addressing substance abuse and addiction to ensure seamless transition out of the hospital and compliance with care.
- **Section 6** illustrates the essential role of a physical therapist in establishing safe and effective postacute care.

This handbook represents our commitment to providing the most thorough care to neurosurgical patients regardless of discipline. This book was a collaborative effort by nurses, nurse practitioners, social workers, physical therapists, and physicians and surgeons, with the common goal of providing optimal patient care. Providing the best clinical care results in the best clinical outcomes. We wish nothing but success for health care workers and speedy recoveries for patients suffering from neurologic ailments. We draw our inspiration for this textbook from the nurses at Thomas Jefferson University Hospital, who take care of neurosurgical patients with the highest degree of professionalism and dedication.

CONTENTS

xi

SECTION 4 **Medical Management of Common Neurosurgical Issues**

SECTION 5 **Complex Issues in Pain Management and Substance Abuse**

SECTION 6 **Posthospitalization Care**

Nursing Management of the Neurosurgical Patient

AN INTERPROFESSIONAL APPROACH

Introduction to Neurosurgery and Medical Management

CHAPTER 1

Preoperative Assessment and Perioperative Bedside Management

Rebecca Jonas, MD ■ René Daniel, MD, PhD, FACP, FHM

Introduction

Before a patient undergoes surgery, providers should complete a thorough preoperative assessment. There are two main objectives when performing a preoperative risk evaluation. The first is to give the surgeons and anesthesiologists insight into the patient's risk for experiencing a heart attack or a stroke in the perioperative period. This analysis evaluates the patient's acute cardiac symptoms, severity of the patient's overall condition, and chronic medical problems. Although past medical history cannot be changed, understanding the patient's chronic comorbidities is important for determining the surgical risk profile and empowering well-informed discussions with the patient and family. The second objective involves optimizing the patient for surgery. This aspect of preoperative care focuses on the treatment of acute medical problems with the intention of improving patient outcomes and minimizing surgical complications.

Pre- and postoperative management is integral to the work performed by nurses who care for neurosurgical patients. Perioperative care encompasses an extensive scope of clinical topics, broadly sharing principles of preoperative risk assessment and mitigation, along with the prevention and management of postoperative complications. Neurosurgical nurses must be familiar with the initial steps of management when postoperative complications arise and feel confident implementing treatment plans in collaboration with the interprofessional care team.

History

Every preoperative assessment includes a medical history and physical exam aimed at establishing an accurate understanding of the patient's risk for adverse perioperative events. The objective is to evaluate the risk of cardiovascular events and other complications that may occur during the perioperative period. This comprehensive assessment includes a history of present illness, past medical history, family history, surgical history, social history, medication history, allergies, and a review of systems (Box 1.1).[1-3]

Physical Exam

A detailed preoperative physical exam should focus on identifying signs of cardiac disease and fluid overload.[1-3]

- Abnormal heart sounds may indicate valvular disease or heart failure.
- Irregular pulses or rapid heart rate may be a sign of an underlying arrhythmia.
- Wheezes in the lungs may signal an acute or chronic lung disease; crackles can be heard when there is fluid overload.

BOX 1.1 ■ Medical History Questions Pertinent to Risk Stratification

Past Medical History

- Does the patient have heart disease? Is the patient being followed by a cardiologist?
- If the patient has had a heart attack in the past, how long ago?
- Does the patient have an abnormal heart rhythm?
- Does the patient have diabetes that requires insulin use?
- Has the patient had a stroke in the past?
- Does the patient have heart failure?
- Does the patient have kidney disease?
- Does the patient have lung disease? Or obstructive sleep apnea?
  - These will be of concern to the anesthesiologist, especially if general anesthesia is used.

Previous Surgeries

- Has the patient had surgeries in the past?
  - If so, were there complications?
- Did the patient tolerate anesthesia well?
- Did the patient have any problems with prolonged bleeding?

Family History

- Did anyone in the patient's family have a heart attack in their 40s?
- Did anyone in the patient's family pass away while driving or swimming?
- Are there bleeding disorders in the patient's family?

Social History

- Does the patient smoke? How long ago did the patient quit?
  - If the patient quit <8 weeks ago, nicotine patches may be appropriate.
- Does the patient use any recreational drugs?
- Does the patient drink alcohol? How much?

Medications

- Does the patient take insulin?
  - If so, the dose will need to be adjusted the day before surgery.
- Does the patient take an ACE inhibitor or ARB?
  - If the patient has any hemodynamic, renal, or electrolyte abnormalities, then these medications need to be held on the day of surgery because they affect how the kidney reacts to fluid shifts and are associated with intraoperative hypotension. However, if no such abnormalities exist and the patient is stable, under some circumstances it may be permissible to continue these medications.[1]
- Does the patient take a thiazide or diuretic?
  - These may need to be held on the day of surgery because they affect how the kidney responds to fluid shifts.
- Does the patient take steroids?
  - Depending on the dose and length of time taking steroids, the patient may require additional steroid supplementation to avoid hypotension perioperatively.
- Does the patient take anticoagulation medicine?
  - These will need to be held to avoid bleeding during and after surgery.
- Does the patient take antiplatelet medicine?
  - These will need to be held to avoid bleeding during and after surgery.

Allergies

- Does the patient have a penicillin allergy?
  - Often, patients are given perioperative antibiotics to avoid infection; thus knowing about an allergy is important.

ACE, Angiotensin-converting enzyme; *ARB,* angiotensin receptor blocker.

- Leg swelling can be seen with heart failure or deep vein thrombosis.
- Distended neck veins may indicate heart failure.
- Excessive skin bruising or petechiae can be warning signs of a bleeding disorder.

Lab Work

Extensive lab workup is not necessary for all patients preoperatively, but in the hospital setting and for patients with multiple medical concerns comprehensive testing may be pursued. For example, based on American Academy of Family Physicians and American College of Cardiology (ACC) guidelines, only patients with a suspected coagulopathy need coagulation labs.[1-3] Because blood loss and large fluid shifts can cause instability during surgery, labs that provide insight into kidney function, swelling, coagulation, and blood counts are often requested prior to surgery. Any abnormalities in platelet count, hemoglobin, or coagulation labs should be corrected according to evidence-based goals prior to surgery to minimize complications. The commonly ordered labs are as follows:

- Prothrombin time/partial thromboplastin time/international normalized ratio: Used to screen for appropriate coagulation function, especially in the surgical setting, as abnormal values can indicate an increased risk of bleeding.
  - If found to be abnormal prior to surgery, medical management may be indicated to ensure surgically safe levels are achieved and maintained.
- Basic metabolic panel: Used to assess kidney function and electrolyte concentrations.
  - An increased creatinine level may indicate kidney disease, which is a risk factor for perioperative cardiovascular events and an increased risk for kidney failure postoperatively.
- Complete blood count: Used to assess hemoglobin level and platelet count to ensure proper perfusion and coagulation.
- Type and screen: Nurses should check to ensure one is active on file before surgery in case a blood product transfusion is needed.
- Blood glucose: These levels are tracked and trended in patients with diabetes to ensure the patient is at goal range, as an increased blood glucose impairs wound healing.

Preoperative Risk Assessment

Sometimes patients require additional cardiac workup with stress testing or cardiac catheterization prior to surgery. These decisions follow an algorithm from the 2014 ACC guidelines on preoperative risk assessment.[1] This algorithm is designed to guide providers when deciding if a patient should be referred for further cardiac testing. This algorithm considers multiple components of a patient's presentation, symptoms, and history.

Assessing Acute Symptoms

Acute symptoms of heart disease are used to determine whether a cardiac workup is needed. A patient who experiences chest pain, tightness, or discomfort during exercise should raise the clinical care team's concern for uncontrolled heart disease. Patients with intermittent palpitations or unexpected syncopal episodes may have an underlying arrhythmia. Patients who demonstrate these symptoms should be asked more questions and an electrocardiogram (ECG) should be obtained. A guideline and an algorithm from Feely et al.[3] can be used to help providers determine if an ECG would be helpful.

Other important considerations include asking patients about orthopnea, paroxysmal nocturnal dyspnea (shortness of breath while sleeping that causes the patient to awaken), and dyspnea on exertion. Any of these symptoms, coupled with lower extremity swelling in the morning, are signs of heart failure and should prompt an echocardiogram, especially if the patient has clinical evidence of fluid overload on exam.

Surgeries are categorized as low, intermediate, or high risk based on the amount of hemodynamic stress a surgery generates for the patient.[4] The level of risk for heart attack and death associated with the procedure is incorporated into the patient's overall risk profile.

Calculating Patient Risk

Patients themselves are also categorized as low, intermediate, or high risk for surgery. That designation is determined by a score derived from information gleaned from the history, physical exam, and lab work. There are several different surgical risk calculators commonly used during a preoperative risk assessment. These include the Gupta perioperative risk index, cardiovascular risk index, revised cardiac risk index (RCRI), and National Surgical Quality Improvement Program risk calculator.[5]

The Gupta and RCRI are commonly used in the inpatient setting and estimate a patient's risk of suffering a heart attack postoperatively. The RCRI is a validated risk score that is broadly utilized due to its sensitivity and simplicity. The RCRI scoring system incorporates the patient's history of coronary artery disease, congestive heart failure, chronic kidney disease when creatinine is >2 mg/dL, treatment of diabetes with insulin, and any history of ischemic stroke. These surgical and medical components contribute to an aggregated score that categorizes the patient's level of risk and estimates the chance of a heart attack or death within 30 days after the surgery.[5]

Metabolic Equivalents

Another helpful tool that providers use to assess a patient's cardiac health is measuring metabolic equivalents (METs).[4] METs are a measure of the energy consumption required for a particular task, and they act as a surrogate marker for how much exercise a patient can tolerate. Here, exercise is used as a proxy for how well a patient's body can tolerate the stress of surgery. If a patient is regularly active, this is an indicator that the patient's heart can handle a particular level of stress. However, a patient who is sedentary, frail, does not exercise, or does not know whether angina occurs with exercise-like activity may require further cardiac evaluation prior to elective surgery. On the other hand, if a patient has comorbidities that present a higher risk for surgery, but the patient can perform vigorous exercise daily without any symptoms of angina, heart failure, or arrhythmia, then that patient would not need additional cardiac workup prior to surgery.

If METs are >4 and there are no other contraindications to surgery, the patient can proceed with surgery. An example of an activity constituting 4 METs is climbing a full flight of stairs. If METs are <4, then the patient may benefit from additional cardiac workup.[1,4]

Postoperative Management

A patient's risk for surgical complications persists in the days following surgery, and different precautions should be taken by the medical team to ensure a smooth postoperative period. A patient remains at risk for heart attack following a procedure and should be monitored for signs and symptoms of ischemia.[6] Nurses should monitor for the most common complications, as described below.

HEART ATTACK

Patients remain at risk after surgery.[6] Often heart attacks will be silent, meaning that the patient does not experience any symptoms. Nurses should be vigilant for complaints of chest tightness, pain, heaviness, and changes in the cardiac features recorded by the telemetry monitor. Nurses should proactively get an ECG and make the care team aware of any concerns with an abnormal change on the telemetry strip.

DELIRIUM

This is common after anesthesia, especially if the patient does not quickly metabolize the anesthetic. Nurses should orient the patient frequently, ensure sleep-wake cycles are consistent, and minimize nighttime disturbances. Medication may be necessary depending on the severity of the delirium.[7]

ASPIRATION

Sometimes a patient has trouble swallowing after surgery due to the process of intubation and extubation needed for general anesthesia. Additionally, a patient may experience delirium after anesthesia. Each of these side effects places the patient at increased risk for aspiration.[8] Nurses should ensure the head of the bed is elevated, aspiration precautions are implemented, and the patient is well positioned, especially when eating, drinking, or taking oral medications. Nurses should observe the patient when swallowing food, fluid, and medications by mouth to ensure the patient is not aspirating or choking. If there is evidence of impaired swallowing function, the nurse or provider team should consult speech-language pathology specialists to conduct a formal bedside swallow assessment and suggest a modified-consistency diet, as needed.

PNEUMONIA

Decreased mobility and postoperative pain can predispose a patient to shallow breathing and atelectasis, thereby putting the patient at risk for pneumonia.[9] A patient should have adequate postoperative pain control to enable mobilization out of bed and participation in physical therapy assessments. Incentive spirometry is critical for preventing atelectasis. Proper use should be taught and encouraged as soon as possible during the perioperative period.

URINARY RETENTION AND URINARY TRACT INFECTION

An indwelling urinary catheter is placed during most surgical procedures. Opioid medications can make it difficult for the patient to urinate postoperatively, but early mobilization and regular stooling will help the patient pass a voiding trial once the catheter has been removed. Indwelling urinary catheters should be removed as soon as possible postoperatively to allow a voiding trial and reduce the risk of developing a catheter-associated urinary tract infection.[10]

POSTOPERATIVE ILEUS AND CONSTIPATION

Nurses should be cognizant of whether the patient is stooling or passing flatus after surgery, and concerns for constipation or ileus should be reported to the provider. Abdominal distention, discomfort, nausea, vomiting, lack of appetite, and inability to pass flatus or stool could be signs of constipation, fecal impaction, or ileus and should be escalated to the physician team. If an ileus is present, bowel rest and intravenous fluids are indicated. Additionally, the medical team may need to place a nasogastric tube. Electrolytes should be closely monitored.[11]

Conclusion

Pre- and postoperative management is integral to the work performed by nurses who care for neurosurgical patients. Preoperative risk assessments are completed by the medical team, but it is important for nurses to understand its purpose and components so that they can partner effectively in the process. Nurses are the frontline caretakers during the perioperative period, and recognizing the signs and symptoms of postoperative complications is essential to protecting patients from adverse outcomes.

References

1. Fleisher LA, Fleischmann KE, Auerbach AD, et al. 2014 ACC/AHA guideline on perioperative cardiovascular evaluation and management of patients undergoing noncardiac surgery: executive summary: a report of the American College of Cardiology/American Heart Association Task Force on Practice Guidelines. *Circulation.* 2014;130(24):2215–2245.
2. King MS. Preoperative evaluation. *Am Fam Physician.* 2000;62(2):387–396.
3. Feely MA, Collins CS, Daniels PR, et al. Preoperative testing before noncardiac surgery: guidelines and recommendations. *Am Fam Physician.* 2013;87(6):414–418.
4. Holt NF. Perioperative cardiac risk reduction. *Am Fam Physician.* 2012;85(3):239–246.
5. Cohn SL, Ros NF. Comparison of 4 cardiac risk calculators in predicting postoperative cardiac complications after noncardiac operations. *Am J Cardiol.* 2018;121(1):125–130.
6. Duceppe E, Parlow J, MacDonald P, et al. Canadian Cardiovascular Society guidelines on perioperative cardiac risk assessment and management for patients who undergo noncardiac surgery. *Can J Cardiol.* 2017;33(1):17–32.
7. Marcantonio ER, Goldman L, Mangione CM, et al. A clinical prediction rule for delirium after elective noncardiac surgery. *JAMA.* 1994;271(2):134–139.
8. Studer P, Räber G, Ott D, et al. Risk factors for fatal outcome in surgical patient with postoperative aspiration pneumonia. *Int J Surg.* 2016;27:21–25.
9. Arozullah AM, Conde MV, Lawrence VA. Preoperative evaluation for postoperative pulmonary complications. *Med Clin North Am.* 2003;87(1):153–173.
10. Jackson J, Davies P, Leggett N, et al. Systematic review of interventions for the prevention and treatment of postoperative urinary retention. *BJS Open.* 2018;3(1):11–23.
11. Schwenk ES, Grant AE, Torjman MC, et al. The efficacy of peripheral opioid antagonists in opioid-induced constipation and postoperative ileus: a systematic review of the literature. *Reg Anesth Pain Med.* 2017;42(6):767–777.

Questions

1. Which of the following is an example of exercise requiring 4 METs?
   a. Walking around the house
   b. Climbing a full flight of stairs
   c. Heavy housework
   d. Heavy yardwork

2. Which of the following includes an example of a low-, medium-, and high-risk surgery (in that order)?
   a. Carotid endarterectomy, endovascular cerebral aneurysm repair, liver transplant
   b. Skull base tumor resection, cataract removal, femoral bypass
   c. Hysterectomy, transurethral resection of the prostate, colonoscopy
   d. Knee replacement, lumbar decompression/fusion, exploratory laparotomy
   e. Breast surgery, abdominal hernia repair, open aortic dissection repair

3. A patient presents for elective surgery without any signs or symptoms of cardiac disease. Which of the following are indications for a preoperative ECG in this patient? (Select all that apply.)
   a. High-risk surgery
   b. Low-risk surgery
   c. Intermediate-risk surgery with at least one RCRI risk factor
   d. Intermediate-risk surgery with no RCRI risk factors

4. Which of these symptoms should prompt further cardiac workup, including echocardiogram? (Select all that apply.)
   a. Orthopnea after running a half marathon
   b. Syncope with concern for underlying cardiac dysrhythmia
   c. Dyspnea on exertion after walking one flight of steps
   d. Fatigue after 8 hours of yardwork
   e. Known varicose veins

5. Common postoperative complications include which of the following? (Select all that apply.)
   a. Heart attack
   b. Urinary tract infection
   c. Pneumonia
   d. Aspiration
   e. Ileus

Answers

1. b

2. e

3. a, c

4. b, c

5. a, b, c, d, e

CHAPTER 2

Nursing Approach to the Neurologic Exam

Rebecca T. Hsu, BS, MD

Introduction

The purpose of the neurologic exam is to ascertain which part of the nervous system might be affected when a neurologic disorder is suspected. Mastering the neurologic exam is integral to catching neurologic emergencies at their onset and monitoring a patient's progress over time through serial exams. Nurses and providers can use the neurologic exam to differentiate and localize lesions of various parts of the brain, including the supratentorial brain (cortex), infratentorial brain (cerebellum, brainstem), spinal cord, peripheral nerves, neuromuscular junction, and muscles. When combined with a thorough history, the neurologic exam is a valuable clinical tool for identifying genuine neurologic emergencies. Furthermore, it can be used to distinguish functional neurologic disorders or malingering from true neurologic pathology.

Outline of the Neurologic Exam

The neurologic exam consists of the following key elements:
- Mental status
- Cranial nerves
- Motor function
- Reflexes
- Coordination
- Sensory
- Gait

Mental Status[1,2]

A. Level of alertness, attention, and cooperation
   - Is the patient awake and alert when providers enter the exam room? Does the patient require auditory or tactile stimulation to awaken? Does the patient fall asleep during the exam? Is the patient cooperative?
      - If a patient is not awake or alert, the degree of stimuli required to wake the patient should be documented.
   - To test concentration, ask the patient to spell *world* forward and backward, count backward from 100 serially by 7s (100, 93, 86, 79, etc.), or name the months of the year backward.
B. Orientation
   - Ask for the patient's full name, location, and date, and the reason for being in the hospital.

- The shorthand for orientation is "alert and oriented" (AAO). When a patient is AAOx3, it is assumed the patient can state their name, location, and date without difficulty. AAOx4 implies that the patient is also situationally aware of the reason for being in the hospital.
- When a patient is AAOx1 or AAOx2, documentation of their exact response is warranted to help track any improvement or decline in exam.

C. Memory
  - There are three components to the memory test: immediate memory, delayed memory, and remote memory.
    - To test recent and delayed memory, give the patient three unrelated words to remember (e.g., *pen, banana, sky*). If the patient can recall the three words immediately, then immediate recall is grossly intact. If the patient can recall the words after 5 minutes, then delayed recall is intact.
    - If a family or friend is nearby, then test remote memory by asking the patient to recall life details that can be corroborated by the visitor, such as date of anniversary, number of children, number of siblings, etc.

D. Language
  - Note the patient's capacity for spontaneous speech.
  - Naming: Ask the patient to name at least three objects.
    - Inability to name or produce spontaneous speech may indicate expressive aphasia, which is caused by damage to an area of the brain called Broca's area, located in the frontal lobe of the dominant hemisphere (usually the left hemisphere).
  - Repetition: Ask the patient to repeat a sentence.
  - Comprehension: Can the patient follow one-step commands (e.g., "Give me a thumbs up with your right hand")? Can the patient follow two-step commands (e.g., "Touch your right ear with your left hand and point to the door")?
    - Ability to produce fluent speech without being able to understand instructions may indicate receptive aphasia, which is caused by damage to an area of the brain called Wernicke's area, located in the temporal lobe of the dominant hemisphere.

Other parts of the mental status exam can be noted or completed in special circumstances. Without having to perform specific exam maneuvers, providers can always take note of the patient's ability to think logically or whether the patient is having any delusions. Impairments in math calculations, inability to recognize fingers, right-left confusion, and inability to write can be caused by damage to the dominant parietal lobe (usually the left parietal lobe).[3] If the patient does not respond to people who are positioned on a particular side of the visual field, this could indicate visual loss or neglect, usually caused by a parietal lesion in the nondominant side (usually the right parietal lobe).[1] Lastly, a patient with lesions in the frontal lobe or language area can have apraxia, which is the inability to follow a motor command or perform daily tasks even when comprehension is intact. To test this, the patient should be asked to perform an imaginary action (e.g., "Pretend to comb your hair"). A patient with apraxia will understand the command but have a hard time carrying it out.

Cranial Nerves

Cranial nerves (CN) are nerves that arise directly from the brain. They control motor functions of the head down to the shoulder, as well as sensation of the face down to the throat. Humans have 12 cranial nerves. Detecting dysfunction in the cranial nerves can help localize a lesion and aid in diagnosis.[4]

A. Olfactory nerve (CN 1) is usually not tested, but it can be noted if the patient is unable to smell.

B. Visual acuity and visual field (CN 2)

- Color vision: Ask the patient to name the color of objects in the room.
- Visual fields: Cover each eye individually and have the patient stare at the examiner's nose. In each visual field quadrant (upper left, upper right, lower left, lower right), the examiner should flash a number using fingers and ask the patient to state the number. Alternatively, the examiner can wiggle the fingers in each visual field quadrant and ask the patient to call out or point every time the wiggling fingers are visible.

C. Pupillary response (CN 2, 3)
- The normal size of a pupil is generally between 2 and 3 mm in the light, 4 and 5 mm initially in the dark, and 6 and 7 mm after settling in the dark for 1 minute. The average difference between pupillary sizes is rarely >0.8 mm.[5]
- Look for a direct response to light (constriction of the pupil being illuminated) and for a consensual response to light (constriction of the opposite pupil).

D. Extraocular movements (CN 3, 4, 6)
- Ask the patient to move the eyes in all directions while keeping the head still. Ask the patient to report any double vision. If reporting double vision, then the patient should cover one eye.
  - If the double vision resolves after one eye is covered, the patient has binocular diplopia.
  - If double vision persists after one eye is covered, the patient has monocular diplopia.
  - If applicable, document which eye movements worsen the double vision.
- Nystagmus is a rhythmic, involuntary, rapid movement of the eyes. Horizontal nystagmus from testing extraocular movements at the extreme is physiologic, meaning that it can be found in healthy individuals.
  - Physiologic nystagmus is fatigable, meaning that it will stop with persistent end gaze. Any persistent, vertical, or direction-changing nystagmus may be concerning and should be documented.[6]

E. Facial sensation and muscles of mastication (CN 5)
- Test sensation in the forehead, cheek, and jaw, and ensure that the sensation is the same on both sides of the face.
  - Division I of CN 5 (V_1), the ophthalmic division, innervates the scalp, forehead, and upper eyelid.
  - Division II of CN 5 (V_2), the maxillary division, innervates the lower eyelid, cheek, and upper lip/teeth.
  - Division III of CN 5 (V_3), the mandibular division, innervates the chin, jaw, lower lip, mouth, and lower teeth/gums.

F. Muscles of facial expression (CN 7)
- Ask patients to raise the eyebrows, squeeze the eyes shut, puff out the cheeks, and smile.
  - Upper motor neuron lesions, such as stroke or brain mass, cause contralateral facial weakness that spares the forehead.
  - Lower motor neuron lesions, such as Bell palsy, cause weakness involving the whole ipsilateral face.

  Lower motor neuron facial weakness does not warrant a stroke alert, whereas a new upper motor neuron facial weakness does.

G. Hearing (CN 8)
- Rub your fingers together by the patient's ear to assess if the patient hears equally well on both sides.

H. Palate elevation and gag reflex (CN 9, 10)
- When the patient says "Ahh," check to see if the palate rises symmetrically and if the uvula is midline.

I. Muscles of articulation (CN 5, 7, 9, 10, 12)
- Assess the quality of a patient's speech. (Is it hoarse, quiet, low or high pitched, or slurred?)

TABLE 2.1 ■ **Medical Research Council Manual Muscle Testing Scale: Most Common Method of Evaluating Muscle**

Grading (out of 5)	Interpretation
0	No contraction
1	Muscle flicker but no movement
2	Movement possible, but not against gravity
3	Movement possible against gravity, but not against resistance
4	Movement possible against some resistance by the examiner (sometimes this category is subdivided into 4–/5, 4/5, and 4+/5)
5	Normal strength

   J. Sternocleidomastoid and trapezius muscles (CN 11)
       ■ This can be tested by asking patients to shrug the shoulders against force or turn the head with force.
           ■ The sternocleidomastoid muscles turn the head contralaterally (e.g., the right sternocleidomastoid muscle turns the head to the left).
   K. Tongue muscles (CN 12)
       ■ Assess for tongue deviation: Ask the patient to stick out the tongue.
       ■ Assess for tongue weakness: Ask the patient to move the tongue from side to side.

Motor Function

   A. Observation
       ■ Describe any involuntary movements, tremors, unusually slow movements (bradykinesia), or any muscle wasting.
   B. Evaluate muscle tone
       ■ Ask the patient to fully relax while you move the patient's limbs and joints to get a sense of rigidity or spasticity (passive muscle examination).
           ■ Rigidity is stiffness that is consistent throughout the movement of the joint regardless of how fast you move the limb (velocity independent).
           ■ Spasticity is stiffness that emerges with fast velocity movements (velocity dependent).
   C. Grading strength of individual muscle groups (Table 2.1)
   D. Pronator drift
       ■ Ask the patient to hold the arms straight ahead with palms up and close the eyes for 10 seconds. Subtle weakness can manifest as an arm rotating inward, known as pronator drift, or dropping downward. Loss of proprioception can manifest by an arm drifting upward.

Reflexes

   A. Deep tendon reflexes (Fig. 2.1)
       ■ Check brachioradialis, brachial, and triceps reflexes in the upper extremities.
       ■ Check patellar and Achilles tendon reflexes in the lower extremities.
       ■ Grade each reflex (Table 2.2).
   B. Pathologic reflexes: If a patient has brisk or overreactive reflexes, check for pathologic reflexes. Presence of these reflexes points to upper motor neuron lesions, such as lesions in the spinal cord or brain. Lesions in the peripheral nerves, neuromuscular junction, and muscles alone will not lead to increased reflexes.

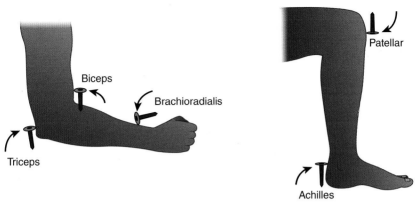

Fig. 2.1 Locations for common deep tendon reflexes.

- Hoffmann reflex: To check for this, hold the patient's hand by the third finger. Flick down on the nail of the third finger. If the first and second fingers contract (or make a C shape), this is a positive Hoffmann reflex.
- Of the population, 0.3–3% have a positive Hoffmann reflex without upper motor neuron injury.[1,7]
- Babinski reflex is also easy to check: Use a tool to scrape the bottom of the foot from the base of the lateral side to the top and medially across (Fig. 2.2). An upgoing toe is a positive Babinski sign.
- A positive Babinski reflex is seen in adults with an upper motor neuron injury.[1,7]

Coordination

The main function of a coordination exam is to test the cerebellum. Ataxia describes abnormal movements in cerebellar disorders.[1,8]

A. Dysmetria. Dysmetria is a discoordination of movement that leads to overshooting (past-pointing) or undershooting with target-oriented movements. Dysmetria can be tested by the following actions:
- Finger-to-nose test: The examiner should hold the pointer finger an arm's length away. Ask the patient to touch the nose with the index finger, then touch the examiner's index finger, going back and forth as rapidly as possible. Perform this test on both arms.
- Heel-to-shin test: Ask the patient to slide the heel from the opposite knee down along the shin and back up to the knee. Perform this test on both sides.

TABLE 2.2 ■ **Grading Scale for Reflexes**

Grade	Interpretation
0	Absent reflex
1+	Trace
2+	Normal
3+	Brisk
4+	Nonsustained clonus (repetitive vibratory movements visible on forced flexion of the wrist or ankle)
5+	Sustained clonus

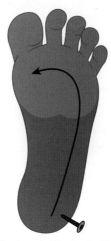

Fig. 2.2   Checking for the Babinski reflex involves stroking the foot from the lower lateral corner to the top and medially across the top.

B. Dysdiadochokinesia. Dysdiadochokinesia is a term describing abnormal alternating movements. Test the coordination of rapid alternating movements by asking the patient to hold one hand palm up while using the other hand to tap the stationary hand, alternating between the palm and the dorsum of the hand. Repeat this test on both hands.

Sensory

The sensory exam tests the body's response to different sensory modalities, including light touch, pain, temperature, vibration, and joint position awareness. Different patterns and locations of sensory loss can pinpoint damage to corresponding parts of the nervous system. Often, unilateral sensory loss is caused by damage in the contralateral brainstem, thalamus, or cortex. Loss of pain and temperature sensation suggests a small-fiber neuropathy. Loss of light touch, vibration, and joint position sensation indicates a large-fiber neuropathy. A "sensory level"—characterized by the bilateral loss of sensation to all modalities below a distinct level—points to a spinal cord lesion.

During each part of the sensory modality exam both distal and proximal aspects of the limbs should be tested. The following are modalities that can be tested as part of the sensory exam[1,9,10]:

A. Light touch: This is tested with a tissue, cotton-tipped swab, or light finger touch.

B. Pain: This can be tested with a needle tip, safety pin, or broken tongue depressor. Ask the patient if the sensation feels sharp or dull. Feeling dullness in response to a sharp tip represents decreased pain sensation.

C. Temperature: This can be tested with a cool piece of metal such as a tuning fork.

D. Vibration: This can be tested with a vibrating tuning fork over a joint, such as a finger or toe joint. Ask the patient to report when the vibration stops. If there is loss of vibration sensation in a distal joint, ascend to a more proximal joint until the patient reports intact sensation.

E. Joint position sense: This should be tested on the toes and fingers first. Take the most distal part of the big toe and move it up or down. Ask the patient to close the eyes and identify whether the joint is being moved up or down. Repeat this process for the most distal finger joint of any finger. If the patient cannot identify the joint's position (i.e., up or down) with eyes closed, then move to a more proximal joint such as the ankle or wrist until the patient can identify the movements correctly.

F. Romberg test: Ask the patient to stand with feet together, then close the eyes. Observe the patient's overall stability of position, and be cautious if the patient begins to fall. This test should not be performed if the patient already has significant instability while standing and cannot control balance even with the eyes open.

Gait

Observe as the patient walks around the room or down the hall. Note the following:
  A. Stance: How far apart are the feet? A wide-based stance and gait can indicate cerebellar disease.
  B. Posture: Is the patient standing straight or stooped?
  C. Stability: Is the patient stable on the feet? Does the patient sway?
  D. Gait: Does the patient lift the feet off the floor? Do the legs swing normally? Are the legs stiff? Do the arms swing?
  E. Turns: Does the patient take more steps to make turns?
  F. Tandem gait: Ask the patient to walk in a straight line, heel to toe, as if walking on a tightrope. A patient with truncal ataxia, which is caused by damage in the cerebellum, will have difficulty with tandem gait. Truncal ataxia presents with a wide-based and unsteady gait.[1]

Abbreviated/Screening Exams

Often neuroscience nurses will not have time to perform a comprehensive neurologic exam, and an abbreviated exam is more practical in many instances. Nurses should be sure to include the following key components when conducting a brief neurologic exam:
  A. Alertness and orientation: Test orientation, insight into illness, and language abilities.
  B. Cranial nerves: Observe size of pupils, reaction to light, visual acuity, movement of eyes, and facial symmetry.
  C. Strength: Examine outstretched hands for signs of pronation or downward drift; the examiner asks the patient to grip the hand for assessment of general flexion muscles (e.g., "Pull me toward you") and general extensor muscles (e.g., "Push me away"). The examiner asks the patient to lift each leg, one at a time, while providing resistance.
  D. Reflexes: Test biceps, brachioradialis, triceps, patellar, and Achilles reflexes.
  E. Sensation: Test either light touch, vibration sense, or position sense (carried by large-fiber nerves) in addition to either pinprick or temperature sensation (carried by small-fiber nerves).
  F. Coordination: Test finger-to-nose and heel-to-shin movements.
  G. Gait: Observe for gait instability.

Coma Exam

Coma is defined as unresponsiveness that is unarousable. Although a detailed mental status exam, including orientation and language, cannot be assessed in comatose patients, other parts of the neurologic exam are integral to assessing the extent of neurologic injury and monitoring progression or improvement of disease.[1,2]
  A. Observation: Observe for signs of cranial trauma, nuchal rigidity, evidence of systemic illness, and evidence of drug use (needle marks, alcohol on breath).
  B. Mental status: Determine the patient's Glasgow Coma Scale score (Table 2.3).
  C. Brainstem reflexes
     ▪ Pupillary light reflex (CN 2, 3): Most of the time, toxic or metabolic causes of coma are associated with normal size and reactive pupils. Blown pupils or pupils that are unresponsive to light can indicate a transtentorial herniation, which is when brain structures shift downward due to excessive pressure buildup.
     ▪ Vision (CN 2): Test by blink to threat. The examiner approaches each visual field quadrant (upper right, upper left, lower right, lower left) with a hand, one eye at a time. If the patient does not respond with a blink when the examiner's hand approaches each visual

TABLE 2.3 ■ **Glasgow Coma Scale (GCS) Used to Score Level of Alertness**

Eye Response		Motor Response		Verbal Response	
Eye opens spontaneously	4	Obeys commands	6	Oriented	5
Eye opens to verbal command	3	Localizes to pain	5	Confused	4
Eye opens to pain	2	Withdraws from pain	4	Inappropriate words	3
No eye opening	1	Flexion response to pain	3	Incomprehensible sounds	2
		Extension response to pain	2	No verbal response	1
		No motor response	1		

A GCS score of ≥13 indicates mild brain injury, 9–12 indicates moderate brain injury, and ≤8 indicates severe brain injury. For further details, visit https://www.glasgowcomascale.org.

quadrant, document this by stating "no blink to threat in each visual field." A patient with a stroke may lose the same visual field quadrant(s) in each eye, whereas a patient with disease in the eye itself will have visual loss only in the corresponding eye.

- Corneal reflex (CN 5, 7): Elicit the corneal reflex by using either a saline bullet (or saline flush) or gauze. Drop saline into each eye and observe if the patient blinks. Alternatively, use a small gauze to gently dab the cornea of each eye. A positive corneal reflex is a blink in response to stimulation of the cornea.
- Oculocephalic maneuver (CN 8): Hold the patient's eyes open and turn the head rapidly from side to side. A patient with an intact oculocephalic reflex will keep the eyes fixated on one spot, whereas an impaired oculocephalic reflex means that the eyes move with the head. This maneuver should not be performed in patients with suspected spinal cord injury.
- Facial symmetry (CN 7): Make note of facial symmetry.
- Gag reflex (CN 9, 10): Gag reflex can be tested by using an oral suctioning tool to suction the back of a patient's throat.
- Cough reflex (CN 9, 10): Cough reflex can be tested using the inline suctioning of an endotracheal tube.

D. Sensory and motor exam: Observe whether there are spontaneous movements. If a patient is comatose, sensory and motor exams are performed at the same time by testing a patient's response to a painful stimulus. Noxious stimuli are applied centrally and peripherally.

- Examples of central noxious stimuli include eliciting the gag and cough reflexes, squeezing the trapezius muscle, sternal rubbing, or pinching skin on the torso.
- Examples of peripheral noxious stimuli include pinching skin on the limbs or applying pressure to the nailbed (the area between the nail and the cuticle) using an object such as a marker/pen.
- If the patient grimaces, then sensation to noxious stimuli is intact in that limb.

The best response a patient can give to a noxious stimulus is to localize the stimulus (i.e., using a limb to attempt to remove the noxious stimulus). A patient can also withdraw, briskly or sluggishly, from the stimulus. In cases of severe brain damage, posturing movements, such as flexor posturing of the arm or extensor posturing, may be observed.

To distinguish posturing from withdrawal, sustain the noxious stimulus. In a withdrawal movement, the patient will attempt to move the limb away from the noxious stimulus. In a posturing movement, no matter where you provide noxious stimuli on the same limb, the patient will exhibit the same movement even if it means moving toward the noxious stimulus.

E. Reflexes
- Deep tendon reflexes
- Plantar reflexes (Babinski)

■ Triple flexion is a reflex seen with brain injuries. It is a spinal reflex that can manifest even in the context of brain death. Triple flexion describes flexion of the hip, knee, and dorsiflexion of the ankle in response to stimulation in the feet. Applying deep pressure to the nailbed of the toe can cause brisk flexion of the hip, knee, and ankle in both withdrawal and triple flexion. Therefore, to distinguish triple flexion from withdrawal, continue to apply deep pressure to the nailbed. In a triple flexion response, the patient's leg will relax into the noxious stimulus within a few seconds. In a withdrawal response, the patient will maintain the flexed position to pull the limb away from the noxious stimulus.

When Functional Neurologic Disorder or Malingering Is Suspected

Psychiatric disorders that subconsciously generate neurologic deficits are also known as functional neurologic disorders.[11] These include:

■ Conversion disorder: A psychiatric illness that causes the patient to have sensory or motor deficits without a focal lesion in the nervous system. Patients with conversion disorder are not feigning their symptoms, and these symptoms can cause significant distress.

■ Somatization disorder: An excessive worry about having one or more serious physical illnesses, manifested by having multiple unexplained symptoms in various body systems. Like conversion disorder, somatization disorder is thought to be associated with traumatic events often occurring in childhood.

There are also psychiatric disorders in which neurologic deficits are consciously generated:

■ Factitious disorder (Munchausen syndrome): This mental illness is characterized as conscious simulation of an illness for the primary purpose of assuming the role of the patient.

■ Malingering: This mental illness is characterized as conscious simulation of an illness for a secondary gain, such as receiving opioid medications, obtaining disability benefits, or evading legal repercussions.

Although extensive testing is sometimes unavoidable when evaluating neurologic deficits that ultimately are caused by psychiatric disorders, there are bedside exam maneuvers that can help differentiate a psychiatric disorder from an organic neurologic disease.[1,12,13] These include:

■ Hand-dropping: If you hold up the hand of a truly comatose patient above the patient's face, the hand will drop straight down when released, even striking the patient's own face in the process. In contrast, most patients who have at least some level of awareness will protect their face, and their arm will swing away when dropped.

■ Giveaway resistance: In true weakness, a patient will exhibit the same degree of weakness throughout a full motion. In psychogenic neurologic disease, strength testing will display variable resistance (i.e., giveaway weakness).

■ Hoover test: In a patient who demonstrates hip extension weakness, keep a hand under the heel of both legs and ask the patient to raise the nonaffected leg with full effort. If the patient can push down with the weak leg more than exhibited during focused testing, this is a positive Hoover sign and indicates that the patient was not giving a best effort during the focused exam. Another way to use the Hoover test is to test hip flexion in the weak leg while keeping a hand under the good heel. If the unaffected leg is not pushing downward into the examiner's hand while the weak leg is being raised, this demonstrates poor effort and signifies a positive Hoover sign.

■ Midline splitting of vibration sense: Vibration is readily conducted through the bone to the contralateral side on the sternum or skull, so splitting of the vibration on one side of the sternum or the forehead is nonphysiologic. When someone has true sensory loss on one side of the body—such as due to a brain or spinal lesion—vibration sense on the forehead or on the sternum should feel equal on both sides.

Conclusion

The neurologic exam is an important tool for determining whether a neurologic disease should be suspected, where a lesion in the neurologic system might be located, when emergency protocols should be activated, and whether someone may have a psychiatric illness leading to neurologic deficits. Nurses play a fundamental role in detecting changes in a patient's neurologic exam and promptly notifying the interprofessional team of their findings can save patients from greater harm. Mastering the neurologic exam is integral to catching neurologic emergencies at their onset and monitoring a patient's progress over time.

References

1. Blumenfeld H. *Neuroanatomy Through Clinical Cases*. 2nd ed. Sinauer Associates; 2018.
2. Posner JB, Plum F, Saper CB, et al. *Plum and Posner's Diagnosis of Stupor and Coma*. Oxford University Press; 2007.
3. Ardila A. Gerstmann syndrome. *Curr Neurol Neurosci Rep*. 2020;20(11):48.
4. Taylor A, Mourad F, Kerry R, et al. A guide to cranial nerve testing for musculoskeletal clinicians. *J Man Manip Ther*. 2021;29(6):376–390.
5. Ettinger ER, Wyatt HJ, London R. Anisocoria: variation and clinical observation with different conditions of illumination and accommodation. *Invest Ophthalmol Vis Sci*. 1991;32(3):501–509.
6. Sekhon RK, Rocha Cabrero F, Deibel JP. *Nystagmus Types*. StatPearls Publishing; 2022.
7. Tejus MN, Singh V, Ramesh A, et al. An evaluation of the finger flexion, Hoffmann's and plantar reflexes as markers of cervical spinal cord compression: a comparative clinical study. *Clin Neurol Neurosurg*. 2015;134:12–16.
8. Mariotti C, Fancellu R, Di Donato S. An overview of the patient with ataxia. *J Neurol*. 2005;252(5):511–518.
9. Salardini A, Biller J, eds. *The Hospital Neurology Book*. McGraw Hill; 2016.
10. Ropper AH, Samuels MA, Klein J. *Adams and Victor's Principles of Neurology*. 11th ed. McGraw-Hill Education; 2019.
11. Ali S, Jabeen S, Pate RJ, et al. Conversion disorder—mind versus body: a review. *Innov Clin Neurosci*. 2015;12(5-6):27–33.
12. Stone J. Functional neurological disorders: the neurological assessment as treatment. *Pract Neurol*. 2016;16:7–17.
13. Stone J, Carson A, Sharpe M. Functional symptoms and signs in neurology: assessment and diagnosis. *J Neurol Neurosurg Psychiatry*. 2005;76(S1):i2–i12.

Questions

1. A 62-year-old male with a history of type 2 diabetes, peripheral neuropathy, and a previous stroke is noted to have a contracted right arm, 3+ reflexes on the right biceps, triceps, and brachioradialis, 3+ reflexes on the right patella, and 4+ reflexes on the right Achilles with sustained clonus. You also note a positive Babinski sign on the right foot. Damage to what part of the nervous system has caused these exam findings?
   a. Brain, from previous stroke
   b. Peripheral nerves, from diabetes
   c. Neuromuscular junction
   d. Muscles

2. A 72-year-old female with chronic obstructive pulmonary disease (COPD), multiple myeloma (currently undergoing evaluation for treatment options), diabetes, and hypertension presents to the hospital with coughing, fever, and increased sputum production. She is treated for community-acquired pneumonia and COPD exacerbation. On day 2 of hospitalization,

she develops numbness below her belly button, leg weakness, and bladder incontinence. What part of the nervous system is affected?
a. Brain
b. Spinal cord
c. Neuromuscular junction
d. Muscles

3. You are taking care of a 33-year-old male who developed severe COVID-19 infection and has required extracorporeal membrane oxygenation in the intensive care unit. He has been in the hospital for 97 days awaiting a lung transplant and is on a heparin drip to prevent clot formation. Usually he is awake, alert, and able to follow all commands. You arrive at 7:00 pm to begin your night shift, and you notice he is unresponsive. You quickly examine his pupils and find they are dilated bilaterally and unresponsive to light. You speak with the daytime nurse and learn that this is a change in the patient's exam. What part of the nervous system is affected?
a. Brain
b. Spinal cord
c. Neuromuscular junction
d. Muscles

4. An 82-year-old patient with hypertension, hyperlipidemia, diabetes, peripheral artery disease, and atrial fibrillation presents with a necrotic right toe. She is awaiting amputation, and her home anticoagulation has been held. On day 3 of her hospitalization, you notice that the left side of her mouth is drooping, which was not present before. She can raise her forehead equally on both sides, and eye closure is symmetric on both sides, but she is unable to lift the left side of her mouth. Should you be concerned?
a. No; occasionally, elderly patients will have transient drooping of the mouth that resolves.
b. No; this sounds like Bell palsy, which does not warrant a stroke alert.
c. Yes; this sounds like a stroke, which requires a stroke alert.
d. Yes; she likely has developed conversion disorder and needs antipsychotic medications immediately.

5. If a patient can lift the left arm against gravity but not against resistance, how would you grade the left arm strength?
a. 1/5
b. 2/5
c. 3/5
d. 4/5
e. 5/5

6. You ask a patient to lift the arms straight out in front with palms up. If the patient has subtle weakness in an arm, what would you notice in that arm?
a. The weak arm will drift upward.
b. The weak arm will pronate.
c. The weak arm will have a tremor.

Answers
1. a
2. b
3. a
4. c
5. c
6. b

Common Procedures and Pathology of the Brain

CHAPTER 3

Management of the Patient With Subarachnoid Hemorrhage

Lauren Malinowski-Falk, MSN, BA, CRNP, AGACNP-BC

Patient Presentation

Subarachnoid hemorrhages (SAHs) are devastating intracranial hemorrhages that represent bleeding in the subarachnoid space of the brain. The bleeds may result from trauma, arteriovenous malformation, intracranial artery dissection, venous perimesencephalic cerebral aneurysms, or amyloid angiopathy. The most common cause of atraumatic SAH is from the rupture of a cerebral aneurysm.[1,2] During an aneurysmal rupture, a patient often experiences sudden onset of "the worst headache of my life," otherwise known as a "thunderclap headache." This is often accompanied by nausea, vomiting, neck stiffness, photophobia, and loss of consciousness. Risk factors for a ruptured aneurysm include smoking, hypertension, high cholesterol, a first-degree relative with cerebral aneurysm, certain genetic conditions, alcohol consumption, and use of sympathomimetic drugs.[1,2] Ruptured cerebral aneurysms are more common in females and patients 40–60 years old.[3] While many people assume that ruptures most often follow intense physical or psychological stress, ruptured aneurysms occur more commonly during activities of daily living.[4]

Physiology and Diagnosis

Many of the effects from SAH arise from the increase in cranial pressure caused by the accumulation of blood volume. When an aneurysm first ruptures, blood expands into the subarachnoid space until the intracranial pressure (ICP) equalizes and tamponades the bleed.[4] This cessation of blood flow allows time for patients to seek help, but many patients die before reaching the hospital.[1] Furthermore, a majority of those who reach the hospital sustain permanent disability from the sequelae of the SAH.[2] The severity of SAH is graded on two scales: the Hunt and Hess score, which is based on clinical presentation; and the modified Fisher score, which is based on the results of neuroimaging (Fig. 3.1).[2]

- Once a patient with clinical symptoms of SAH presents to the hospital, the gold-standard diagnosis of SAH is through a noncontrast computed tomography (CT) scan of the head. A positive scan shows blood surrounding the basal cisterns of the brain.[1] If the head CT is inconclusive, patients may undergo a lumbar puncture, CT angiogram (CTA), or magnetic resonance imaging (MRI) (Fig. 3.2).
- A lumbar puncture is used to test the cerebrospinal fluid (CSF) for the presence of red blood cells (RBCs) or xanthochromia (bilirubin from broken-down RBCs), particularly in the last few tubes of CSF.[1,3] Blood products that are present in the first few tubes of CSF could be related to a traumatic puncture.
- A CTA is a noninvasive scan that highlights vascular anatomy and detects aneurysms using contrast dye.[3] Limitations include any findings of incidental aneurysms that are not related to the SAH and an inability to detect small culprit aneurysms.[3]

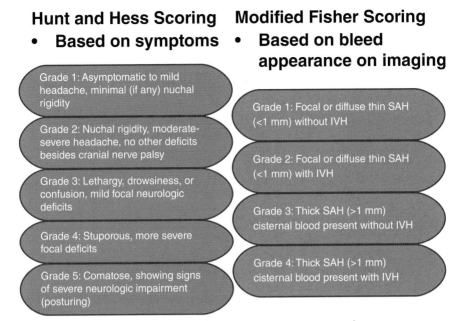

Hunt and Hess Scoring
- ### Based on symptoms

Grade 1: Asymptomatic to mild headache, minimal (if any) nuchal rigidity

Grade 2: Nuchal rigidity, moderate-severe headache, no other deficits besides cranial nerve palsy

Grade 3: Lethargy, drowsiness, or confusion, mild focal neurologic deficits

Grade 4: Stuporous, more severe focal deficits

Grade 5: Comatose, showing signs of severe neurologic impairment (posturing)

Modified Fisher Scoring
- ### Based on bleed appearance on imaging

Grade 1: Focal or diffuse thin SAH (<1 mm) without IVH

Grade 2: Focal or diffuse thin SAH (<1 mm) with IVH

Grade 3: Thick SAH (>1 mm) cisternal blood present without IVH

Grade 4: Thick SAH (>1 mm) cisternal blood present with IVH

Fig. 3.1   Different methods of diagnosis of subarachnoid hemorrhage *(SAH)*. *IVH*, Intraventricular hemorrhage.

- MRIs are most useful in patients who have experienced a delay in presenting to the hospital.[3] They have a high sensitivity for detecting the presence of blood and are often more sensitive for detecting prior hemorrhage.[1,5] However, performing an emergent MRI may be precluded by time, patient tolerance, clinical status, and MRI availability.[5]

Management

Blood pressure (BP) management is the cornerstone of SAH care. Before an aneurysm is surgically secured, nurses should prioritize treating hypertension, which, if present, causes an increased risk of rerupture/rebleed. Patients who rerupture have a much higher risk of death and neurologic dysfunction than patients with a single rupture.[4] Due to the variability in BPs that occurs during SAH, patients should be initially managed in the intensive care unit (ICU). BP goals should be maintained using short-term titratable intravenous (IV) BP agents,[2] such as nicardipine, labetalol, clevidipine, and esmolol.[1] BP parameters are often specific to the institution and neurosurgeon but are targeted to balance the risk of hypoperfusion with the risk of aneurysm rerupture.[1]

In addition to blood pressure management, nurses should ensure that patients with SAH maintain adequate circulating blood volume and a positive fluid balance. Overall, maintaining higher hemoglobin levels and a state of euvolemia can improve functional outcomes.[2] The presence of subarachnoid blood often results in impaired cerebral blood flow and oxygen delivery to the brain. Anemia also reduces oxygen delivery to the brain, so having a higher hemoglobin level ensures that the brain can tolerate the reduction in cerebral blood flow that occurs during SAH.[2]

- To maintain a positive fluid balance, nurses should be responsible for strict intake/output monitoring. They should calculate both IV and oral (PO) intake and measure the urine output of each void. Incontinent patients should have a Foley or external catheter placed to facilitate accurate measurements.

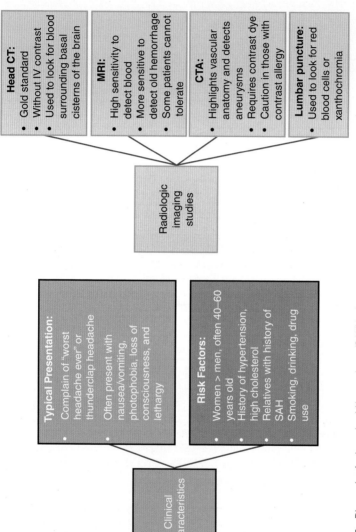

Fig. 3.2 Diagnosis of subarachnoid hemorrhage *(SAH)* is done through clinical symptoms and radiologic imaging. *CT,* Computed tomography; *CTA,* CT angiogram; *IV,* intravenous; *MRI,* magnetic resonance imaging.

- Nurses should also consider insensible losses, which are bodily fluids lost from the respiratory system, skin (such as excessive sweating), and water in stool.[6] They are not easily measured, but if noted in excessive amounts, they should be reported to the provider, as they can impact a patient's overall fluid balance.

Negative fluid balances should be corrected using IV fluid boluses and encouraging increased PO intake/free water flushes with tube feeds.

Vasospasms

Patients with SAH are at increased risk for vasospasm, defined as the acute narrowing of cerebral arteries causing cerebral ischemia.[2] Vasospasms occur when the subarachnoid blood irritates the cerebral vessels of the brain. The risk of vasospasm peaks within 7–10 days of the initial bleed and resolves 14–21 days after the bleed.[1,4] As a result, patients with SAH often remain in the ICU during most of their hospital stay so nurses can do frequent neuro exams and monitor closely for any strokelike symptoms that would indicate vasospasm is occurring.[2] Furthermore, these patients should undergo twice-daily transcranial doppler (TCD) ultrasound. TCD ultrasound measures the velocity of blood in the arteries, allowing for early detection of vasospasm even before any changes in neurologic status are detected. Once the peak vasospasm window is over, TCD ultrasound should be continued daily and usually end on postbleed day 21.

To reduce the risk of vasospasm, patients with SAH should be started on nimodipine immediately upon diagnosis. Nimodipine is a calcium channel blocker that has been shown to decrease the risk of cerebral ischemia and improve neurologic outcomes.[1,4] It is available in pill or liquid form for easy administration—orally or through a feeding tube. Nimodipine should be administered as 60 mg every 4 hours for 21 days after the initial bleed. Alternatively, the medication can be ordered as 30 mg every 2 hours if the patient's BP decreases excessively during treatment because this can negatively impact the cerebral perfusion pressure (CPP).[2] When administering nimodipine for the first time, nurses should begin with a 30-mg dose and monitor its effect on the patient's BP. If vasospasm occurs, nimodipine will not alter the overall incidence or severity, but administration should be continued.[4]

Patients who develop cerebral vasospasm can undergo medical or surgical therapy to reduce the risk of delayed cerebral ischemia (DCI) and improve cerebral perfusion.[4]

- "Triple H" therapy is used to medically reduce the risk of injury from DCI and improve blood flow through narrowed vessels in vasospasm.[7] The three Hs include inducing hypertension (by using fluid boluses or vasopressors), hemodilution (by utilizing blood transfusions to maintain higher hemoglobin levels), and hypervolemia (by ensuring the patient has a positive fluid balance).
  - However, recent research has shown that inducing hypervolemia may increase the risk of adverse medical complications, such as pulmonary edema, myocardial ischemia, and cerebral edema.[8] Furthermore, maintaining a state of euvolemia, as opposed to hypervolemia, was found to be more effective in preventing the development of cerebral vasospasms.[8]
  - "Triple H" therapy is therefore shifting to hypertension, hemodilution, and euvolemia.

Surgical therapy is reserved for vasospasms that persist despite medical therapy. Treatment options in this category include chemical management with an intraarterial infusion of a vasodilatory agent and mechanical management with balloon angioplasty to expand the narrowed vessel.[4,7]

Hydrocephalus

Hydrocephalus is the abnormal accumulation of CSF in the brain, and it occurs when normal CSF flow is blocked or when the body is unable to reabsorb CSF properly.[9] Symptoms include but are not limited to nausea, vomiting, altered mental status, and headache.[10] Hydrocephalus can develop after subarachnoid bleeding when thick blood blocks the normal flow of CSF through the subarachnoid cistern surrounding the arteries at the base of the brain.[4] ICP can increase in the setting of hydrocephalus due to expanding ventricular size, and this often is coupled with a sudden change in the patient's level of consciousness or a sudden decline in clinical stability.[4] In patients with hydrocephalus, ICP, and CPP should be monitored, especially if the patient has a fluctuating neurologic exam.[11] These patients may undergo the placement of an external ventricular drain (EVD). EVDs have the dual purpose of continuously monitoring ICP and simultaneously draining CSF and blood products that have inappropriately accumulated in the ventricles.[12] If left undrained, excess blood products in the subarachnoid space cause inflammation and irritation of the brain tissue. Using EVDs to facilitate the removal of blood products can prevent cerebral vasospasm and delayed infarctions.[12]

When managing an EVD, nurses should ensure that the drain remains level with the tragus of the patient's ear (which is a landmark for the intraventricular foramen), and they should follow the specific draining parameters designated by the neurosurgeon. To help reduce ICP, nurses should keep the patient's head in neutral position with the head of the bed (HOB) at >30 degrees to promote jugular venous outflow, while also working to control the patient's pain and nausea.[3,13]

Open drains are set to a specific pressure goal, and when the pressure in the brain exceeds that goal, CSF is automatically removed into the drainage system. This method typically is used when the patient is very symptomatic and there is a greater urgency to clear blood and improve the CPP.[12] Nurses should caution patients and their families not to alter their head position, raise the HOB, or attempt to mobilize when the drain is open. This may result in ventricular collapse from overdrainage, reflux in the system, and risk of central nervous system infection.[13] Overdrainage can generate a drastic change in pressure, thereby increasing the chance of rerupturing the aneurysm.[12] Open EVDs display a flat line when transduced on a cardiac monitor.

Alternatively, closed drains require manual manipulation by the nurse to drain CSF (Fig. 3.3). This is performed by unclamping the drain when the ICP rises above the set pressure goal. EVDs that are clamped/closed will display the ICP on the cardiac monitor if they are properly zeroed to the monitor and level with the tragus of the ear (Fig. 3.4). Patients can move freely when an EVD is clamped without the risk of overdrainage, but the ICP indicated on the cardiac monitor will not be accurate unless the EVD is leveled. Closed EVDs should have a peaked triphasic waveform when transduced on a cardiac monitor.

Over time, the neurosurgery team will attempt to wean patients from the EVD with a clamp trial, which involves gradually weaning the EVD parameters, usually over several days, until the nurse is instructed to stop draining CSF. During the trial, nurses will need to continue frequent neurologic exams to ensure the patient does not exhibit symptoms of hydrocephalus. They will also need to monitor the patient for the inability to self-regulate their ICP. Often patients will undergo serial head CT (HCT) scans to be certain that the ventricles do not increase in size, thus reassuring providers that the body can properly regulate ICP on its own. Successfully passing the clamp trial (no hydrocephalus seen on HCT despite the cessation of drainage over several days and no decrease in level of consciousness) indicates that normal CSF flow and ICP self-regulation have been restored, and the EVD can be removed.[12] While attempting clamp trials early in the course of management can lower the risk of ventriculostomy-related infection and reduce length of stay in the ICU, EVDs should not be removed while the patient is in the vasospasm window.[12] Patients with chronic symptomatic hydrocephalus and a failed clamp trial will require the placement of a ventriculoperitoneal shunt (VPS) for permanent CSF flow management.[4]

Ventriculoperitoneal Shunt

Patients with SAH and a failed EVD clamp trial will require placement of a VPS to prevent hydrocephalus (Fig. 3.5). A VPS has four components: a proximal catheter, one-way valve, reservoir, and

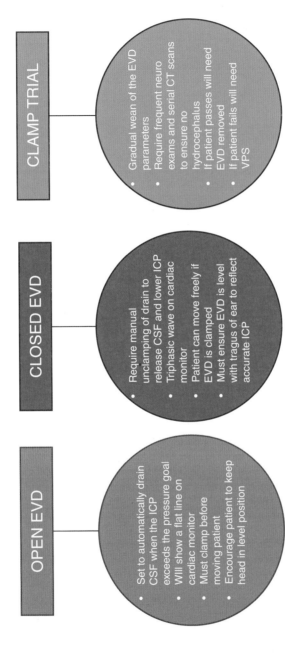

Fig. 3.3 Difference between external ventricular drain (*EVD*) orders and clamp trial. *CSF*, Cerebrospinal fluid; *CT*, computed tomography; *ICP*, intracranial pressure; *VPS*, ventriculoperitoneal shunt.

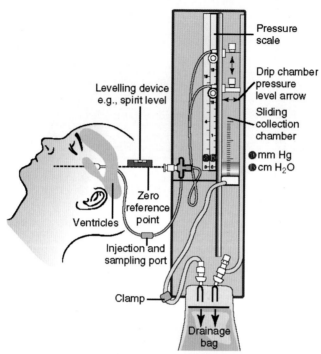

Fig. 3.4 Sample external ventricular drain *(EVD)* setup, used to ensure adequate drainage of cerebrospinal fluid *(CSF)* when intracranial pressure *(ICP)* exceeds the recommended threshold. (From Urden L, Stacy K, Lough M. *Priorities in Critical Care Nursing.* 9th ed. Elsevier; 2023.)

distal catheter.[9] The distal catheter runs under the skin and most commonly ends in the peritoneal cavity, though it can also terminate in the pleural space or atrium if there are contraindications to placement within the abdomen.[10] The VPS is programmed to remove CSF from the brain when the pressure exceeds a set level. When this occurs, CSF drains down to the distal catheter, where it is absorbed and excreted by the body. If the valve is programmable, then the amount of CSF removed from the brain can be easily adjusted to alleviate symptoms. If a VPS is placed when the patient is young and still growing, the proximal and/or distal catheter will migrate from their original positions; thus the shunt must be monitored regularly for the need for revision.[9] The most common complications of VPS placement include infection, shunt obstruction/occlusion, overdrainage, and peritoneal complications.

- Infection: If a shunt infection is confirmed (whether by cultures obtained from the shunt reservoir or head imaging in the context of clinical indicators of infection), standard management includes removal of the infected hardware, conversion to an EVD, and initiation of IV antibiotics.[10] The patient will need to undergo daily CSF cultures to monitor for infection while on antibiotics, and only once the infection is cleared can the shunt be replaced.
- Obstruction/occlusion: Patients with shunt obstruction will develop symptoms of hydrocephalus because CSF cannot be regulated properly and will accumulate in the brain. In addition to symptoms, these patients will have dilated ventricles on HCT and elevated opening pressure if a lumbar puncture is performed.[9] If the exact location of the obstruction is pinpointed, the patient may need only that particular component of the shunt replaced, not the entire shunt.[10]

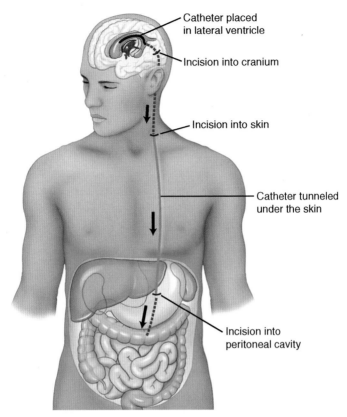

Catheter placed
in lateral ventricle

Incision into cranium

Incision into skin

Catheter tunneled
under the skin

Incision into
peritoneal cavity

Fig. 3.5 Placement of ventriculoperitoneal shunt, extending from the brain to abdomen. (From Shiland BJ. *Mastering Healthcare Terminology*. 7th ed. Elsevier; 2022.)

- Overdrainage: Shunts that are overdraining can lead to subdural collections and hemorrhages due to the tearing of bridging veins in the brain.[9] These collections, if small enough, can be absorbed over time, but can also lead to neurologic compromise, edema, and brain compression if left to grow.[10] If discovered early, the valve setting can be readjusted to ensure proper CSF drainage and resolution of symptoms without causing expansion or addition of subdural collections.
- Peritoneal complications: Because the VPS deposits CSF into the peritoneal space, patients may develop fluid collections at the end of the distal catheter. This commonly causes abdominal pain, distention, and even a palpable mass.[10] These collections may be reabsorbed by the body without intervention, but an abdominal washout and shunt revision may be necessary in cases where infection is suspected.[9]

Treatment

Patients with SAH due to a ruptured aneurysm require prompt repair of the aneurysm either by surgical clipping or endovascular intervention. Treatment is designed to minimize the risk of rebleeding, and the modality utilized is determined by the aneurysm's location and configuration.[14] Regardless of surgical clipping versus endovascular intervention, patients will undergo a diagnostic angiogram. Diagnostic angiograms involve the administration of contrast dye to visualize blood flow of the brain. This procedure can check for narrowed lumens, abnormal anatomy, and any areas of blood extravasation from ruptured aneurysms. Once an aneurysm is treated, patients require regular follow-up diagnostic angiograms to ensure continued cessation of blood flow into the aneurysm.

- Endovascular intervention is less invasive but may be impractical in the case of tortuous vascular anatomy.[3] During the procedure a catheter is inserted into the arterial system (via the femoral or radial artery) and carefully advanced until it reaches the aneurysm.
  - Coil: This procedure involves depositing metal coils directly into the lumen of the aneurysm, which prevents blood from flowing into the aneurysm and stimulates thrombus formation.[4] Metal coils are the preferred treatment in cases of acute SAH because they do not require the initiation of an antiplatelet agent, which could increase the risk of rebleeding.
  - Stent: Aneurysm flow diversion using a pipeline embolization device (PED) avoids entering the aneurysm itself.[15] A wire-mesh stent is placed directly into the artery next to the aneurysm, thereby blocking blood flow into the aneurysm and allowing it to shrink over time. However, patients with PEDs are at increased risk of thromboembolic events from platelet aggregation to the stent, so these patients are placed on antiplatelet therapy (e.g., aspirin/clopidogrel).
  - Stent and coil: Some aneurysms are very large or have a complicated shape. These complex aneurysms may require a combination of stent and coil therapy to redirect blood flow and prevent it from filling the aneurysm.[16]
  - Woven EndoBridge (WEB) device (Microvention/Terumo): This modality is best for wide-necked aneurysms. It involves placing a mesh device entirely within the aneurysm's pouch, causing blood flow stasis and thrombosis. This treatment eliminates the need for antiplatelet therapy.[16]
- Surgical clipping is an invasive procedure in which the skull is opened and the subarachnoid space exposed to gain access to the aneurysm. A titanium clip is applied at the base of the aneurysm to obstruct blood flow into the aneurysm without compromising otherwise normal cerebral blood flow.[4] Clip ligation has been shown to be more durable than coil embolization in ensuring cessation of blood flow into the aneurysm.[14]

Special Considerations for Endovascular Procedures

Before a patient undergoes an endovascular procedure, nurses should obtain a baseline neurologic and extremity pulse exam. The patient's distal pulses should be marked and the amplitude noted. Documenting a preprocedure baseline exam enables nurses to quickly detect changes or additional deficits postprocedurally, which could indicate further bleeding in the brain or stent/coil failure.[14] Unfortunately, the endovascular approach has been associated with a wide range of access site complications, but documenting pulses allows for early recognition of decreased blood flow to the accessed extremity.[17]

Contrast Complications

During an endovascular procedure, patients receive IV contrast to highlight the vascular anatomy of the brain. Nurses and physicians must take caution in patients with a history of renal dysfunction or IV contrast allergies. Patients with renal dysfunction may benefit from increased fluid intake to promote adequate excretion of the contrast dye. Nurses should proactively discuss fluid management pre- and postprocedurally with the physician team, including indications for IV fluids and a goal volume and rate of infusion. Lab monitoring postprocedurally is also necessary in some cases to be certain that no damage to the kidney has occurred. Additionally, patients with contrast allergies should receive steroids (e.g., prednisone or methylprednisolone), antihistamines, and acetaminophen preprocedurally to minimize the risk of an allergic reaction.[14] Usually these medications are scheduled to be administered the day before (13 and 7 hours before) and the day of the procedure (1–2 hours before). Nurses should request medical prophylaxis for any patient with an IV contrast sensitivity or an allergy to shellfish. Nurses must ensure these premedications are administered correctly, on time, and not held for any reason.

Access Site Complications

The cerebral vasculature can be accessed through either the femoral or the radial artery.[14] The femoral approach requires the patient to remain on flat bedrest until adequate hemostasis is achieved, whereas the radial approach allows for immediate activity out of bed. Access site complications are more common with insufficient compression and early ambulation.[17] Thus nurses must frequently monitor the catheter insertion site for bleeding, the extremity's color for any mottling or dusky appearance, and the distal pulses for any decrease in amplitude.

- The most common complication is a hematoma at the catheter insertion site from inadequate hemostasis. A hematoma indicates bleeding below the skin. If detected, nurses should apply firm pressure to the insertion site and notify the physician team. Patients should limit movement in the affected extremity until hemostasis is obtained.
- Another potential adverse outcome of femoral artery catheter insertion is retroperitoneal hematoma (RPH). Symptoms of RPH include severe back and lower quadrant abdominal pain, lower extremity pain, and suprainguinal tenderness.[17] RPH can be diagnosed with CT imaging. Management of RPH includes fluid resuscitation for hypotension, blood transfusion for severe anemia, and bedrest.[17] Many RPH will eventually self-tamponade and resolve without invasive intervention, but large-volume and unresolving RPH may need surgical intervention.
- Patients may also develop a pseudoaneurysm, which is an injury to the artery causing a leakage of blood. These are typically associated with increased bruising at the insertion site, and they are monitored through ultrasound imaging. Small pseudoaneurysms often close on their own, but larger pseudoaneurysms may require treatment with a thrombin injection into the aneurysmal sac. Ultimately, stasis of blood flow into the pseudoaneurysm leads to thrombosis of the site.[17]

Conclusion

SAH are devastating intracranial hemorrhages consisting of bleeding in the subarachnoid space of the brain. Patients who sustain SAH often describe sudden onset of "the worst headache of my life," otherwise known as a thunderclap headache. Headache may be accompanied by nausea, vomiting, neck stiffness, photophobia, and loss of consciousness. Patients with SAH require prompt diagnosis, typically through CT scan, and early repair in cases of a ruptured aneurysm. Ruptured aneurysms are commonly treated with surgical clipping or endovascular intervention. Core principles of management include BP control and triple H therapy to ensure continued cerebral blood flow especially if vasospasm occurs. Cerebral vasospasm occurs when blood in the subarachnoid space irritates the cerebral vasculature, causing narrowing of the arteries and leading to brain ischemia. Patients with SAH may require EVD placement for continuous ICP monitoring and drainage of CSF and blood products that have accumulated in the ventricles. Unfortunately, many patients die or sustain permanent disability from SAH. Nurses need to understand the intricacies and rationale behind the various scans, procedures, and medications involved in managing SAH, as well as what to do if complications arise. Neuroscience nurses play a vital role in decreasing morbidity, minimizing the disabling impact of adverse sequelae, and reducing the hospital length of stay.

References

1. Dubosh NM, Edlow JA. Diagnosis and initial emergency department management of subarachnoid hemorrhage. *Emerg Med Clin North Am.* 2021;39(1):87–99.
2. Boling B, Groves TR. Management of subarachnoid hemorrhage. *Crit Care Nurse.* 2019;39(5):58–67.
3. Marcolini E, Hine J. Approach to the diagnosis and management of subarachnoid hemorrhage. *West J Emerg Med.* 2019;20(2):203–211.
4. Lawton MT, Vates GE. Subarachnoid hemorrhage. *N Engl J Med.* 2017;377(3):257–266.
5. Morgenstern LB, Hemphill III JC, Anderson C, et al. Guidelines for the management of spontaneous intracerebral hemorrhage: a guideline for healthcare professionals from the American Heart Association/ American Stroke Association. *Stroke.* 2010;41(9):2108–2129.
6. McNeil-Masuka J, Boyer TJ. *Insensible fluid loss*: StatPearls Publishing; 2022.
7. Sokolowski JD, Chen CJ, Ding D, et al. Endovascular treatment for cerebral vasospasm following aneurysmal subarachnoid hemorrhage: predictors of outcome and retreatment. *J Neurointerv Surg.* 2018;10(4):367–374.
8. Daou BJ, Koduri S, Thompson BG, et al. Clinical and experimental aspects of aneurysmal subarachnoid hemorrhage. *CNS Neurosci Ther.* 2019;25(10):1096–1112.
9. Ferras M, McCauley N, Stead T, et al. Ventriculoperitoneal shunts in the emergency department: a review. *Cureus.* 2020;12(2).
10. Paff M, Alexandru-Abrams D, Muhonen M, et al. Ventriculoperitoneal shunt complications: a review. *Interdiscip Neurosurg.* 2018;13:66–70.
11. Diaz B, Elkbuli A, Wobig R, et al. Subarachnoid versus nonsubarachnoid traumatic brain injuries: the impact of decision-making on patient safety. *J Emerg Trauma Shock.* 2019;12(3):173–175.
12. Chung DY, Mayer SA, Rordorf GA. External ventricular drains after subarachnoid hemorrhage: is less more? *Neurocrit Care.* 2018;28(2):157–161.
13. Sakamoto VT, Vieira TW, Viegas K, et al. Nursing assistance in patient care with external ventricular drain: a scoping review. *Rev Bras Enferm.* 2021;74(2):e20190796.
14. Ringer AJ, Lopes DK, Boulos AS, et al. Current techniques for endovascular treatment of intracranial aneurysms. *Sem Cerebrovasc Dis Stroke.* 2001;1(1):39–51.
15. Ihn YK, Shin SH, Baik SK, et al. Complications of endovascular treatment for intracranial aneurysms: management and prevention. *Interv Neuroradiol.* 2018;24(3):237–245.
16. Pierot L, Wakhloo AK. Endovascular treatment of intracranial aneurysms: current status. *Stroke.* 2013;44(7):2046–2054.
17. Oneissi M, Sweid A, Tjoumakaris S, et al. Access-site complications in transfemoral neuroendovascular procedures: a systematic review of incidence rates and management strategies. *Oper Neurosurg (Hagerstown).* 2020;19(4):353–363.

Questions

1. Francheska was just diagnosed with a subarachnoid hemorrhage and is frustrated that she cannot get anything strong for her pain. How can you help her?
   a. Reinforce that you cannot give her strong opioids because you do not want to cause a change in mental status that could be mistaken for a worsening bleed.
   b. Ensure that the patient has her HOB raised and neck midline to promote venous drainage and decrease ICP.
   c. Discuss with the provider different oral options of pain medicine you can give her that will help manage any symptoms contributing to her headache.
   d. All of the above are correct.

2. Brooklyn is intubated and sedated after requiring an EVD placement for her subarachnoid hemorrhage diagnosis. She is due for nimodipine, but you remember that her blood pressure dropped the last time she got 60 mg. What should you do?
   a. Hold this dose; it is more important that her BP remains stable.
   b. Request that the doctor insert a temporary feeding tube for her to get the medicine now that she is NPO.

    c. Ask the provider to order her doses as 30 mg every 2 hours instead of 60 mg every 4 hours.

    d. Both b and c are correct.

3. Harper just came back from an angiogram through her right femoral artery. When she returned you marked her distal pulses and assessed the groin to be soft and dry. One hour later the patient calls you in because her right leg is tingly, and it is found to be mottled on assessment. What should you do?

    a. Sit the patient up and help her ambulate to improve the blood flow in her right leg.

    b. Keep the patient flat, apply pressure to any groin hematoma, and call the surgeon immediately.

    c. Apply a heating blanket to the leg and reassess in 30 minutes.

    d. Remind the patient that she must remain on flat bed rest, then reassess the groin site when she is able to sit up.

4. Austin presented to the hospital after the worst headache of her life and was found to have a subarachnoid hemorrhage. She has a BP goal of mean arterial pressure (MAP) <90 mm Hg. She has an arterial line placed, and you notice that her MAPs are in the 50s. What should you do?

    a. Check a manual BP to ensure her arterial BPs are accurate.

    b. Make no changes; her MAP is within goal.

    c. You know that a low MAP means her overall CPP is low, so suggest the provider order a fluid bolus or IV vasopressor to help increase her BP.

    d. Both a and c are correct.

5. Liam is a 24-year-old male admitted for possible SAH. He has an allergy to shellfish (anaphylaxis) but is ordered a CTA brain with IV contrast to assess his bleed. What should you do as the bedside nurse?

    a. Because imaging is the gold standard of diagnosis, take the patient as ordered hoping that this time he has a mild reaction to the dye.

    b. Ask the provider to order a steroid prep for him.

    c. Preemptively call an RRT to the CT scan suite to prepare for a possible allergic reaction.

    d. Keep telling the CT scan personnel that you are busy and refuse to take the patient until shift change.

Answers

1. d

2. d

3. b

4. d

5. b

CHAPTER 4

Pathophysiology and Nursing Management of Brain Bleeds

Lauren Malinowski-Falk, MSN, BA, CRNP, AGACNP-BC

Introduction

The brain is composed of a complex system of blood, cerebrospinal fluid (CSF), and brain matter (gray and white). According to the Monro-Kellie hypothesis, the total pressure generated by the brain matter, CSF, and blood volume must remain constant and therefore is tightly regulated within the cranial vault.[1] When one of these components increases, the others must decrease to maintain a stable intracranial pressure (ICP). Brain bleeds are detrimental because they result in an increase of blood volume circulating in the cranial vault. Due to the relative rigidity of the skull and cranial vault, even small increases in blood volume can lead to increased ICP and possible herniation (when brain tissue is pushed through structures and openings in the skull).[1] Patients who experience a rapid increase in ICP can develop Cushing triad, which is characterized by[2]:

- Elevated blood pressure (BP)
- Decreased heart rate
- Irregular breathing

Brain bleeds can be spontaneous or traumatic. There are three protective layers of the brain: the pia mater, arachnoid mater, and dura mater. The bleed type is characterized by the location of the bleed, and the Glasgow Coma Scale (GCS) is used to grade the severity of the bleed (Fig. 4.1)[3]:

- A mild brain injury is defined as a GCS score of 13–15.
- A moderate brain injury is defined as a GCS score of 9–12.
- A severe brain injury is defined as a GCS score of 3–8.
    - Lower GCS scores are associated with rapid rises in ICP, increased edema of the brain matter, and blockages of CSF flow that can result in hydrocephalus.[4]

Regardless of severity, all patients with brain bleeds need close hemodynamic monitoring and frequent neurologic exams. Neuroscience nurses need to be trained in how to manage these patients and how to recognize concerning signs and symptoms. Patient outcomes largely depend on the type, morphology, and location of the bleed, along with other associated injuries, but knowledgeable and experienced nursing care correlates directly with better outcomes overall.[3,5]

Types of Brain Bleeds

EPIDURAL HEMATOMA

An epidural hematoma is an arterial bleed located between the dura mater layer of the brain and the skull. It does not cross suture lines of the brain.[2] These bleeds expand rapidly, and most often they result from traumatic head injuries.[2] Patients with epidural hematomas typically present with an initial loss of consciousness immediately after injury, followed by a lucid recovery period with a complete recovery of consciousness (which occurs during bleed expansion), and then develop

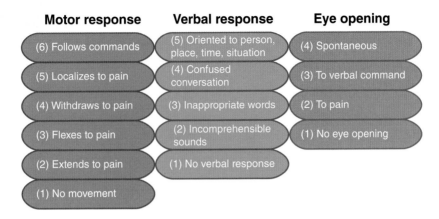

Total score= Eye opening + verbal response + motor response
Mild brain bleed score: 13-15
Moderate brain bleed score: 9-12
Severe brain bleed score:3-8

Fig. 4.1 Glascow Coma Scale scoring.

rapid neurologic deterioration.[2] The extent of neurologic deficit depends on the degree of expansion of the hematoma.

SUBDURAL HEMATOMA

A subdural hematoma (SDH) is a bleed that occurs between the dura and arachnoid space of the brain, which results from tearing of the bridging cortical veins from the surface of the brain to the dural sinuses.[6-8] SDH is most often caused by traumatic injury but can occur from bleeding disorders, vascular malformations, after cranial surgery, or spontaneously. Elderly patients in particular are predisposed to SDH due to age-related atrophy of the brain, which stretches the bridging veins of the brain and makes them more susceptible to tearing.[8] SDH can be characterized as acute, acute-on-chronic, or chronic, depending on the age of the blood seen on computed tomography (CT) imaging.[9]

INTRACRANIAL HEMORRHAGE

An intracranial hemorrhage (ICH) is a severe type of stroke that results in hemorrhage directly within the brain structure. These bleeds cause mass effect (when the increased blood volume causes increased pressure in the brain, and leads to secondary pathological effects) and disruption of the cerebral tissue.[4] While most of these bleeds stop spontaneously, sometimes the hematoma expands, causing increased brain edema and midline shift.[4] The two major risk factors for ICH are systemic hypertension and cerebral amyloid angiopathy, in which amyloid plaques are deposited in the vessels of the brain.[4]

- Providers typically use an ICH bleeding scale to grade bleed severity and predict the patient's overall 30-day mortality risk.[10] The scale, which generates scores ranging from 0–6, incorporates the following features[10]:
  - Patient's GCS score (zero points for GCS 13-15, one point for GCS 5-12, and two points for GCS 3-4)
  - Patient's age (one point if >80 years old)
  - Presence of infratentorial blood (at the brainstem or cerebellum) (one point if present)

- ICH volume on CT imaging (one point if >30cc)
- Presence or absence of intraventricular hemorrhage (IVH) (one point if present)

INTRAVENTRICULAR HEMORRHAGE

IVH is a bleed located within the ventricles of the brain. The ventricles are fluid-filled cavities that help protect and cushion the brain. An IVH can be primary (confined to the ventricles) or, more commonly, secondary (originating as an extension of an ICH).[5] IVH will interfere with the normal flow of CSF in the brain, which can lead to hydrocephalus. Patients with hydrocephalus will have a decreased level of consciousness (Figs. 4.2 and 4.3).

Initial Management of Brain Bleeds

Patients with brain bleed typically present with a severe headache, vomiting, and some degree of altered neurologic function. The nurse's initial role is to elicit a detailed history from the patient or a family member. This history should include the time of symptom onset, any trauma or precipitating events, the patient's past medical history, and a medication list.[5] When a brain bleed is the clinical concern, neuroimaging is the gold standard of diagnosis, starting with a CT scan of the head without contrast.[9] Once a brain bleed is formally diagnosed, pursuing medical or surgical management depends on bleed size, extent of midline shift, GCS score, and neurologic symptoms.[2]

However, while preparing for imaging and awaiting a formal diagnosis, nurses caring for these at-risk patients should not neglect the patient's airway, breathing, and circulation (ABCs). Hemodynamic stabilization through ventilatory and cardiovascular support is always the priority and should precede further efforts at diagnosis and treatment of a bleed.[5] Without first achieving clinical stabilization, rapid decline can ensue as the patient progresses through the devastating sequela of a brain bleed.

Medical Management of Brain Bleeds

Medical management of brain bleeds is often trialed for patients with minimal symptoms and those with radiographically small-sized bleeds. The principles of medical management are:
- Monitoring for bleed progression
- Preventing bleed progression
- Avoiding potential complications

ICP MANAGEMENT

Unless contraindicated, patients with brain bleeds should be positioned with the head of the bed (HOB) at ≥30 degrees to facilitate venous drainage.[9] Care should be taken to ensure there is no apparatus near or around the neck (such as a constrictive C-spine collar) that could obstruct venous drainage.[9] Patients with increased ICP may be prescribed intravenous mannitol or hypertonic saline to help lower ICP and reduce edema in the brain.

BP CONTROL

Patients with brain bleeds often present with severe hypertension, which increases the risk of rerupture and rebleeding. Due to the variability that may be encountered throughout the course of a brain bleed, BP usually is best managed by using short-term titratable BP agents.[1] Nurses should keep in mind that the ideal cerebral perfusion pressure (CPP) to ensure adequate blood

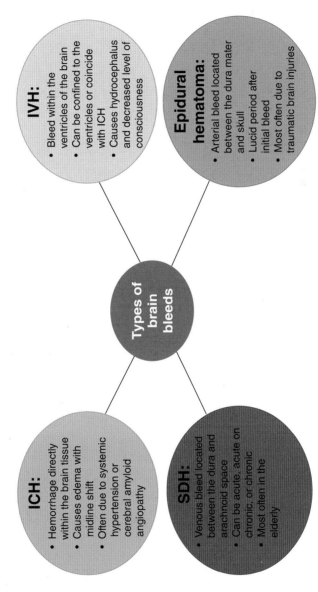

Fig. 4.2 Types of brain bleeds and their distinguishing characteristics. *ICH*, Intracranial hemorrhage; *IVH*, intraventricular hemorrhage; *SDH*, subdural hematoma.

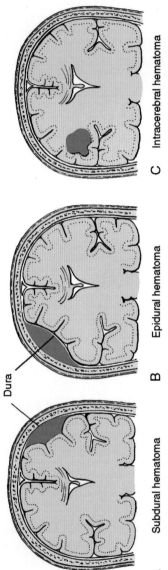

Fig. 4.3   Differences between subdural hematoma (A), epidural hematoma (B), and intracranial hemorrhage (C) in the brain tissue. (From Black JM, Hawks JH. *Medical-Surgical Nursing: Clinical Management for Positive Outcomes.* 8th ed. Saunders; 2009.)

A   Subdural hematoma   B   Epidural hematoma   C   Intracerebral hematoma

Dura

flow to the brain is ~60 mm Hg.[4] Strategies to optimize CPP through BP control often overlap with those aimed at reducing ICP.[9]

- The calculation for CPP: Mean Arterial Pressure (MAP) – ICP.

ANTICOAGULATION

Anticoagulation use can increase the risk of hematoma expansion, unfavorable outcomes, and death.[4] Patients on anticoagulants should have those medications held immediately, and if possible, reversal agents should be administered. Nurses should inform the provider immediately about any use of anticoagulants or antiplatelet agents when obtaining the patient's medical history and attempt to note when the patient last received the medication.

NEUROLOGIC EXAMS

The easiest way to monitor for neurologic changes is through frequent and consistent physical exams. Any change in neurologic exam, such as decreased consciousness, orientation, motor function, or pupils that are dilated or poorly responsive, should be reported to the provider without delay. These changes can indicate rising ICP, possible rebleeding, new or worsening hydrocephalus, or impending herniation.[9]

IMAGING

CT scans are used to monitor for bleed expansion, increased brain edema, midline shift, or other worsening conditions that may prompt surgical intervention.[11] In the acute bleed period, CT imaging is done regularly, often every 6–12 hours during the first 24-hour period, to evaluate bleed stability. After stability has been established, CT imaging is reserved for assessment of any changes in neurologic function detected by bedside physical exam.

PAIN CONTROL

While patients with brain bleeds often experience severe headache, typical pain management modalities, such as IV opioids, should be avoided. Opioids can decrease a patient's level of consciousness, potentially masking other changes in neurologic function and thereby preventing prompt recognition of a clinically significant change in neurologic status.[1] Oral opioids can be administered with caution, but nurses should make a concerted effort to use alternative methods of pharmacologic and nonpharmacologic pain control.

SEIZURE PROPHYLAXIS

Seizures can occur due to the presence of blood and edema in the brain. They can cause hemodynamic instability, increase the body's metabolic demand, and increase ICP.[9,12] Patients with brain bleeds may be initiated on seizure prophylaxis before actual seizure activity is detected, but this practice often is neurosurgeon dependent.[8] Antiepileptic medication may be titrated off in the absence of seizure activity or continued for a duration determined by the neurosurgeon. Often patients with decreased mental status that is thought to be out of proportion to the severity of brain injury may be placed on electroencephalogram monitoring to catch both clinical and subclinical seizure activity.[5]

BLOOD GLUCOSE MANAGEMENT

Hyperglycemia has been linked to an increased risk of mortality and poor outcomes in all patients, with or without a history of diabetes.[5] Marked episodes of hyper- and hypoglycemia should be avoided. Blood glucose checks should occur regularly, and abnormal levels should be reported to the provider for further evaluation and management.

FEVER MANAGEMENT

Patients with brain bleeds should be kept afebrile, as fever is associated with poor outcomes and the development of cerebral ischemia.[1] Additional attempts should be made to stop shivering because shivering increases the body's metabolic demand and decreases brain tissue oxygenation.[1]

IMMOBILITY

Patients who develop brain bleeds are at a higher risk of complications from immobility. These patients should have antithrombotic stockings placed and prophylactic doses of anticoagulation administered to help prevent the formation of blood clots. These prophylactic doses should be prescribed only when the bleed has proven to be stable and the patient is out of the window for bleed recurrence.[5] In addition, patients should be repositioned at frequent intervals to prevent pressure injuries, and they should be mobilized as soon as possible.[5]

Surgical Management of Brain Bleeds

Surgical intervention is utilized to manage larger bleeds in patients with neurologic symptoms (Fig. 4.4).[8] Large bleeds cause brain compression, brain shifting, increased ICP, and ischemia of brain tissue.[9] Surgical intervention is aimed at decreasing ICP, improving CPP, limiting mechanical compression of the brain, and minimizing the harmful effects of extravasated blood, but surgeons should take the operative risk of cutting through uninjured brain tissue into consideration in a thoughtful risk-benefit analysis.[5] It is important to note that the medical therapies detailed in the preceding section still apply when a patient is undergoing surgical intervention.

BURR HOLE IRRIGATION FOR SDH

The gold standard surgical intervention for SDH is burr hole irrigation with drain placement.[9] Continued drainage through the insertion of subdural drains has been found to decrease the rate of bleed recurrence, to aid in the evacuation of residual fluid, and to promote brain reexpansion.[8] Patients with drains should remain supine in bed with the HOB flat to prevent postoperative pneumocephalus (air in the intracranial space), which can cause increased pressure and midline shift of the brain.[13] Residual fluid collections are common, and it may take several months to achieve complete resolution of SDH.[8]

MIDDLE MENINGEAL ARTERY EMBOLIZATION FOR SDH

Meningeal artery embolization is used for patients with intractable SDH who require lifelong anticoagulation/antiplatelet therapy. Embolization is performed via a catheter that is threaded endoscopically through the femoral artery. The procedure releases pellets into the artery, sealing off the artery and preventing further blood flow into the SDH. Stopping the blood flow is thought to lead to hematoma resolution and allow for the resumption of anticoagulation/antiplatelet therapy.[9] In addition to neurologic exams, patients need femoral access site monitoring with distal pulse checks during the postoperative period.

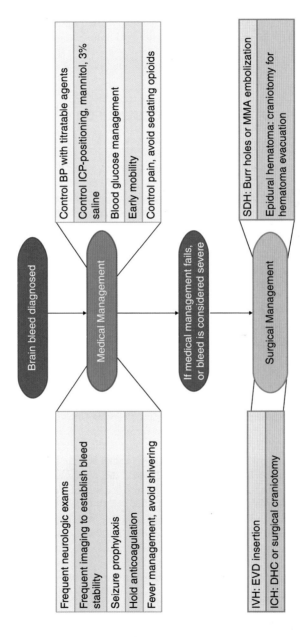

Fig. 4.4 Medical and surgical management techniques. *BP*, Blood pressure; *DHC*, decompressive hemicraniectomy; *EVD*, external ventricular drain; *ICH*, intracranial hemorrhage; *ICP*, intracranial pressure; *IVH*, intraventricular hemorrhage; *MMA*, middle meningeal artery; *SDH*, subdural hematoma.

CRANIOTOMY FOR ICH

Surgical management of ICH can entail either an open craniotomy for hematoma evacuation or a decompressive hemicraniectomy. A hematoma evacuation involves accessing the hematoma through the dissection, retraction, and manipulation of brain tissue, which risks damaging healthy brain tissue in the process.[4] Neurosurgical decompression is reserved for patients with significant midline shift, large hematoma, and refractory ICP >20 mmHg despite maximum medical therapy.[3,4] This surgery involves removing the skull bone flap on the side of the brain with the bleed. The flap remains off to allow a safe outlet for the brain to safely swell and expand in response to the injury, without the risk of herniation and death.

EXTERNAL VENTRICULAR DRAIN PLACEMENT FOR IVH

IVH requires the placement of an external ventricular drain (EVD) to allow for drainage of CSF, monitoring of ICP, administration of medications, and CSF sampling.[14] If present, coagulopathy and thrombocytopenia should be treated before device insertion, and CT imaging should always be performed after EVD placement.[5] Postprocedure imaging protocols verify that the device is in the correct location of the brain and that the placement did not cause any additional bleeding. One of the major complications that can occur with EVD placement is infection, which can lead to ventriculitis. Insertion and manipulation of EVDs require sterile technique. Nurses are responsible for protecting the sterility and integrity of the EVD system, in part by ensuring that the EVD is manipulated as little as possible.[14] If ventriculitis occurs, nurses should anticipate drawing daily CSF cultures to test for successful eradication of infection with antibiotics.

Conclusion

Brain bleeds are devastating events for patients to experience. They increase the overall amount of circulating blood in the cranial vault, ultimately leading to increased ICP. If left untreated, increased ICP can cause rapid deterioration of the patient's neurologic function and ultimately result in brain herniation and death. Brain bleeds are characterized based on the location of the bleed, while the patient's GCS score is used to classify the severity of the bleed. Epidural hematomas are rapidly expanding arterial bleeds, whereas SDHs are slow venous bleeds. Intracranial hemorrhages occur directly within the brain structure, whereas intraventricular hemorrhages occur within the ventricles of the brain and interfere with the normal flow of CSF in the brain.

From diagnosis to discharge, nurses play an essential role in the management of patients with brain bleeds. Medical management without surgical intervention is often trialed for patients with minimal symptoms and radiographically small-sized bleeds; it is crucial to preventing bleed progression and avoiding potential complications. Surgical interventions are reserved for radiographically larger bleeds that risk causing brain compression, brain shifting, and ischemia of brain tissue. Patients with a brain bleed need close hemodynamic monitoring and frequent neurologic exams. Changes in neurologic status can indicate progression of the bleed and should always be discussed with the provider without delay. Caring for patients with a brain bleed can be a complex task. The stakes are high, so it is of the utmost importance that neuroscience nurses be knowledgeable and expertly trained in the management of these patients, with the ultimate goal of improving outcomes and saving lives.

References

1. Boling B, Groves TR. Management of subarachnoid hemorrhage. *Crit Care Nurse*. 2019;39(5):58–67.
2. Khairat A, Waseem M. *Epidural hematoma*: StatPearls Publishing; 2022.
3. Diaz B, Elkbuli A, Wobig R, et al. Subarachnoid versus nonsubarachnoid traumatic brain injuries: the impact of decision-making on patient safety. *J Emerg Trauma Shock*. 2019;12(3):173–175.

4. de Oliveira Manoel AL. Surgery for spontaneous intracerebral hemorrhage. *Crit Care*. 2020;24(1):45.
5. Morgenstern LB, Hemphill III JC, Anderson C, et al. Guidelines for the management of spontaneous intracerebral hemorrhage: a guideline for healthcare professionals from the American Heart Association/American Stroke Association. *Stroke*. 2010;41(9):2108–2129.
6. Bordia R, Le M, Behbahani S. Pitfalls in the diagnosis of subdural hemorrhage–mimics and uncommon causes. *J Clin Neurosci*. 2021;89:71–84.
7. Al-Mufti F, Mayer SA. Neurocritical care of acute subdural hemorrhage. *Neurosurg Clin N Am*. 2017;28(2):267–278.
8. Mehta V, Harward SC, Sankey EW, et al. Evidence based diagnosis and management of chronic subdural hematoma: a review of the literature. *J Clin Neurosci*. 2018;50:7–15.
9. Srivatsan A, Mohanty A, Nascimento FA, et al. Middle meningeal artery embolization for chronic subdural hematoma: meta-analysis and systematic review. *World Neurosurg*. 2019;122:613–619.
10. Cheung RTF, Zou LY. Use of the original, modified, or new intracerebral hemorrhage score to predict mortality and morbidity after intracerebral hemorrhage. *Stroke*. 2003;34(7):1717–1722.
11. Cooper SW, Bethea KB, Skrobut TJ, et al. Management of traumatic subarachnoid hemorrhage by the trauma service: is repeat CT scanning and routine neurosurgical consultation necessary? *Trauma Surg Acute Care Open*. 2019;4(1):e000313.
12. Lawton MT, Vates GE. Subarachnoid hemorrhage. *N Engl J Med*. 2017;377(3):257–266.
13. Fomchenko EI, Gilmore EJ, Matouk CC, et al. Management of subdural hematomas, part II: surgical management of subdural hematomas. *Curr Treat Options Neurol*. 2018;20(8):34.
14. Sakamoto VT, Vieira TW, Viegas K, et al. Nursing assistance in patient care with external ventricular drain: a scoping review. *Rev Bras Enferm*. 2021;74(2):e20190796.

Questions

1. Petra walked into the emergency department complaining of a severe headache after a bicycle accident. You are about to take her to CT scan when she suddenly gets very sleepy, will only open her eyes to sternal rubbing, and is unable to sustain conversation. What is your priority?
   a. Rush her to CT scan yourself; it is the only way to ensure prompt diagnosis.
   b. Check her bag to ensure she did not take her own pain medicine.
   c. Request respiratory staff to come to bedside and prepare for intubation.
   d. Dim the light in the room and let her rest.

2. Rocco has an EVD with an order to keep his ICP <15 mm Hg. The drain is level with the tragus of his ear and has been zeroed for accuracy. What do you need to do to prevent any complications?
   a. Drain as much as possible so that you can avoid going into his room frequently.
   b. Ensure proper hand hygiene when manipulating the EVD and sterile technique when drawing cultures to prevent infection.
   c. Restrain the patient early—who knows when he may get agitated and attempt to pull out the drain.
   d. Teach the family how to drain off CSF in case Rocky's ICP rises while you are stuck in another room.

3. Dylan was transported to the hospital by EMS, unconscious after an ATV accident. His mother is at bedside and appears very concerned. According to her, Dylan had an initial loss of consciousness at the scene, then a lucid period where he seemed completely normal, followed by another rapid loss of consciousness. Dylan is getting his CT now. What type of bleed is he likely to have?
   a. SAH
   b. SDH
   c. IVH
   d. Epidural hemorrhage

4. You walk into the room to complete your initial assessment of Mary, who is a 45-year-old female presenting with ICH and IVH. She does not open her eyes until you rub her sternum. She moans when you ask her questions. When you pinch her right shoulder, she uses her left arm to push you away. What is her GCS score?
   a. 12
   b. 5
   c. 9
   d. Unable to assess

5. Madeline is a 34-year-old female with a past medical history of a deep venous thrombosis, now treated with anticoagulation. She is on postoperative day 1 following a decompressive hemicraniectomy for ICH with edema. This morning you notice that she has been restarted on her apixaban. What should you do?
   a. Administer the medication as ordered.
   b. Hold the medicine until you check with the provider that the timing of starting anticoagulation is appropriate, considering the risk of bleed expansion.
   c. Administer half the dose, and if there is no change in her neurologic exam, administer the remainder of the dose in a few hours.
   d. Override subcutaneous heparin from the storage unit to administer this medication instead.

Answers

1. c

2. b

3. d

4. c

5. b

CHAPTER 5

Nursing Management of the Patient With Acute Ischemic Stroke

Naomi Owusu Acheampong, MSN, CRNP   Elise Lambertson, MSN, CRNP

Introduction

According to the Centers for Disease Control and Prevention, stroke is the fifth leading cause of death in the United States. Each year, ~795,000 people experience a new or recurrent stroke, and of all stroke cases, 87% are ischemic in nature.[1] Ischemic strokes occur when there is inadequate perfusion of the brain, causing neuronal death and irreversible damage. There are several common risk factors for ischemic stroke, including hypertension, diabetes, hyperlipidemia, smoking, obesity, and a sedentary lifestyle. Reperfusion therapy is an important component of the treatment for acute ischemic stroke (AIS). Thrombolytics, such as intravenous (IV) recombinant tissue plasminogen activator (r-tPA) and tenecteplase (TNK), along with endovascular interventions such as mechanical thrombectomy (MT) with a retrievable stent, are the gold standard for the management of AIS. Reperfusion aims to rapidly restore cerebral blood perfusion and prevent further brain tissue injury. A thorough understanding of acute stroke evaluation, blood pressure management in the setting of AIS, reperfusion modalities, and the risks and complications associated with reperfusion interventions is essential to delivering expert nursing care and optimizing a patient's recovery.

Acute Stroke Evaluation

For patients already in a health care facility, management of stroke begins with a stroke alert to initiate an emergent interprofessional assessment. This commonly involves the bedside nurse and a neurologist, internist, radiologist, critical care personnel, and pastoral care, but the exact members of the stroke alert team may vary across institutions and types of facilities. Nurses should activate a stroke alert when there is a sudden change of mental status, cranial nerve exam, motor strength exam, and/or pattern of speech. Nurses can also activate a stroke alert when a new patient is brought into the hospital with a reported change in neurologic status. Critical information gathered during the evaluation includes when the patient was last seen at their neurologic baseline, their medical and surgical history, current medications, blood pressure, and glucose level. Furthermore, it is important to rule out other medical conditions, such as hypoglycemia or seizure, which can mimic stroke. This comprehensive assessment will help a neurologist determine if the patient is a candidate for thrombolytic therapy.

Patients presenting with AIS should be assessed using the National Institutes of Health Stroke Scale (NIHSS). The NIHSS is a scored list of neurologic features and functions that may be impacted by stroke, including level of consciousness, language, neglect, visual deficits, extraocular movement, motor strength, ataxia, changes in speech, and sensory loss (Fig. 5.1).[2] Using the NIHSS, patients are assessed and assigned a score that indicates a clinical measure of neurologic

Ia—Level of consciousness	0 = Alert; keenly responsive
	1 = Not alert, but arousable by minor sitimulation
	2 = Not alert; requires repeated sitimulation
	3 = Unresponsive or responds only with reflex
Ib—Level of consciousness questions: What is your age? What is the month?	0 = Answers two questions correctly
	1 = Answers one question correctly
	2 = Answers neither questions correctly
Ic—Level of consciousness commands: Open and close your eyes Grip and release your hand	0 = Performs both tasks correctly
	1 = Performs one task correctly
	2 = Performs neither task correctly
2—Best gaze	0 = Normal
	1 = Partial gaze palsy
	2 = Forced deviation
3—Visual	0 = No visual lost
	1 = Partial hemianopia
	2 = Complete hemianopia
	3 = Bilateral hemianopia
4—Facial palsy	0 = Normal symmetric movements
	1 = Minor paralysis
	2 = Partial paralysis
	3 = Complete paralysis of one or both sides
5—Motor arm Left arm Right arm	0 = No drift
	1 = Drift
	2 = Some effort against gravity
	3 = No effort against gravity
	4 = No movement
6—Motor leg Left leg Right leg	0 = No drift
	1 = Drift
	2 = Some effort against gravity
	3 = No effort against gravity
	4 = No movement
7—Limb ataxia	0 = Absent
	1 = Present in one limb
	2 = Present in two limbs
8—Sensory	0 = Normal; no sensory loss
	1 = Mild-to-moderate sensory loss
	2 = Severe-to-total sensory loss
9—Best language	0 = No aphasia; normal
	1 = Mild-to-moderate aphasia
	2 = Severe aphasia
	3 = Mute; global aphasia
10—Dysarthria	0 = Normal
	1 = Mild-to-moderate dysarthria
	2 = Severe dysarthria
11—Extinction and inattention	0 = No abnormality
	1 = Visual, tactile, auditory, spatial, or personal inattention
	2 = Profound hemi-inattention or extinction
Score = 0–42	

Fig. 5.1 National Institutes of Health Stroke Scale (NIHSS). (Modified from National Institute of Neurological Disorders and Stroke. *NIH Stroke Scale*. NIH; 2023.)

deficit, ranging from 0 (no deficit) to 42 (maximum possible deficit). The NIHSS is used to help physicians and nurses gauge the severity of a stroke, guide appropriate treatment, and predict patient outcomes.

Regardless of stroke severity and whether acute intervention is indicated, patients should undergo a comprehensive evaluation to determine the cause of stroke and the extent of their stroke burden. Acute stroke evaluation includes a variety of imaging studies and laboratory testing (described next; Box 5.1).

BOX 5.1 ■ Stroke Evaluation

- General assessment
- Vital signs
- Noncontrast computed tomography (CT) head
- CT angiography head and neck
- CT perfusion
- Magnetic resonance imaging brain
- Echocardiogram
- Electrocardiogram
- Complete blood count, chem 7, hemoglobin A1C, troponin, lipid panel, blood glucose
- Toxicology screen
- Pregnancy test in women of childbearing age
- Other studies based on the patient's comorbidities and clinical presentation

---

Data from Powers WJ, Rabinstein AA, Ackerson T, et al. 2018 guidelines for the early management of patients with acute ischemic stroke: a guideline for healthcare professionals from the American Heart Association/American Stroke Association. *Stroke*. 2018;49(3):e46-e110.

Imaging studies include the following[3]:
- Magnetic resonance imaging of the brain is obtained to confirm AIS and to identify the full extent of the stroke.
  - This also reveals any hemorrhagic transformation of the stroke bed.
- Computed tomography angiography or magnetic resonance angiography head and neck is used to evaluate intracranial and extracranial vessels.
  - These studies help to identify any atherosclerotic disease that may have contributed to the stroke.
- A carotid duplex ultrasound is a noninvasive test used to screen for carotid artery disease.
  - Findings of significant stenosis or occlusion may lead to additional neurosurgical intervention.
- Echocardiogram is used to investigate cardiac sources for stroke, such as patent foramen ovale, atrial appendage thrombus, and valvular abnormalities.

Laboratory testing is aimed at identifying uncontrolled vascular risk factors that could lead to an ischemic stroke. These tests typically include:
- Lipid panel: focusing on low-density lipoprotein and triglycerides
- Hemoglobin A1C
- Comprehensive metabolic panel
- Coagulation studies

Blood Pressure Management

Hypertension is a risk factor for ischemic strokes, and blood pressure (BP) management is an important part of caring for patients with stroke. Providers must understand the risks and benefits of treatment in the acute care setting. Overall, while severely elevated BP over time can lead to a stroke, after a stroke occurs, the brain requires a certain level of BP to be maintained to achieve adequate perfusion. In fact, rapidly lowering BP during the acute phase of ischemic stroke may worsen the patient's clinical outcome by causing hypoperfusion of the brain and the vascular territory affected by the stroke.

Permissive hypertension is a strategy that promotes adequate perfusion of the ischemic penumbra in the context of AIS. The ischemic penumbra is defined as the part of an ischemic stroke that is at risk of progressing to complete infarction and is located around the core of the stroke. In the

TABLE 5.1 ■ AHA/ASA Recommendations for BP Management in Acute Ischemic Stroke

1. Patients eligible for treatment with IV thrombolytics or other acute reperfusion intervention and SBP >185 mm Hg or DBP >110 mm Hg should have BP lowered before the intervention. A persistent SBP >185 mm Hg or a DBP >110 mm Hg is a contraindication to IV thrombolytic therapy. After reperfusion therapy, keep SBP <180 mm Hg and DBP <105 mm Hg for at least 24 hours.
2. Patients who have other medical indications for aggressive treatment of BP should be treated.[a]
3. For those not receiving thrombolytic therapy, BP may be lowered if it is markedly elevated (SBP >220 mm Hg or DBP >120 mm Hg). A reasonable goal would be to lower BP by ~15% during the first 24 hours after onset of stroke.
4. In patients who are hypotensive, the cause of hypotension should be sought. Hypovolemia and cardiac arrhythmias should be treated and in exceptional circumstances, vasopressors may be prescribed in an attempt to improve cerebral blood flow.

[a]Different treatment options may be appropriate in patients who have comorbid conditions that may benefit from rapid reductions in BP such as acute coronary events, acute heart failure, aortic dissection, or preeclampsia/eclampsia.

AHA, American Heart Association; *ASA*, American Stroke Association; *BP*, blood pressure; *DBP*, diastolic BP; *IV*, intravenous; *SBP*, systolic BP.

Data from Adams Jr HP, del Zoppo G, Alberts JM, et al. Guidelines for the early management of adults with ischemic stroke: a guideline from the American Heart Association/American Stroke Association Stroke Council, Clinical Cardiology Council, Cardiovascular Radiology and Intervention Council, and the Atherosclerotic Peripheral Vascular Disease and Quality of Care Outcomes in Research Interdisciplinary Working Groups: the American Academy of Neurology affirms the value of this guideline as an educational tool for neurologists. *Stroke.* 2007;38(5):1655–1711.

penumbra, brain tissue is still salvageable. Permissive hypertension is used during the first 24–48 hours after the ischemic event. After that time period, providers should initiate a gradual lowering of BP parameters. The final BP goal is patient specific and determined by the presence of intracranial stenosis and coexisting medical conditions. Specific management of high BP should be individualized and based on factors such as the patient's history of hypertension, candidacy for thrombolytic therapy, location of the large vessel occlusion, and whether there is collateral blood flow.[4]

- For patients who do not receive thrombolytics and have no other contraindications, permissive hypertension allows for a systolic BP up to 220 mm Hg and diastolic BP up to 120 mm Hg.[5]
- The American Heart Association recommends that patients who are eligible for thrombolytic therapy be treated to a goal systolic BP <185 mm Hg and diastolic BP <110 mm Hg before the administration of thrombolytics[3] (Table 5.1).
  - After thrombolytic therapy, systolic BP should be kept <180 mm Hg and diastolic BP <105 mm Hg.[3]

Interventions for the Emergent Treatment of Acute Ischemic Stroke

Arterial recanalization and cerebral reperfusion have been shown to help restore brain function when performed shortly after AIS.[6] The primary goal of treatment is to optimize perfusion and avoid secondary brain injury.[4] It is important for neurologic nurses to understand the principles of thrombolytic medications and mechanical thrombectomy to provide optimal care for patients before and after interventions.

Thrombolytic Therapy: r-tPA and TNK

Thrombolytic therapy is used to stimulate clot breakdown and restore cerebral circulation, effectively limiting the extent of brain injury caused by an ischemic stroke. To be a candidate for

TABLE 5.2 ■ **Inclusion and Exclusion Criteria for IV Thrombolytic Treatment of Acute Ischemic Stroke**

Inclusion Criteria	Exclusion Criteria
• Diagnosis of ischemic stroke causing measurable neurologic deficit • Treatment within 4.5 hours of symptom onset (IV r-tPA between 3 and 4.5 hours is not FDA approved)	• Current intracranial hemorrhage • Subarachnoid hemorrhage • Active internal bleeding • Recent (within 3 months) intracranial or intraspinal surgery or serious head trauma • History of intracerebral hemorrhage • Bleeding diathesis (platelet count <100,000 and therapeutic anticoagulation) • Current severe uncontrolled hypertension • Infective endocarditis • Aortic arch dissection • Intraaxial intracranial neoplasm • GI malignancy or GI bleed within 21 days

Additional exclusion criteria between 3 and 4.5 hours:
- Age >80 years
- Severe stroke (NIHSS >25)
- History of diabetes and prior stroke
- Taking an oral anticoagulant regardless of INR

FDA, Food and Drug Administration; *GI,* gastrointestinal; *INR,* international normalized ratio; *IV,* intravenous; *NIHSS,* National Institutes of Health Stroke Scale; *r-tPA,* recombinant tissue plasminogen activator.
Data from de los Rios la Rosa F, Khoury J, Kissela BM, et al. Eligibility for intravenous recombinant tissue-type plasminogen activator within a population: the effect of the European cooperative acute stroke study (ECASS) III trial. *Stroke.* 2012;43(6):1591–1595.

thrombolytic therapy with r-tPA or TNK, patients must be evaluated within 4.5 hours of the onset of symptoms and have a neurologic deficit measured by the NIHSS (Table 5.2).[2] Thrombolytics have been shown to successfully improve patients' functional outcomes only when administered within 4.5 hours of symptom onset.[4] Given this specific time frame, it is of the utmost importance that family members and nurses note precisely when the patient was last at their neurologic baseline. Furthermore, activating a stroke alert as early as possible will ensure that a patient has the best chance of being eligible for maximum reperfusion therapy. Eligible patients should receive thrombolytic treatment without delay even if mechanical thrombectomy also is under consideration.[7]

The guidelines in Table 5.2 highlight important inclusion and exclusion criteria for treatment with thrombolytics. Before starting thrombolytic therapy, a noncontrast CT scan of the brain is required to rule out intracranial hemorrhage. Giving r-tPA or TNK when there is cerebral hemorrhage present can lead to devastating and life-threatening consequences.[2]

- r-tPA (Alteplase) dosing: 0.9 mg/kg IV, not to exceed 90 mg total dose. Administer 10% of the total dose as an initial IV bolus over 1 minute and the remainder infused over 60 minutes.
- TNK (Tenecteplase) dosing: 0.25 mg/kg, not to exceed 25 mg as a single bolus.[8]

Due to the risk of cerebral hemorrhage associated with thrombolytic therapy itself, thrombolytic infusions should be immediately discontinued if there is any change in the patient's neurologic exam during treatment, the physician should be notified, and the staff should prepare the patient for a STAT head CT. Postthrombolytic nursing care is aimed at the prevention and early detection of complications within the first 24 hours after thrombolytic infusion. Vital signs and neurologic exam should be checked every 15 minutes for 2 hours, followed by every 30 minutes for 6 hours, then every hour for 16 hours. During this time, patients should not be given any anticoagulation therapy (e.g., warfarin, apixaban, rivaroxaban, or heparin) or antiplatelet medications (e.g., aspirin or clopidogrel). It is important to avoid nasogastric tubes, unnecessary blood draws, and invasive lines if possible because the patient is at a higher risk of bleeding after receiving thrombolytic medications.

Signs and symptoms of neurologic deterioration include new or worsening neurologic deficits, headache, nausea and vomiting, change in level of consciousness, lethargy, sedation, confusion, and agitation. If any of these develop, nurses should immediately notify the physician team for further evaluation. Nurses must also identify and report any evidence of angioedema, such as swelling of the tongue. At the end of the 24-hour postthrombolytic monitoring period, a noncontrast CT scan of the brain should be obtained to screen for cerebral hemorrhage.[6,9,10]

Mechanical Thrombectomy

MT is a procedure performed by an interventional neurologist or neurosurgeon. It is the standard of care for patients with ischemic strokes caused by large vessel occlusions, mostly localized in the anterior circulation. The anterior circulation of the brain is supplied by the internal carotid arteries, and it consists of the middle cerebral artery and anterior cerebral artery. Occlusions within this vascular network can be seen on CT angiogram/perfusion images.[6,9,10]

MT begins with the insertion of a catheter into the femoral or radial artery. This catheter is passed through to the carotids and advanced until it reaches the thrombus (blood clot) that has caused the stroke. Using CT imaging guidance, a stent retriever is inserted into the catheter and advanced beyond the thrombus, where it is expanded to stretch the arterial walls and allow increased blood flow before being retrieved (i.e., pulled backward), thereby removing the clot. Unlike thrombolytic therapy, which has a strict 4.5-hour time frame for administration, MT can be done for patients with a large vessel occlusion within 6–24 hours of initial stroke symptom onset regardless of whether they also received thrombolytic therapy.

Nursing management postthrombectomy should prioritize early detection of neurologic decline and catheter site problems (Box 5.2). Following MT, patients often are admitted to a neurologic intensive care unit for close surveillance of their neurologic status and to monitor for hemorrhagic conversion and mass effect.[3] Postprocedurally, nurses should assess the catheter

---

BOX 5.2 ■ Postmechanical Thrombectomy Management

- Check blood pressure and neurologic exam every 15 minutes for 2 hours, followed by every 30 minutes for 6 hours, then every hour for 16 hours.
- Assess and monitor the groin/wrist catheter insertion site and the distal extremities, including their circulation, pulses, capillary refill, skin color, sensation, and motor function.
- Monitor for access site complications such as arterial spasm, pain, swelling, bruising, erythema, bleeding, hematoma, pulsatile mass, and drainage from the puncture site.

Data from Rodgers ML, Fox E, Abdelhak A, et al. Care of the patient with acute ischemic stroke (endovascular/intensive care unit-postinterventional therapy): update to 2009 comprehensive nursing care scientific statement: a scientific statement from the American Heart Association. *Stroke.* 2021;52(5):e198-e210.

insertion site (femoral or radial) and check circulation in the distal extremities. Complications related to catheter insertion include retroperitoneal hemorrhage, pseudoaneurysm, arterial occlusion neuropathy, and infection. Vital signs and neurologic exams should be checked at the same interval as patients who have received thrombolytics.

Conclusion

Nursing management of stroke requires strong foundational knowledge of the topic, attentive clinical assessments, and diligent adherence to evidence-based protocols. Neurologic nurses should know the inclusion and exclusion criteria for receiving thrombolytic therapy, medication dosage and infusion protocols, and how best to care for patients in the postthrombolytic period. They are in the best position to detect any changes in status and advocate for proper stroke care. Protocolized vital signs and neurologic exams are critical to prevention and early detection of complications, and nurses should ensure that all members of the interprofessional team remain cognizant of the risk of bleeding and take appropriate measures to minimize the chances of causing harm. If any signs or symptoms of neurologic deterioration are noted, nurses should immediately alert the physician or stroke alert team so that timely assessment and interventions can be performed.

Caring for patients who have undergone MT follows the same guidelines as r-tPA, even when r-tPA was not administered. Frequent nursing assessment of the catheter insertion site is important for the identification of postprocedural complications, which may include hematoma, bleeding, pulsatile mass, swelling, or drainage. It is important that nurses examine the pulses and circulation distal to catheter access sites, noting the capillary refill, skin color, temperature, and motor function of the extremities.[5] Any abnormal findings should be reported immediately to the physician team. A thorough understanding of stroke management and a collaborative communicative approach with patients, their families, and the care team can help maximize a patient's recovery after a devastating ischemic event.

References

1. Virani SS, Alonso A, Aparicio HJ, et al. Heart disease and stroke statistics—2021 update: a report from the american heart association. *Circulation*. 2021;143(8):e254–e743.
2. Meyer BC, Hemmen TM, Jackson CM, et al. Modified national institutes of health stroke scale for use in stroke clinical trials: prospective reliability and validity. *Stroke*. 2002;33(5):1261–1266.
3. Powers WJ, Rabinstein AA, Ackerson T, et al. 2018 guidelines for the early management of patients with acute ischemic stroke: a guideline for healthcare professionals from the American Heart Association/American Stroke Association. *Stroke*. 2018;49(3):e46–e110.
4. Rabinstein AA. Treatment of acute ischemic stroke. *Continuum*. 2017;23(1):62–81.
5. Rodgers ML, Fox E, Abdelhak T, et al. Care of the patient with acute ischemic stroke (endovascular/intensive care unit-postinterventional therapy): update to 2009 comprehensive nursing care scientific statement: a scientific statement from the American Heart Association. *Stroke*. 2021;52(5):e198–e210.
6. Molina CA. Reperfusion therapies for acute ischemic stroke: current pharmacological and mechanical approaches. *Stroke*. 2011;42(1):S16–S19.
7. Oliveira-Filho J, Samuels OB. Mechanical thrombectomy for acute ischemic stroke. *UpToDate*. Retrieved February 8, 2022.
8. Parsons M, Spratt N, Bivard A, et al. A randomized trial of tenecteplase versus alteplase for acute ischemic stroke. *N Engl J Med*. 2012;366(12):1099–1107.
9. SPS3 Study Group, Benavente OR, Coffey CS, et al. Blood-pressure targets in patients with recent lacunar stroke: the sps3 randomised trial. *Lancet*. 2013;382(9891):507–515.
10. Nogueira RG, Jadhav AP, Haussen DC, et al. Thrombectomy 6–24 hours after stroke with a mismatch between deficit and infarct. *N Engl J Med*. 2018;378(1):11–21.

Questions

1. A patient is admitted to the hospital with an acute ischemic stroke. Which of the following should be obtained during her workup?
   a. Noncontrast head CT
   b. ECG
   c. Lipid panel
   d. Both a and c
   e. All the above

2. A patient presents with left facial droop that started 5 hours ago and is diagnosed with an acute ischemic stroke. His BP is 202/108 mm Hg, and his family asks why he has not received more treatment to lower the blood pressure. How should the nurse respond?
   a. He will likely receive r-tPA, and it is best to wait until after the infusion to lower the blood pressure.
   b. His blood pressure is too high and should be lowered to a systolic BP <180 mm Hg and diastolic BP <105 mm Hg.
   c. Permissive hypertension is recommended to promote thrombus breakdown.
   d. His blood pressure is high, but for now it is within an acceptable range to promote cerebral perfusion.

3. A 56-year-old patient arrives in the emergency department with hemiparesis and dysarthria that started 2 hours ago. Which of the following would exclude this patient from receiving r-tPA?
   a. The presence of hemiparesis
   b. Systolic BP 180 mm Hg
   c. Brain tumor resection 2 months ago
   d. Gastrointestinal bleed 5 months ago

4. A patient who presented with an acute ischemic stroke received r-tPA. How frequently should the patient's vital signs and neurologic exam be monitored after receiving r-tPA?
   a. Every 15 minutes for 2 hours, then every 30 minutes for 6 hours, then hourly for 16 hours
   b. Every 15 minutes for 1 hour, then every 30 minutes for 3 hours, then hourly for 20 hours
   c. Every 15 minutes for 2 hours, then every 30 minutes for 4 hours, then hourly for 6 hours
   d. Every 15 minutes for 3 hours, then every 30 minutes for 4 hours, then hourly for 5 hours

5. A patient is admitted to the neurologic intensive care unit after undergoing a mechanical thrombectomy. Which of the following should the nurse assess?
   a. Catheter insertion site
   b. Distal extremity pulses and circulation
   c. Vital signs
   d. Neurologic exam
   e. All the above

Answers

1. e

2. d

3. c

4. a

5. e

CHAPTER 6

Nursing Management of the Patient With a Brain Tumor

Michael P. Baldassari, BA, MD ▪ Nikolaos Mouchtouris, MD
▪ Ellina Hattar, MD ▪ Christopher J. Farrell, MD

Introduction

Of all neurosurgery patients, patients with brain tumors are perhaps the most complex and varied in terms of their disease process, neurologic exam, preoperative planning, postoperative care, and prognosis. Nursing care for these patients is similarly varied and requires an in-depth understanding of a wide range of disease protocols. Preoperative management includes optimization of patients for the procedure, while perioperative and postoperative phases focus on management of complications that may arise from both surgery and prolonged hospital stay. Nurses should understand the most common pathways of brain tumor care to maximize patient recovery and limit complications.

TYPES OF BRAIN TUMORS

Brain tumors are broadly categorized by their location relative to brain tissue. Intraaxial tumors arise from cells within the brain tissue; extraaxial tumors arise from the tissues surrounding the brain, such as the dura or peripheral nerves. Radiographic features are typically able to discern whether a brain tumor is intra- or extraaxial (Fig. 6.1).

Brain tumors may also be categorized as either benign or malignant. This determination must be made by a pathologist after examining surgically obtained tumor tissue. However, clinical factors and radiographic features often provide many clues as to whether a particular brain tumor is benign or malignant. See Table 6.1 for a list of the most common brain tumors and their broad categories.[1]

TYPES OF NEUROSURGICAL PROCEDURES FOR BRAIN TUMORS

Neurosurgical procedures for brain tumors are categorized by the goal of the procedure being performed. The goal of a biopsy procedure is to obtain enough representative tissue for pathologic exam and genetic testing, which are needed to guide further treatment. Biopsies can be conducted via stereotactic localization with a needle or via open craniotomy and excision. Tumor resections involve opening the skull via craniotomy or craniectomy and removing as much of the tumor as is safely possible. The goal of surgical resection is often twofold: The first is to relieve mass effect and tumor burden; the second is to obtain a tissue diagnosis, such as in biopsy procedures. In both biopsy and resection surgeries, pathologic exam is usually performed immediately on a frozen sample, then later on preserved/processed tissue, which can be tested to produce a final pathologic diagnosis.[2]

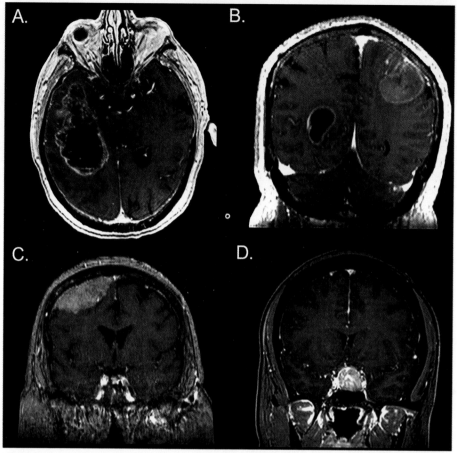

Fig. 6.1 Common brain tumors on magnetic resonance imaging, postcontrast. (A) Glioblastoma (grade 4 astrocytoma), ring-enhancing lesions with irregular borders. (B) Breast adenocarcinoma metastases, varying appearance (cystic vs homogenous), appearing at white/gray matter junction. (C) Meningioma—peripheral, typically homogenous enhancing mass causing mass effect against the cortex, arising from dura. (D) Pituitary macroadenoma—enhancing mass in sella, between optic nerves and carotid arteries.

Biopsy

In general, biopsies offer a less invasive way of diagnosing a tumor, and they often precede more invasive procedures of tumor removal. Tissue diagnosis is an invaluable step in the care of most patients with brain tumors. In some cases, radiographic features and clinical presentation could be so definitive that a neurosurgeon is confident proceeding with resection without a biopsy. This is often the case for meningiomas, schwannomas, pituitary macroadenomas, and some metastases/primary brain cancers. However, there are certain situations in which a biopsy must precede total resection. For example, for central nervous system (CNS) lymphoma or germinoma, the tumor must be pathologically identified as such before treatment, as these tumors are not treated with total resection. CNS lymphoma is treated with systemic methotrexate, and germinoma is treated with radiation. If an intraoperative frozen section of these tumors is suggestive of either of these tumor types, further resection is aborted in favor of the respective nonsurgical treatment option.

TABLE 6.1 ■ Common Intraaxial and Extraaxial Brain Tumors

Intraaxial	Extraaxial
Central nervous system lymphoma	Colloid cyst
Central neurocytoma	Cranial nerve schwannoma
Craniopharyngioma	Dermoid cyst
Dysembryoplastic neuroepithelial tumor	Epidermoid cyst
Ependymoma	Hemangiopericytoma
Ganglioglioma	Meningioma
Germinoma	Metastasis
Glioblastoma	
Hemangioblastoma	
Lipoma	
Low-grade astrocytoma	
Medulloblastoma	
Metastasis	
Oligodendroglioma	
Pilocytic astrocytoma	
Pineoblastoma	
Pineocytoma	
Pituitary adenoma	
Pleomorphic xanthoastrocytoma	
Subependymoma	
Teratoma	

If the frozen section were to return with a diagnosis of likely glioma, for example, a neurosurgeon would proceed with maximal safe resection.[3]

Craniotomy/Craniectomy

Craniotomy is the most well-known neurosurgical treatment option for brain tumors. It involves opening the skin, exposing the skull, creating a window through the skull with a drill, opening the overlying dura, then performing dissection and tumor removal. Cranial windows can be either a small burr hole or a larger window created by removing a section of the skull, called a bone flap. Burr hole exposures are adequate for needle biopsy of tumors or some endoscopic surgeries that involve passing an endoscope through the brain cortex into the cerebrospinal fluid (CSF)–filled ventricles. Open craniotomies, which produce a bone flap, are used for larger exposures that require two-handed dissection and a larger surgical corridor. After craniotomy procedures, the bone flap is usually replaced and fixed with titanium plates and screws, or a titanium mesh is used instead of the original bone flap. There are certain situations in which the bone is left off and the opening in the skull is left open. In this situation the procedure is referred to as a craniectomy rather than a craniotomy.[4]

Endoscopy

A craniotomy typically requires a long reach with significant dissection and retraction of normal anatomy to create an adequate corridor. Certain common tumors are in anatomic regions that are more difficult to access through standard craniotomy approaches. For example, pituitary adenomas and craniopharyngiomas affect regions of the skull base behind the optic chiasm called the sellar and suprasellar regions. Modern surgical treatment of pituitary adenomas is conducted by both neurosurgeons and otorhinolaryngologists, who access and remove the tumor using long and narrow instruments through the nose with the help of an endoscopic camera. Endoscopic instruments can be used to access any deep-seated lesion, whether it is through the nose or a craniotomy/burr hole.[5]

Common Treatment Pathways

Although the clinical course for patients with a brain tumor is often tailored to the patient, some of the most common tumor types will follow a predetermined treatment pathway. Most patients with a brain tumor in the hospital will be experiencing one or several of the steps of these common pathways; however, it is important to understand that many brain tumors do not fit into these broad categories. For example, metastatic brain tumors are typically resected to relieve mass effect, while further treatment course will depend on the primary cancer identity. Also, patients who are enrolled in clinical trials may have different clinical courses or medical requirements when compared to typical patients with the same disease.

GLIOBLASTOMA (GRADE 4 ASTROCYTOMA)

Glioblastoma (GBM) is the most common primary malignant brain tumor and has a thoroughly studied treatment pathway also known as the Stupp protocol. In 2005, a research team published an optimized treatment pathway to maximize progression-free survival in GBM patients, which is still widely accepted as standard of care.[6] Once GBM is suspected on imaging, the patient will undergo surgery to remove as much of the tumor as possible, known as maximal safe resection. After surgery, the tissue is examined, and the final pathology report is completed, along with certain genetic markers that have implications for response to therapy. Then, after a 2–4-week recovery period, the patient begins a 6-week treatment course of temozolomide chemotherapy and concomitant radiotherapy. Once this stage is complete, the patient undergoes a 4-week recovery period, then begins adjuvant maintenance temozolomide without radiotherapy. Despite this process, patients with GBM have a median progression-free survival of only 15 months.[7]

LOW-GRADE GLIOMA (GRADES 1–3 ASTROCYTOMA)

Although grade 4 gliomas are the most common type of primary brain cancer, other, less aggressive gliomas are relatively commonly encountered. Low-grade gliomas typically carry a better prognosis than GBM, but survival varies significantly by genetic subtype and multiple other factors. Grade 3 gliomas have a median survival of 3–5 years, and grade 2 median survivals of 8 years. Grade 1 gliomas are usually cured by surgery alone and have a 96% survival rate at 5 years from surgery.[8] Although there is some disagreement about the best adjuvant therapy between the different subtypes of glioma, the first step in treatment involves histopathologic diagnosis and maximum safe resection.

- Patients with grade 1 tumors are generally followed with serial imaging and require no adjuvant therapy.
- Patients with grade 2 tumors sometimes will undergo adjuvant chemotherapy and radiation depending on prognostic factors including age, extent of resection, and genetic biomarkers.
- Patients with grade 3 tumors almost always require adjuvant chemotherapy (temozolomide) and radiation, although the interval and dosing of these treatment methods vary.

METASTASES

The most common type of brain tumor is metastasis from a primary tumor somewhere else in the body. The most common primary cancer sites that metastasize to the brain include lung, breast, and melanoma.[9] Metastases have a variable appearance on imaging but tend to occur at the gray-white matter junction of the cortex. Brain metastases grow quickly, so patients often present after hemorrhage or due to extensive edema around the tumor. The role of surgery for brain metastasis varies depending on size, number of metastases, and prior treatments; however, highly symptomatic lesions are usually considered for surgical removal.

If considering surgical resection for a lesion that is causing minimal symptoms, a computed tomography (CT) scan of the chest, abdomen, and pelvis is usually performed prior to the neurosurgical procedure. If systemic imaging shows no obvious source of metastasis, a peripheral lesion or lesion in a non-eloquent area is usually biopsied, as tissue diagnosis may reveal a tumor type that is amenable to chemotherapy, radiation, or monoclonal/immunotherapy. When multiple brain metastases occur, it is often reasonable to perform a resection on the largest or most symptomatic lesion and leave the smaller, asymptomatic lesions for treatment with other modalities. Patients will typically undergo radiation after their resection to prevent recurrence. Multiple lesions can be treated by stereotactic radiosurgery; however, whole brain radiation is also an option when the intracranial metastatic tumor burden is extensive.[10]

MENINGIOMA

Meningioma is the most common benign brain tumor in the adult population, accounting for ~33% of all diagnosed brain tumors.[11] Meningiomas are typically operated on only when they become symptomatic or are demonstrated to be growing. If they are incidentally identified, neurosurgeons may opt for conservative imaging surveillance. For smaller tumors exhibiting growth or for tumors in areas of the brain difficult to access without causing surgical morbidity, such as the cavernous sinus region, the patient may undergo radiosurgery to halt the progression of the tumor. If this is unsuccessful in stopping the growth of the meningioma, the neurosurgeon may then choose to take the patient to the operating room (OR) for the progressive tumor.

The goal of surgery on meningiomas is gross total resection, with removal of all adjacent dura from which the tumor originated. However, some meningiomas, particularly those affecting the skull base, major vessels, and cranial nerves, may be difficult to resect in their entirety. Recurrence of meningiomas can be predicted by the extent of resection. Follow-up of postoperative meningioma patients will involve monitoring for recurrence, particularly if gross total resection was not achieved on postoperative imaging. It is important to note, however, that >15% of meningiomas behave in a more aggressive manner with high rates of recurrence and in approximately 1% of situations have a malignant course.[12] Pathology diagnosis is still important for prognostic purposes and to guide adjuvant therapies such as radiation.

SELLAR TUMORS

Most sellar tumors arise along an area of the skull base that is easily accessed through an endonasal endoscopic approach. The most common types of tumors that occur in this region include pituitary adenomas and craniopharyngiomas. Both tumors are benign and may be cured by complete resection. Pituitary adenomas can be either secretory or nonsecretory depending on which pituitary cell type they originated from. If secretory, they will secrete the hormone corresponding to their cell of origin. As sellar tumors grow, they press against the posterior aspect of the optic chiasm resulting in the classic physical exam finding of bitemporal hemianopsia. Sellar tumors are typically removed electively except when they present with hemorrhage (apoplexy) and an acute change in exam typically in the form of sudden onset headache and/or visual deficit diplopia, in which case they are removed emergently. Postoperative nurses need to monitor these patients for evidence of CSF leak, because inadequate closure of the intradural space may lead to the development of meningitis.[13]

POSTERIOR FOSSA TUMORS

Common tumors that affect the posterior fossa include metastasis, glioma, meningioma, schwannoma, ependymoma, and epidermoid/dermoid cysts. Performing surgery in this anatomic region is particularly dangerous due to the higher relative density of arteries, venous sinuses, and cranial nerves. Also, the posterior fossa is a smaller space when compared with the rest of the brain, so changes in pressure or small amounts of edema can have dangerous consequences. CSF flows from the brain into the posterior fossa through a thin outflow tract called the cerebral aqueduct. If surgery is performed in posterior fossa, the cerebellum could swell from direct tissue manipulation or stroke around the surgical area. If swelling occurs, the cerebral aqueduct could become occluded, and the patient could potentially suffer acute obstructive hydrocephalus, which is a neurosurgical emergency. In general, there is a low threshold for repeat imaging with any changes in exam.

Another complication after posterior fossa surgery is the development of a pseudomeningocele, which is a CSF filling of the epidural space over the surgical bed. This would present as excessive, ballotable incisional swelling. To reduce the chances of hydrocephalus and pseudomeningocele formation, patients are kept with their head of bed (HOB) elevated to reduce intracranial pressure (ICP). Headwraps are utilized to provide support to the incision for 24–72 hours until it heals, minimizing the risk of pseudomeningocele formation. Depending on the extent of the surgery, many neurosurgeons will opt to leave the bone flap off after a posterior fossa tumor resection.[14]

Preoperative Period

The preoperative period for patients with a brain tumor revolves around operative clearance and surgical planning. Patients should obtain preoperative cardiac risk stratification and blood work to assess electrolytes, hemoglobin, coagulation profile, and tumor markers (in certain situations).

SPECIAL LAB VALUES

In patients with concern for metastasis (i.e., have a known primary), particular lab values may be drawn to monitor the tumor burden of the respective primary. Such values include carcinoembryonic antigen, carbohydrate antigen 19, prostate-specific antigen, and vitamin D. Other tumors, such as germinoma, teratoma, and choriocarcinoma, may present with systemically measurable tumor markers, such as beta-human chorionic gonadotropin, alpha-fetoprotein, and/or placental alkaline phosphatase.[15] For patients with pituitary tumors it is imperative to check a full pituitary function panel to determine which cell type the pituitary tumor originated from. In the specific case of a prolactin-secreting pituitary tumor, the first-line treatment is a dopamine agonist medication, such as bromocriptine or cabergoline. Such medications have been proven effective in treating these prolactinomas and can obviate the need for surgery.[16] Patients with other pituitary adenomas (such as thyroid-secreting or nonsecretory tumors) may need preemptive endocrine replacement therapy.

ANTICOAGULATION/ANTIPLATELETS

Patients who have conditions that warrant anticoagulation or antiplatelets will likely be asked to stop taking these medications prior to surgery. It is of the upmost importance to confirm that patients have stopped taking these medications as instructed when they arrive for surgery. Patients who are admitted to the hospital will often be ordered medical deep venous thromboembolism (DVT) prophylaxis. Patients undergoing craniotomy should have this prophylactic medication paused by midnight prior to the procedure.[17] For common antiplatelet and anticoagulation medications, see Table 6.2.

TABLE 6.2 ■ Common Preoperative Anticoagulation and Antiplatelets

Generic	Trade Name	Category
Warfarin	Coumadin	Anticoagulant
Rivaroxaban	Xarelto	Anticoagulant
Apixaban	Eliquis	Anticoagulant
ASA 81 mg	Baby Aspirin	Antiplatelet
ASA 325 mg	Full Aspirin	Antiplatelet
Clopidogrel	Plavix	Antiplatelet
Ticagrelor	Brilinta	Antiplatelet

IMAGING

All preoperative patients with a brain tumor must undergo a series of brain imaging for operative planning. Head CT is typically the first study performed and is responsible for identifying the lesion in question. In most scenarios, the CT is followed up by magnetic resonance imaging (MRI) of the brain with and without contrast. The typical ring-enhancing lesions can only be seen when comparing pre- and postcontrast MRI. Peritumoral edema must be identified on either MRI T2 or fluid-attenuated inversion recovery sequences. If a patient has concern for bony involvement, a dedicated CT is obtained of the region in question (sinus, skull base, etc.). If an intraaxial tumor is affecting either eloquent language or motor regions, the neurosurgeon could potentially order a functional MRI (fMRI) to delineate these regions prior to surgery. Pending the results of the fMRI, surgical resection may be performed awake for cortical brain mapping, which tells the surgeon which areas of the brain are safe to remove and which must be left behind.

Patients with concern for metastasis will invariably undergo imaging of the body to determine if a possible primary tumor exists. Usually this body imaging is a CT of the chest, abdomen, and pelvis or potentially a positron emission tomography scan. If extensive bony metastases are noted, a nuclear medicine radioisotope scan may be ordered as well. If there is a mass in an easily accessible location, and the brain metastasis is not causing significant symptoms or edema/mass effect, then the neurosurgeon may opt to not proceed with cranial surgery and defer to a biopsy of the systemic mass for pathology.[18]

ANTIEPILEPTICS

Patients with tumors affecting the supratentorial region are at increased risk for seizures, especially those tumors that directly impact the cortex or medial temporal lobes. Any manipulation of the brain cortex (either by the brain tumor or the neurosurgeon) could potentially lead to hyperactivity, which can generate epileptic discharges. Due to this risk, seizure prophylaxis, which commonly includes levetiracetam 500 mg twice daily (BID) or lacosamide 100 mg BID, is usually prescribed.[19] Symptoms of seizures include staring, altered mental status, forced gaze deviation, uncontrollable jerking movements, and sensory changes. If a patient is possibly seizing or has an altered mental status after a possible unwitnessed seizure, the physician should be notified, and lorazepam 2 mg should be administered intravenously (IV) to abort the seizure. Cranial electroencephalogram may be initiated with the goal of documenting epileptic activity.[20]

STEROIDS

Dexamethasone is the quintessential steroid used by neurosurgeons to control peritumoral edema. Compared to other steroids, dexamethasone is more active in the CNS while causing fewer neuropsychiatric side effects. Also, oral (PO) and IV dosing is in a 1:1 ratio, which is useful in outpatient to inpatient transitions. Starting dose is typically 4 mg every 6 hours, but clinical presentation and surgeon preference will cause this value to vary. Dexamethasone may be used for both intra- and extraaxial tumors. When parenchymal edema is present, dexamethasone can lessen the symptoms associated with edema.[21]

In patients suspected of having CNS lymphoma, steroids must be avoided. The pathway for CNS lymphoma first involves a biopsy of the brain tumor, as this will guide treatment and prognosis. If steroids are given, a CNS lymphoma tumor will rapidly and significantly decrease in size without curing the disease. If the tumor changes morphology and size between the preoperative imaging and the image-guided biopsy procedure, the accuracy and yield of the biopsy could be jeopardized.[22] Once CNS lymphoma is confirmed on biopsy, high-dose steroids may be used to reduce mass effect and tumor burden.

Patients who are on a chronic steroid regimen will sometimes need stress-dose steroids before and after undergoing surgery to prevent adrenal insufficiency. In these patients, cranial procedures for tumor removal are considered major surgery; therefore 100 mg of hydrocortisone should be administered on the day of surgery, with another 100 mg administered on postoperative day 1.[23] In the tumor population many patients are already receiving adequate steroid dosing, which incidentally meets this requirement. A 0.75-mg dose of dexamethasone is equivalent to 20 mg of hydrocortisone. Patients who are already taking >4 mg of dexamethasone daily will meet stress-dose requirements, and additional hydrocortisone is not indicated.

Most patients will continue their preoperative steroid dosing for several days postop and then begin a taper. Patients with meningiomas or other benign tumors will likely taper their dexamethasone to off, while malignant brain tumors may taper to a lower dose but continue that indefinitely. Much of the dosing is subject to surgeon preferences, side effects, and individual medical factors. While on steroids, patients should be closely monitored for hyperglycemia via serial point-of-care glucose measurements.[24]

Perioperative Period

Postoperative complications are likely to present in the first 24–48 hours after surgery. Consistent and thorough neurologic exams, as well as the optimization of all bodily systems, can prevent minor and/or devastating complications and improve overall outcomes. Most postoperative patients with a brain tumor are brought to the neuro-intensive care unit (NICU) for at least 1 day for perioperative management. The postoperative course in the NICU will vary from patient to patient, but patients may stay in the NICU for extended periods if they require mechanical ventilation, external ventricular drain (EVD) placement, pressor requirement, and administration of medications via central line access.

NEUROLOGIC SYSTEM

Once the patient is brought from the OR to the NICU, close monitoring of the patient's neurologic status should begin immediately with serial neurologic exams. Most patients will be positioned supine, with the HOB raised to >30 degrees. In patients at risk for increased postoperative ICP, the HOB should be elevated to >45 degrees. Patients who undergo larger craniotomies may come to the NICU with subgaleal Jackson-Pratt (JP) drains and a headwrap. The JP drains are often kept to suction and removed 1–2 days after the surgery, pending decreasing output. It is important for nurses to note the consistency and color of the drain output. If CSF is suspected in the drain (thin consistency, high volume, mostly clear or blood tinged), there may be a communication with the drain and the subdural space, and the physician should be notified. The headwrap will typically remain in place until the attending neurosurgeon clears it for removal. Typically, patients with a posterior fossa tumor will have their headwraps stay on longer than patients with a supratentorial tumor, but this varies by surgeon preference.[25]

Common complications include hemorrhage into the surgical bed, surgically induced stroke, seizure, and hydrocephalus. Hemorrhage and postsurgical stroke are more common after intra-axial brain tumor resection. Signs of a hemorrhage include sudden headache, altered mental status, and examination findings consistent with herniation (e.g., blown pupil and hemiparesis).[2] A change in neurologic exam may indicate a surgically induced stroke. The location of the surgery will impact which stroke symptoms the patient will have.

- If a brain tumor close to the motor strip is removed, a surgical stroke may produce a contralateral focal motor deficit.
- If a brain tumor in the temporal or occipital lobes is removed, a surgical stroke may produce a visual field deficit.

It is important, however, to distinguish between new surgical stroke deficits, preexisting neurologic deficits, and deficits expected from the specific surgery performed. For example, ipsilateral cerebellar tumors and posterior fossa surgery commonly cause dysmetria. If this is noted on postoperative exam, it is important to know whether this finding predated surgery or was only present immediately after surgery. Imaging may only be warranted if the symptom is new or significantly worsened from pre- or postoperative exam.

Patients who undergo tumor resections in the posterior fossa (e.g., cerebellum, brainstem) or midbrain (e.g., pineal region) are at risk for acute hydrocephalus. Here, postsurgical swelling can occlude the normal outflow of the CSF through the cerebral aqueduct. Symptoms of hydrocephalus include headache, altered mental status, and persistent decreased wakefulness. A head CT is used to check for postoperative hydrocephalus, and if present, the patient may need bedside EVD placement. In fact, many patients with a high suspicion of developing postoperative hydrocephalus will preemptively undergo EVD placement in the OR. Hydrocephalus must always be suspected in patients with leptomeningeal metastasis. In this case, the occlusion of the arachnoid granulations by cancer cells can cause the intracranial space to accumulate CSF. Patients with leptomeningeal hydrocephalus may require EVD, lumbar drain, or palliative ventriculoperitoneal shunt placement.[26]

CARDIAC SYSTEM

Close cardiac monitoring is important in postoperative patients with a brain tumor. Mean arterial pressure (MAP) should remain at <100 to reduce the chance of postoperative hemorrhage. In the NICU a nicardipine or labetalol titratable infusion should be used in most scenarios, but control with as-needed (PRN) medications may be adequate in many cases. Arrhythmias are common in postoperative patients. When noted on telemetry, an immediate 12-lead electrocardiogram (ECG) should be obtained, and the physician should be notified. The physician may order lab work to test the patient's electrolytes and replete any abnormalities.[27]

Patients with high preoperative risk stratification of postoperative cardiac events should undergo close cardiac monitoring by telemetry. Patients on home anticoagulation or antiplatelets for prior stroke, coronary artery disease/stents, or atrial fibrillation will likely be holding their respective medication for surgery. These patients are thus additionally hypercoagulable beyond standard postoperative hypercoagulability. Any symptoms of myocardial infarction (chest pain, dyspnea, radiating pain, and/or nausea) should prompt an ECG and serial troponin blood tests. Patients with congestive heart failure are also at increased risk of exacerbation after surgery. Neurosurgery procedures may require the use of mannitol or liberal fluid administration, which can lead to fluid imbalances. Therefore clinical volume status should be frequently assessed on all patients with a brain tumor.

If there is concern for a major arterial injury during a neurosurgical procedure, the patient may be ordered increased MAP parameters to help support perfusion of the potentially stenotic/spastic artery. The patient may require a titratable pressor infusion to reach the target MAP. The neurosurgeons are responsible for communicating the target MAP, type of pressor to be used, and the expected duration of the MAP goal. Patients who have increased MAP parameters are at increased risk of hemorrhage, and the care team should monitor for symptoms of postoperative hemorrhage.

PULMONARY SYSTEM

All patients undergoing brain tumor resection are intubated for their procedure. Most patients will be extubated after the procedure in the OR; however, some patients whose mental status does not improve quickly enough after surgery may come to the NICU still intubated. This is a common occurrence after a particularly long surgery or after a surgery where significant complications, such as massive hemorrhage, air embolism, metabolic disturbance, or seizure, have occurred. If coming out of the OR late in the day, most patients will remain intubated overnight and will be sedated accordingly.

Dexmedetomidine is a common option for sedation because its effects can be held temporarily to obtain a neurologic exam, and its intensity is easily titratable.[28] Propofol may be used for patients who require deeper sedation. Significant agitation should be avoided, as it can transiently increase blood pressure and precipitate hemorrhage in the postoperative patient. Once extubated, patients should be closely monitored for oxygen requirements and taught to use an incentive spirometer to avoid postoperative atelectasis.

Due to the immobility associated with surgery, nursing and physician staff should be on high alert for pulmonary embolism (PE). Signs of PE include sudden-onset sharp chest pain, tachypnea, and increasing oxygen requirements. When a patient is sedated and/or intubated, these symptoms could be masked. If there is sufficient concern for PE, physicians may order a STAT CT angiography of the pulmonary vessels.[29]

RENAL/GENITOURINARY/ENDOCRINE SYSTEMS

Patients who undergo brain tumor surgery are also at an increased risk for issues related to the renal and genitourinary systems. Patients may have received a dye load for CT or MRI imaging, they could have a significant fluid imbalance, or their tumor may be affecting their electrolyte homeostasis (i.e., pituitary tumors). Patients should have regular lab work to monitor for kidney injury, and Foley catheters should be removed as soon as possible to reduce the risk of infection.

Pituitary tumors can obliterate some or all functions of the pituitary gland. Patients who have undergone endoscopic surgery to remove a tumor affecting the pituitary gland should be very closely monitored for aberrations in cortisol, sodium homeostasis, input and output trends, and thyroid function. Endocrinologists may be involved in the patient's care to replace the hormones otherwise lost to pituitary resection. Steroids may be prescribed to replace cortisol, levothyroxine may be used to replace thyroid hormone, and DDAVP may be used to replace antidiuretic hormone.[30]

Serious complications of pituitary surgery are diabetes insipidus (DI) and syndrome of inappropriate secretion of antidiuretic hormone (SIADH).[31] Immediately postop, DI can lead to massive urine output and hypernatremia, especially if the patient is unable to drink enough water to compensate for fluid losses. If SIADH occurs, the patient is at an increased risk for seizures due to the hyponatremia that results from the retention of free water.

Postoperative glucose control may be challenging in the neurosurgical subpopulation. NPO status, liberal postoperative steroid use, and possible preoperative diabetic comorbidities may complicate the management of blood glucose. Tight blood glucose control has been linked to improved surgical incision healing and reduced risk for surgical site infection.[24] Point-of-care glucose measurements should be obtained on all postoperative patients, and deviations from normoglycemia should be communicated to the care team. As a rule of thumb, two serial blood glucose levels of >300 will warrant the immediate administration of a titratable insulin infusion.

GASTROINTESTINAL SYSTEM

Adequate nutrition is important in the postoperative recovery process of patients with a brain tumor. Patients should be encouraged to eat as soon as they can tolerate PO intake after postoperative imaging is obtained. Postoperative imaging has the theoretical risk of showing an anomaly that requires further urgent operative intervention.[32] Many patients complain of postanesthesia nausea. First-line treatment for nausea includes prochlorperazine, ondansetron, and transdermal scopolamine patches; second-line treatment includes promethazine or trimethobenzamide. Regular ECG monitoring is important to monitor for QT prolongation when using these medications. Patients should also have frequent metabolic panels done to determine the presence of any electrolyte abnormalities from persistent vomiting.

It is also important to determine whether postoperative nausea is a symptom of the neurosurgical procedure, a side effect from anesthesia, or from postsurgical hydrocephalus. Procedures involving potential trauma to the vestibular nerves (acoustic neuroma resection) or cerebellum (posterior fossa tumor resection) can cause iatrogenic nausea. If the patient has nausea and an altered mental status, or if nausea occurs in a delayed fashion after surgery, a physician should be notified immediately.[33]

HEMATOLOGIC/ONCOLOGIC SYSTEMS

Patients who undergo brain tumor surgery will usually have postoperative labs drawn the following morning. If the estimated blood loss from surgery was high (e.g., if there was a large venous sinus injury), labs may be drawn immediately after surgery. In general, the hemoglobin goal is >7, and any value <7 would prompt a transfusion of packed red blood cells. Furthermore, white blood cell (WBC) count and platelet count should be monitored. WBC could be artificially elevated by administration of steroids or due to infection. Platelet count is usually maintained at >100,000 to avoid excessive bleeding intra- and postoperatively.

INFECTIOUS DISEASE

Postoperative mild fevers are common in the first 24–48 hours after surgery and can be controlled with acetaminophen. Atelectasis or pneumonia can cause a fever. A chest x-ray and sputum culture can be used to confirm the diagnosis, and incentive spirometry should be encouraged. If pneumonia is suspected, the patient can be started on empiric antibiotics. Urinary tract infections (UTIs) are more common in female patients and those who have a Foley catheter in place. UTIs typically occur 3–5 days postoperatively. A urinalysis and urine culture are used for diagnosis, and the treatment is typically a short course of antibiotics. A fever that occurs 5–6 days after surgery can be related to superficial thrombophlebitis or DVT, both of which can be diagnosed by ultrasound. DVTs may prompt anticoagulation therapy or an inferior vena cava filter placement.

It is important for nursing staff to examine the cranial incision multiple times per day to monitor for surgical site infection. Signs of developing infection include erythema, pus, drainage, periincisional swelling, and separation of incision edges. It is also important to examine sites where drains may have exited the skin, as these are potential sources of infection as well. Incisional infections can be treated medically with antibiotics or surgically with wound washout procedures. Infection control is of the utmost importance in patients recovering from brain tumor surgery because infections can easily track down to the subdural space and cause meningitis or encephalitis. An MRI brain, with and without contrast, can determine the depth of the infected tissue and guide prognosis.[34]

Washout procedures are aimed at removing all infected tissue and may involve removing all hardware in the surgical bed. Infectious disease physicians will determine a final course of antibiotics based on OR cultures and sensitivities. If extensive enough, the patient may require a 6-week course of IV antibiotics.[35]

PROPHYLAXIS

Mechanical prophylaxis should be initiated immediately postoperatively and continue for the duration of the admission. Studies have proven it is safe to restart DVT prophylaxis as soon as 24 hours after an intracranial procedure.[36] Enoxaparin is typically preferred over subcutaneous heparin for patients with known malignancy. Antibiotic prophylaxis is also common in the postoperative period. Typically this includes a short 1- or 2-day course of IV antibiotics.

DISPOSITION

Patients with a persistent functional deficit should be evaluated by physical therapy, occupational therapy, and physical medicine and rehabilitation if their rehabilitation needs are extensive. Medical oncology and radiation oncology should be consulted for patients with malignant brain tumors to determine the role of chemotherapy and radiation therapy in the future care of the patient. A restart plan for a patient's anticoagulation and antiplatelet medications should also be determined prior to discharge. Incisions may be closed with absorbable sutures, nonabsorbable sutures (i.e., nylon), or staples. Nonabsorbable sutures or staples are typically removed 14 days postoperatively. If the patient is discharged prior to this date, the sutures or staples should be removed at a predetermined outpatient visit with surgical staff. Prior to discharge, nurses should help ensure follow-up with the neurosurgeon is arranged and the patient understands any need for future imaging.

Conclusion

The clinical course of patients with a brain tumor is complex and varied. Nursing care for these patients is similarly varied and requires an in-depth understanding of the wide range of disease protocols and pathways. Nurses need to be aware of the nuances of pre-, peri-, and postoperative care to maximize patient recovery. Nurses are responsible for close monitoring and are often the first to notice neurologic changes or symptoms concerning infection and complications. By understanding the protocols and pathways, nurses are in the best position to provide thorough education to patients, to continue their recovery in the outpatient setting, and to understand further steps in their care.

References

1. McNeill KA. Epidemiology of brain tumors. *Neurol Clin.* 2016;34(4):981–998.
2. Haybaeck J, von Campe G, Hainfellner JA. Der schnellschnitt in der neuropathologie [Rapid frozen sections in neuropathology]. *Pathologe.* 2012;33(5):379–388.
3. Bonosi L, Marrone S, Benigno UE, et al. Maximal safe resection in glioblastoma surgery: a systematic review of advanced intraoperative image-guided techniques. *Brain Sci.* 2023;13(2):216.
4. Chughtai KA, Nemer OP, Kessler AT, et al. Post-operative complications of craniotomy and craniectomy. *Emerg Radiol.* 2019;26(1):99–107.
5. Shim KW, Park EK, Kim DS, et al. Neuroendoscopy: current and future perspectives. *J Korean Neurosurg Soc.* 2017;60(3):322–326.
6. Stupp R, Mason WP, van den Bent MJ, et al. Radiotherapy plus concomitant and adjuvant temozolomide for glioblastoma. *N Engl J Med.* 2005;352(10):987–996.
7. Omuro A, DeAngelis LM. Glioblastoma and other malignant gliomas: a clinical review. *JAMA.* 2013;310(17):1842–1850.

8. Ostrom QT, Cote DJ, Ascha M, et al. Adult glioma incidence and survival by race or ethnicity in the United States from 2000–2014. *JAMA Oncol.* 2018;4(9):1254–1262.

9. Johnson JD, Young B. Demographics of brain metastasis. *Neurosurg Clin N Am.* 1996;7(3):337–344.

10. Patchell RA, Tibbs PA, Regine WF, et al. Postoperative radiotherapy in the treatment of single metastases to the brain: a randomized trial. *JAMA.* 1998;280(17):1485–1489.

11. Wiemels J, Wrensch M, Claus EB. Epidemiology and etiology of meningioma. *J Neurooncol.* 2010;99(3):307–314.

12. Yang SY, Park CK, Park SH, et al. Atypical and anaplastic meningiomas: prognostic implications of clinicopathological features. *J Neurol Neurosurg Psychiatry.* 2008;79(5):574–580.

13. Fang C, Zhu T, Zhang P, et al. Risk factors of neurosurgical site infection after craniotomy: a systematic review and meta-analysis. *Am J Infect Control.* 2017;45(11):e123–e134.

14. Bullock MR, Chesnut R, Ghajar J, et al. Surgical management of posterior fossa mass lesions. *Neurosurgery.* 2006;58(3):S47–S55; discussion Si–iv.

15. Duffy MJ. Tumor markers in clinical practice: a review focusing on common solid cancers. *Med Princ Pract.* 2013;22(1):4–11.

16. Molitch ME. Diagnosis and treatment of pituitary adenomas: a review. *JAMA.* 2017;317(5):516–524.

17. Alshehri N, Cote DJ, Hulou MM, et al. Venous thromboembolism prophylaxis in brain tumor patients undergoing craniotomy: a meta-analysis. *J Neurooncol.* 2016;130(3):561–570.

18. Kotecha R, Gondi V, Ahluwalia MS, et al. Recent advances in managing brain metastasis. *F1000Res.* 2018;7:F1000 Faculty Rev-1772.

19. Chandra V, Rock AK, Opalak C, et al. A systematic review of perioperative seizure prophylaxis during brain tumor resection: the case for a multicenter randomized clinical trial. *Neurosurg Focus.* 2017;43(5):e18.

20. Ajinkya S, Fox J, Houston P, et al. Seizures in patients with metastatic brain tumors: prevalence, clinical characteristics, and features on EEG. *J Clin Neurophysiol.* 2021;38(2):143–148.

21. Jessurun CAC, Hulsbergen AFC, Cho LD, et al. Evidence-based dexamethasone dosing in malignant brain tumors: what do we really know? *J Neurooncol.* 2019;144(2):249–264.

22. Grommes C, DeAngelis LM. Primary CNS lymphoma. *J Clin Oncol.* 2017;35(21):2410–2418.

23. Hockey B, Leslie K, Williams D. Dexamethasone for intracranial neurosurgery and anaesthesia. *J Clin Neurosci.* 2009;16(11):1389–1393.

24. Lee P, Min L, Mody L. Perioperative glucose control and infection risk in older surgical patients. *Curr Geriatr Rep.* 2014;3(1):48–55.

25. Winston KR, McBride LA, Dudekula A. Bandages, dressings, and cranial neurosurgery. *J Neurosurg.* 2007;106(6):S450–S454.

26. Lamba N, Fick T, Nandoe Tewarie R, et al. Management of hydrocephalus in patients with leptomeningeal metastases: an ethical approach to decision-making. *J Neurooncol.* 2018;140(1):5–13.

27. Conner AK, Briggs RG, Palejwala AH, et al. The safety of post-operative elevation of mean arterial blood pressure following brain tumor resection. *J Clin Neurosci.* 2018;58:156–159.

28. Tasbihgou SR, Barends CRM, Absalom AR. The role of dexmedetomidine in neurosurgery. *Best Pract Res Clin Anaesthesiol.* 2021;35(2):221–229.

29. Epstein NE. A review of the risks and benefits of differing prophylaxis regimens for the treatment of deep venous thrombosis and pulmonary embolism in neurosurgery. *Surg Neurol.* 2005;64(4):295–301 discussion 302.

30. Higham CE, Johannsson G, Shalet SM. Hypopituitarism. *Lancet.* 2016;388(10058):2403–2415.

31. Hoorn EJ, Zietse R. Water balance disorders after neurosurgery: the triphasic response revisited. *NDT Plus.* 2010;3(1):42–44.

32. Stumpo V, Staartjes VE, Quddusi A, et al. Enhanced recovery after surgery strategies for elective craniotomy: a systematic review. *J Neurosurg.* 2021:1–25.

33. Audibert G, Vial V. Nausées et vomissements postopératoires en neurochirurgie (chirurgie infra-et supratentorielle) [Postoperative nausea and vomiting after neurosurgery (infratentorial and supratentorial surgery)]. *Ann Fr Anesth Reanim.* 2004;23(4):422–427.

34. Narayan M, Medinilla SP. Fever in the postoperative patient. *Emerg Med Clin North Am.* 2013;31(4):1045–1058.

35. Conen A, Raabe A, Schaller K, et al. Management of neurosurgical implant-associated infections. *Swiss Med Wkly.* 2020;150:w20208.

36. Shaikhouni A, Baum J, Lonser RR. Deep vein thrombosis prophylaxis in the neurosurgical patient. *Neurosurg Clin N Am.* 2018;29(4):567–574.

Questions

1. A 23-year-old male is postop day 1 from an endoscopic resection of a large pituitary adenoma. The patient is neurologically and hemodynamically stable and is not complaining of any new symptoms other than extreme thirst and mild headache. He has been drinking >12 small cups of water per hour. He has a Foley catheter in place that has been requiring repeated emptying of dilute urine. Although he is producing 350–500 cc of urine per hour, his overall fluid balance is roughly even. What is this patient's most likely diagnosis?
   a. Syndrome of inappropriate antidiuretic hormone (SIADH)
   b. Physiologic compensation for fluid depletion during surgery
   c. Hypocortisolemia
   d. Diabetes insipidus
   e. Acute kidney injury

2. A 54-year-old female is admitted to the intermediate ICU to undergo preoperative testing and clearance prior to a craniotomy to remove a large incidental meningioma. She has a history of hyponatremia, which was corrected prior to undergoing surgery. On arrival she is neurologically intact. Her labs show no abnormalities, and her electrolytes are within normal limits. Overnight, while NPO, the patient is noted be having a generalized tonic-clonic seizure in bed. What is the most appropriate order of response?
   a. Obtain bedside glucose level, take patient to CT scanner, call neurosurgery.
   b. Secure patient, notify neurosurgery, administer the standing dose of Keppra that is already ordered.
   c. Notify neurosurgery, administer Ativan 2 mg IV until seizures stop, load with an antiepileptic drug of choice, obtain head CT, repeat basic metabolic panel.
   d. Administer prophylactic dose of Keppra immediately, monitor for repeat seizures, notify neurosurgery if seizures occur again.
   e. Call neurology to begin continuous electroencephalogram, administer Ativan 2 mg IV if repeat seizures noted on monitoring.

3. A 64-year-old female presents as an outpatient to the neurosurgery office. She was experiencing intermittent episodes of confusion over the past several weeks but complains of no other symptoms other than a mild persistent headache. While feeding her grandson last week she realized she was lifting the spoon to a telephone on the wall next to where the child was sitting. She undergoes MRI of the brain with and without contrast, and her neurosurgeon informs her that she has a large ring-enhancing lesion. The neurosurgeon says that while he cannot be certain until the tumor tissue is examined under a microscope, her most likely diagnosis is glioblastoma. What is the most likely plan for this patient, and what is her median survival?
   a. Biopsy and tissue diagnosis, chemotherapy indefinitely; median survival 15 years
   b. Biopsy and tissue diagnosis, radiotherapy indefinitely; median survival 15 months
   c. Maximal safe resection; median survival 3–5 years
   d. Maximal safe resection and tissue diagnosis, chemotherapy and radiotherapy, maintenance chemotherapy; median survival 15 months
   e. Maximal safe resection and tissue diagnosis, chemotherapy and radiotherapy for 6 weeks, maintenance chemotherapy indefinitely; median survival 8 months

4. A 70-year-old male is brought to the ICU after undergoing a suboccipital craniectomy for removal of a cerebellar metastasis. His surgery was reportedly uncomplicated, and he quickly recovered from anesthesia in the unit. His only complaint is a moderate headache that is well controlled by PRN pain medications. His neurologic exam is stable, with only significant

dysmetria on finger-to-nose testing on the right side. Two days after surgery he becomes gradually more agitated overnight, eventually requiring wrist restraints. In the morning he seems sleepier than usual. The incision looks swollen and fluctuant. What is the most likely finding, and acute concern?

a. Delirium

b. Pseudomeningocele with obstructive hydrocephalus

c. Superficial skin infection with incisional swelling

d. Epidural abscess formation

5. A 62-year-old female underwent resection of a brain metastasis to the left parietal lobe yesterday. She is recovering in the ICU and is found to be newly weak on the right side. The neurosurgery team is immediately notified, and a STAT head CT is ordered. The imaging shows no hemorrhage in the surgical bed, and there are no obvious signs of stroke. Her exam does not change relative to normal variations in her blood pressure. Continuous electroencephalogram is applied, but there is no sign of seizure activity. What is the most likely cause of this patient's symptoms, and which treatment would be most effective?

a. Hydrocephalus; external ventricular drain

b. Cerebral edema; dexamethasone

c. Stroke; tissue plasminogen activator

d. Surgical stroke; increase MAP for perfusion

Answers

1. d

2. c

3. d

4. b

5. b

CHAPTER 7

Nursing Management of the Patient With a Headache Disorder

Aniket Natekar, MD, MSc

Introduction

Headache episodes can be one of the most difficult symptoms to treat in the inpatient setting. Patients with headache disorders often require a comprehensive, multifaceted approach to management. Furthermore, these patients face unique challenges when receiving inpatient treatment due to psychological stress from refractory headache pain and the inadequacy of care that they may have received prior to hospitalization. Successful treatment of headache disorders often requires a combination of pharmacologic and nonpharmacologic therapies. To determine which therapeutic modalities are best for a patient, nurses and physicians must understand the etiology of common headache disorders and which strategies have proven to be the most efficacious. The neurologic nurse should understand that patients suffering from headache disorders are suffering from a disease, such as one would suffer from hypertension, hyperlipidemia, or depression. Bearing this in mind, it is incorrect to say that patients have "headaches"; rather, they have "headache attacks."

Common Headache Disorders

It is important to understand the difference between the numerous types of headache disorders. Each type has its own optimal treatment stratagem, which plays an influential role in achieving the best possible outcome. In the case of hemicrania continua and paroxysmal hemicrania, for example, indomethacin helps to resolve the headache. On the other hand, pain management for patients suffering from a cluster headache involves administering 100% oxygen through a nonrebreather mask, flowing at 15 L/min for 15 minutes while the patient is sitting upright with the head bent down to maximize oxygen delivery. Understanding the typical presentation and specific treatments of different types of headache disorders helps to save countless hours and resources when caring for patients.[1]

The most common headache disorders are tension-type headache, migraine headache, and cluster headache, one of the trigeminal autonomic cephalalgias (TACs). Table 7.1 summarizes the differences between tension-type headache and migraine headache. Migraine is the second most common form of headache and can be challenging to treat because it is often refractory to many treatment modalities. The third edition of the *International Classification of Headache Disorders* outlines the diagnostic criteria of all major headache diagnoses. To qualify for a diagnosis of migraine without aura, patients must exhibit the following[2]:

A. At least five attacks fulfilling criteria B–D

B. Headache attacks lasting between 4 and 72 hours (untreated or unsuccessfully treated)

C. Headache with at least two of four characteristics:
   a. Unilateral location
   b. Pulsating quality
   c. Moderate or severe pain intensity
   d. Aggravation by or causing avoidance of routine physical activity (such as walking around)

TABLE 7.1 ■ Tension-Type and Migraine Headaches: Clinical Features and Treatment Options

Categories	Tension-Type Headache	Migraine Headache
Characteristics	• At least 10 episodes occurring <1 day/month on average (<12 days/year) to classify as infrequent • Episodes for at least 15 days/month for >3 months for chronic version • Mild or moderate intensity • Pressing/tightening quality • Not aggravated by physical activity • Similar medical management to migraine	• Can be with or without aura • Aura typically precedes pain by 15 minutes–1 hour • Aura can be visual, auditory, olfactory, or sensory resembling seizure aura • Aggravated by physical activity
Location	Bilateral location, typically in temple and forehead region	Any location around head, typically unilateral but can be bilateral
Duration	Hours to days	4–72 hours but can be longer or shorter
Associated Symptoms	• Absence of nausea/vomiting • Can only have one of photophobia, phonophobia, or mild nausea	Aura, nausea, vomiting, photophobia, phonophobia, memory issues, irritability, difficulty with concentration
Preventive Medications	• Tricyclic antidepressants, SNRIs, SSRIs • Anticonvulsants (topiramate, valproic acid, zonisamide, lamotrigine) • CGRP inhibitors (galcanezumab, fremanezumab, erenumab) • Gabapentin may be used but not as effective as modalities listed above	
Abortive Medications	• NSAIDs and acetaminophen for infrequent episodes • Triptan medications → can be repeated 2 hours after first dose • DHE → can be used if others don't work but not within 24 hours of triptan administration • Gepant medications (rimegepant, ubrogepant) • Neuroleptic medications (prochlorperazine, chlorpromazine, promethazine, metoclopramide, haloperidol)	

CGRP, Calcitonin gene-related peptide; *DHE,* dihydroergotamine; *NSAIDs,* nonsteroidal antiinflammatory drugs; *SNRI,* selective norepinephrine reuptake inhibitors; *SSRI,* selective serotonin reuptake inhibitors.

D. During an attack, the patient must experience at least one of the following:

    a. Nausea and/or vomiting

    b. Photophobia and phonophobia

E. Not better accounted for by another diagnosis (e.g., subarachnoid hemorrhage, tumor)

TACs comprise multiple headache disorders that involve the trigeminal nerve system and are characterized by both unique and overlapping clinical features (Table 7.2). Of the TACs, cluster headache is most frequently encountered. In cases of short unilateral neuralgiform headache with conjunctival tearing (or SUNCT), conjunctival injection (bloodshot eyes) and lacrimation (tearing) are present. Patients who suffer from short unilateral neuralgiform headache with autonomic symptoms (or SUNA) may have injection or lacrimation but not both simultaneously. Autonomic symptoms usually occur on the same side as the headache and can include conjunctival injection, tearing, nasal congestion, facial sweating, miosis/ptosis (eye drooping), and palpebral edema (eyelid swelling).[3]

TABLE 7.2 ■ Trigeminal Autonomic Cephalalgias: Comparison of Characteristics and Treatments

Categories	Cluster Headache	Paroxysmal Hemicrania	Short Unilateral Neuralgiform Headache with Conjunctival Tearing (SUNCT) and Short Unilateral Neuralgiform Headache with Autonomic Symptoms (SUNA)	Hemicrania Continua
Sex Predominance	Male (4:1)	No (1:1)	Female (1.7:1)	Female (2:1)
Pain Characteristic	Stabbing	Stabbing/throbbing	Stabbing/burning	Stabbing, burning, throbbing, or aching
Severity	Excruciating	Excruciating	Severe to excruciating	Mild to severe
Site	Orbital or temporal	Orbital or temporal	Orbital or temporal	Orbital, frontal, and/or temporal
Typical Attack Frequency	1 every other day to 8 daily	5–40 daily	1–200 daily	Continuous (with exacerbations)
Attack Duration	15–180 minutes	2–30 minutes	1 second–10 minutes	Months to years (untreated)
Autonomic Features?	Yes	Yes	Yes (conjunctival injection and lacrimation prominent in SUNCT)	Yes
Restlessness/Agitation?	Yes	Yes	Sometimes	Yes
Associated Migrainous Features?	Yes	Yes	Rare	Frequent
Triggers	Alcohol	Stress, exercise, alcohol	Tactile stimuli (touching face, shaving, brushing teeth)	Alcohol
Indomethacin Responsive?	No	Yes	No	Yes
Abortive Treatment	Triptans, oxygen	None	Intravenous lidocaine for debilitating symptoms	None
Preventive Treatment	Verapamil Glucocorticoids Galcanezumab Lithium	Indomethacin	Lamotrigine Oxcarbazepine Topiramate Gabapentin	Indomethacin

Commonly Used Medications for Abortive Treatment

TRIPTANS

The triptan category of medications includes sumatriptan, rizatriptan, frovatriptan, zolmitriptan, naratriptan, and eletriptan. Across the spectrum of triptans, available formulations include nasal spray, intramuscular (IM) injections, sublingual tablets, and oral (PO) tablets. Triptans are 5-HT1B/1D receptor agonists that induce vasoconstriction and reduce afferent signal transduction, both of which serve to decrease pain. Triptans are more effective when given earlier in an attack.[4] Contraindications to treatment with triptans include coronary artery disease, history of stroke or transient ischemic attack (TIA), peripheral vascular disease, and chronically uncontrolled high blood pressure.

ERGOT DERIVATIVES

Dihydroergotamine (DHE) is a selective 5-HT1B/1D receptor agonist that promotes vasoconstriction and inhibits the release of calcitonin gene-related peptide (CGRP) from trigeminal afferent neurons, thereby reducing pain signal propagation during a migraine episode. DHE is available as a nasal spray, IM injection, or an intravenous (IV) infusion. If taken early in the headache course, it is an effective abortive medication and has low rates of recurrent headache within 24 hours of use.[5] There is also low risk for developing a medication overuse headache, which makes DHE a great option for someone with frequent attacks. DHE is effective for patients with allodynia (a type of neuropathic pain), but it does not work for hemiplegic migraine and should not be used within 24 hours of taking a triptan. Prior to prescribing DHE, a pregnancy test and urine drug screen should be completed. These tests ensure that there will be no risk to a fetus and no rebound hypertension triggered by concurrent cocaine or amphetamine use. Like triptans, contraindications to treatment with DHE include coronary artery disease, history of stroke or TIA, peripheral vascular disease, and chronically uncontrolled high blood pressure.[6]

NEUROLEPTIC MEDICATIONS

This category of medications consists of dopamine-modulating agents, most of which are dopamine D2-receptor antagonists. Though primarily used to treat nausea, neuroleptic medications are also very effective at treating headaches. Medications in this category include chlorpromazine, prochlorperazine, metoclopramide, promethazine, and haloperidol. Chlorpromazine can cause hypotension, so it is important that nurses monitor the patient's blood pressure before and after administration in the inpatient setting.[7] Metoclopramide is safe to use during pregnancy but has high rates of dystonic reactions, and long-term use is associated with parkinsonism.[8] These adverse effects can be countered with diphenhydramine or benztropine. Promethazine causes fewer dystonic reactions and generally is better tolerated. Haloperidol also has a high rate of dystonic reactions, which can be treated with benztropine. Frequent and chronic use of haloperidol can be associated with drug-induced parkinsonism.[9]

The typical approach to treatment with neuroleptic medications is to start at the lowest dose and pretreat with diphenhydramine 25 mg PO each day. In the inpatient setting, these medications are usually scheduled for administration every 8 hours and continued for the duration of hospitalization to assist with pain reduction and prevention once other medications wear off[10] (Table 7.3).

GEPANT MEDICATIONS

Additional abortive medications currently available for headache management are ubrogepant and rimegepant. These are CGRP receptor antagonists, and early clinical trials demonstrated superior clinical efficacy compared to placebo, without cardiovascular side effects.[11] In fact, gepant

TABLE 7.3 ■ Neuroleptic Medications: Lowest Doses, Interval Dosing, and Special Considerations

	Prochlorpe-razine	Chlorpromazine	Metoclo-pramide	Promethazine	Haloperidol
Lowest Dose	5 mg	25 mg	5 mg	25 mg	1 mg
Dosing Interval	8 hours	8 hours	8 hours	8 hours	8 hours
Special Considerations	Has risk of dystonic reactions	Causes hypotension— great to use with dihydroergotamine	Increased risk of dystonic reactions	Least risk of dystonic reactions	Great for refractory nausea

medications are generally well tolerated and have almost no side effects. They are also unlikely to cause medication overuse headache, and rimegepant was US Food and Drug Administration approved in 2020 as a preventive medication for chronic migraine. Thus gepant agents are a great alternative for patients who cannot take ergot or triptan medications due to the side effects or other contraindications. Unfortunately, gepant medications are expensive and may not be available for use in the inpatient setting because they are not yet commonly included on hospital pharmacy formularies. Nevertheless, if patients are prescribed a gepant medication as an outpatient and can provide their own supply, then these medications can be brought to the hospital and used as needed while patients are hospitalized as a nonformulary alternative.[11]

CGRP and Its Importance to Headache

CGRP is a potent vasodilatory neuropeptide that triggers trigeminovascular inflammation, eventually causing peripheral and central pain sensitization that contributes to migraine pathogenesis.[11] CGRP is increased during a migraine attack and has therefore become a target of preventive treatment.

CGRP INHIBITORS

Galcanezumab, fremanezumab, and erenumab are administered subcutaneously every 30 days, and each requires refrigeration for storage.[12] Erenumab acts by blocking the CGRP receptor, while galcanezumab and fremanezumab bind the CGRP molecule directly.[12] The half-life for these medications is between 27 and 31 days, and patients may need 3 months of treatment before noticing any improvement.[12] Galcanezumab is prescribed as a 240-mg loading dose, followed by 120 mg as a monthly maintenance dose. Fremanezumab is available as 225 mg monthly or 675 mg every 3 months, and erenumab can be dosed as 70 or 140 mg monthly. These medications have been approved for the treatment of chronic migraine, and galcanezumab has also been approved for the treatment of episodic migraine.[13,14]

Patients should not miss any scheduled doses of their prescribed CGRP inhibitor while they are hospitalized. Often this means that the patient or family must bring the medication from home so that it can be administered by nurses in the hospital. Fortunately, CGRP inhibitors do not interact with other medications and are safe for use while in the hospital. However, they are contraindicated in pregnancy due to a theoretical risk to the fetus, and they must be stopped at least 6 months prior to planning pregnancy. If the prescribing provider wants to switch between the CGRP inhibitors, there should be a gap of 1 month between the last dose of one inhibitor and the first dose of the next to allow for a washout period.[14]

Antiepileptic Medications in Headache

Epilepsy and migraine are believed to share some pathophysiologic mechanisms, including a dysfunction of voltage-gated sodium and calcium channels, along with an imbalance between gamma-aminobutyric acid–mediated inhibition and excitatory glutamate-mediated transmission.[15] Patients who suffer from migraine are at higher risk of epilepsy compared to the general population. Given their overlapping pathophysiologic features and patient populations, some antiepileptic medications can be leveraged for the treatment of headache. Valproic acid and topiramate have proven to be effective for migraine prophylaxis.[15]

Valproic acid often is not recommended as the first choice due to side effects associated with long-term use and its risk for teratogenicity in pregnancy. Furthermore, valproic acid is a CYP-450 enzyme inhibitor, which may delay metabolism of other medications. Valproic acid levels need to be checked every 3–6 months to ensure that the dose is therapeutic.[10]

In comparison, topiramate does not require frequent monitoring and is better tolerated overall. Topiramate can cause weight loss, which may also improve migraine symptoms. It is important to note that topiramate doses ≥200 mg daily can increase the metabolism of birth control agents; however, if there are no drug-drug interactions, patients should continue their prescribed birth control regimen.[16,17]

Antidepressants and Headache

During a migraine attack, serotonin levels and dopamine levels decrease. As a result, selective serotonin reuptake inhibitors (SSRIs), selective norepinephrine reuptake inhibitors (SNRIs), and tricyclic antidepressants (TCAs) have been shown to help with migraine and headache prevention.[18] These types of medications may be particularly beneficial in patients who have both headache disorders and depression. Commonly used SSRIs include fluoxetine and paroxetine, whereas the SNRIs are duloxetine, desvenlafaxine, and venlafaxine. Duloxetine and venlafaxine have also been shown to be helpful in vestibular migraine.[19,20] Because SSRIs and SNRIs increase the risk of serotonin syndrome when used in conjunction with DHE or triptans, nurses should monitor closely for symptoms that may indicate an adverse effect (e.g., tachycardia, tachypnea, sweating, irritability, manic behavior, restlessness, rigidity). In theory, SSRIs and SNRIs can increase the patient's risk of bleeding, so they should be used cautiously in patients who have thrombocytopenia or active bleeding.[21] If these medications are administered in the inpatient setting, nurses should be attentive for signs and symptoms of bleeding. Common TCAs used in migraine prophylaxis include amitriptyline and nortriptyline.[18] Between the two, nortriptyline is less sedating and usually better tolerated; often it is the preferred option. Nurses must bear in mind that TCAs also induce anticholinergic side effects (e.g., dry mouth, dry eyes, confusion, hallucinations, tachycardia, blurred vision, decreased sweating, constipation, urinary retention).

Blood Pressure Medications and Headache

Beta blockers and angiotensin-converting enzyme (ACE) inhibitors are commonly prescribed for headache prophylaxis. Propranolol, metoprolol, and candesartan have the most evidence to support their use for this purpose.

BETA BLOCKERS

Beta blockers work by stabilizing blood vessels and limiting vasodilatory activity, reducing nervous system excitability, and modulating serotonin.[22] Beta blockers have the added benefit of treating comorbid anxiety and/or hypertension. The American Headache Society supports the use of propranolol, metoprolol, nadolol, timolol, and atenolol as agents for headache prophylaxis.[23] Between metoprolol and propranolol, the latter is typically more effective and has greater evidence supporting its use for the treatment of headache. Propranolol has been found to be superior in treating episodic migraine and can reduce chronic migraine frequency by at least 50% and by at least 1.5 headache days per month.[24] In the inpatient setting, these medications may be held in the context of hypotension, shock, or if patients are at risk for hypotension. In the outpatient setting, patients should regularly monitor their blood pressure.

ACE INHIBITORS AND ANGIOTENSIN II RECEPTOR ANTAGONISTS

The renin-angiotensin system has multiple factors involved in migraine pathophysiology. Individuals with migraine tend to have increased ACE activity, thus ACE inhibitors and angiotensin II receptor antagonists can serve as preventive medications.[25] This is by blocking ACE receptors, thus increased ACE levels have no benefit. In addition to controlling blood pressure, ACE inhibitors increase vascular tone and stimulate vasoconstriction.[25] They also inhibit free radicals, which generates an antioxidant effect.[25] Angiotensin II leads to the increased expression of nitric oxide synthase, so angiotensin II receptor antagonists act to reduce inflammation.

Of these medications, candesartan at a dose of 16 mg has the most compelling evidence for headache prophylaxis. This can be dosed at night to help avoid any orthostatic hypotension. Patients who are prescribed ACE inhibitors or angiotensin II receptor antagonists should have their blood pressure monitored regularly, and their renal function should be checked periodically due to the increased risk of renal dysfunction. These medications should be avoided in patients with hypotension or who are at risk for hypotension.

Special Considerations for New-Onset Headache

When a patient presents with a new-onset headache, it is important to ensure that there is not a life-threatening cause of the headache. Ruling out emergencies should be the priority for any patient with a concerning finding on examination, and for patients who meet any of the following criteria[26]:

- Systemic symptoms, including fever
- History of neoplasm
- Neurologic deficits, such as decreased consciousness
- Sudden or abrupt onset
- Age >65 years
- Change in pattern or recent onset of new headache
- Positional headache
- Precipitated by sneezing, coughing, or exercise
- Papilledema
- Progressive headache and atypical presentations
- Pregnancy or puerperium
- Painful with autonomic features
- Posttraumatic onset of headache
- Pathology of immune system such as human immunodeficiency virus
- Medication overuse or new drug at onset of headache

Once emergent and life-threatening causes of headache have been ruled out, providers can proceed with treating the headache itself, as needed. When managing headache pain, it is best to avoid opiate medications unless a separate indication has been diagnosed (e.g., intracranial hemorrhage) or if other classes of medications are contraindicated. In most cases, the combination capsule of acetaminophen-butalbital-caffeine is considered a safe medication for the treatment of headaches in the inpatient setting. However, butalbital (a barbiturate agent) can lead to physiologic dependence and fatal withdrawal effects if stopped too quickly. Excessive use of an acetaminophen-butalbital-caffeine combination pill also causes medication overuse headache. Consequently it is not recommended for long-term outpatient therapy.[26]

Conclusion

Treating patients who suffer from headache disorders can be challenging but rewarding when successful outcomes are achieved. There are numerous options for treating headache disorders, including various medications and distinct medication classes. It is important for nurses to remember that there are many different types of headache disorders. Recognizing the correct type can help the interprofessional team tailor their treatment more precisely rather than treating all headache episodes in the same way. Furthermore, anxiety and depression can coexist with headache disorders, and they should be addressed with equal importance to other physical ailments. Empathetic treatment can encourage patients to engage to a greater extent if they believe that their feelings and symptoms are validated when discussing their pain. Clear and proactive communication between patients and the interprofessional team is key to delivering effective care. Acquiring a better understanding of headache disorders and their treatment modalities will empower nursing staff to treat their patients with expertise and compassion.

References

1. Tobin J, Ford JH, Tockhorn-Heidenreich A, et al. Annual indirect cost savings in patients with episodic or chronic migraine: post-hoc analyses from multiple galcanezumab clinical trials. *J Med Econ.* 2022;25(1):630–639.
2. International Headache Society. *Migraine without aura criteria. IHS classification ICHD-3.* IHS; 2022.
3. International Headache Society. *Trigeminal autonomic cephalalgias. IHS classification ICHD-3.* HIS; 2022.
4. Rothrock J, Friedman D. *Triptan therapy for acute migraine.* American Headache Society; 2018.
5. American Migraine Foundation. *Dihydroergotamine (DHE) for migraine treatment.* AMF; 2021.
6. Center for Drug Evaluation and Research. *Drug approvals and databases* (DHE 45). Food and Drug Administration; 2008.
7. Kaur-Mann S, Marwaha R. *Chlorpromazine.* StatPearls Publishing; 2022.
8. Tiyani FL, Agbor VN, Njim T. Metoclopramide induced acute dystonic reaction: a case report. *BMC Res Notes.* 2017;10(1):32.
9. Lewis K, O'Day CS. *Dystonic reactions.* StatPearls Publishing; 2023.
10. Marmura MJ, Hou A. Inpatient management of migraine. *Neurol Clin.* 2019;37(4):771–788.
11. Natekar A, Sahu M, Yuan H, et al. Migraine preventive therapies in development. *Pract Neurol.* 2019:54–57.
12. Edvinsson L, Haanes KA, Warfvinge K, et al. CGRP as the target of new migraine therapies—successful translation from bench to clinic. *Nat Rev Neurol.* 2018;14(6):338–350.
13. Asghar MS, Becerra L, Larsson HB, et al. Calcitonin gene-related peptide modulates heat nociception in the human brain—an fMRI study in healthy volunteers. *PLoS One.* 2016;11(3):e0150334.
14. Rome T. *Comparing CGRP blockers for migraine prevention.* Migraine Warriors; 2019.
15. Shahien R, Beiruti K. Preventive agents for migraine: focus on the antiepileptic drugs. *J Cent Nerv Syst Dis.* 2012;4:37–49.
16. McClellan J, Kowatch R, Findling RL, et al. Practice parameter for the assessment and treatment of children and adolescents with bipolar disorder. *J Am Acad Child Adolesc Psychiatry.* 2007;46(1):107–125.
17. Mayo Clinic. Topiramate (oral route) precautions. *Drugs and Supplements.* Mayo Clinic; 2023.
18. Burch R. Antidepressants for preventive treatment of migraine. *Curr Treat Options Neurol.* 2019;21(4):18.
19. Salviz M, Yuce T, Acar H, et al. Propranolol and venlafaxine for vestibular migraine prophylaxis: a randomized controlled trial. *Laryngoscope.* 2016;126(1):169–174.
20. Vuralli D, Yildirim F, Akcali DT, et al. Visual and postural motion-evoked dizziness symptoms are predominant in vestibular migraine patients. *Pain Med.* 2018;19(1):178–183.
21. Paton C, Ferrier IN. SSRIs and gastrointestinal bleeding. *BMJ.* 2005;331(7516):529–530.
22. National Headache Foundation. *Beta blockers.* NHF; 2007.

23. American Headache Society. The American Headache Society position statement on integrating new migraine treatments into clinical practice. *Headache.* 2019;59(1):1–18.
24. Jackson JL, Kuriyama A, Kuwatsuka Y, et al. Beta-blockers for the prevention of headache in adults, a systematic review and meta-analysis. *PLoS One.* 2019;14(3):e0212785.
25. Nandha R, Singh H. Renin angiotensin system: a novel target for migraine prophylaxis. *Indian J Pharmacol.* 2012;44(2):157–160.
26. Do TP, Remmers A, Schytz HW, et al. Red and orange flags for secondary headaches in clinical practice: SNNOOP10 list. *Neurology.* 2019;92(3):134–144.

Questions

1. You are caring for a 24-year-old patient with asthma and obesity (body mass index ≥30) who presented with a 6-month history of headache. The patient was admitted to the hospital, and evaluation for life-threatening causes of headache was normal. The patient has asthma as well. Which of the following medications would be the best choice for this patient?
   a. Propranolol
   b. Topiramate
   c. Valproic acid
   d. Venlafaxine

2. You evaluate a patient in clinic who has hypertension and migraine, for which the patient is already prescribed propranolol. After some discussion, the advanced practice provider wants to prescribe candesartan in addition to propranolol because the patient has not noticed any improvement in headache. What would be the appropriate next step?
   a. Agree with this management. Prescribe the medication without any additional counseling.
   b. Counsel the patient to check blood pressure regularly.
   c. Consider switching from propranolol to candesartan.
   d. Recommend regular follow-up.
   e. b, c, and d

3. You are caring for a patient who has a headache disorder. She is a full-time student at a local university and has no other medical problems, but she does inform you that she is taking an oral contraceptive pill. While she isn't trying to get pregnant, she is planning on having children soon. Additionally, she lets you know that there are some concerns for bone health in her family. Of the following medications, which would be the least appropriate to prescribe for this patient?
   a. Valproic acid
   b. Topiramate
   c. Propranolol
   d. Candesartan

4. Your patient is admitted to the hospital for brain surgery, and, coincidentally, due for her monthly CGRP injection medicine. The patient is worried about missing her dose, and subsequent worsening headaches. What do you suggest to her?
   a. Ask the provider to substitute the medication for an oral SNRI while she is hospitalized.
   b. Advise patient to continue to hold the medication until she leaves the hospital.
   c. Ask the patient if she can have family bring it in so she can get her dose.
   d. Tell the patient that you will give her increased amounts of opioids to help with headache pain.

5. Your patient is being monitored in the neurosurgical ICU after a successful clipping of her brain aneurysm. The patient's medication list includes amlodipine, fluoxetine, and eletriptan. You went to assess your patient, and you noticed that she was having increased restlessness,

tachycardia, sweating, and seemed rigid. In addition to notifying the provider, what do you anticipate?

a. This is likely due to the aneurysm repair, and the patient should be monitored with frequent neurologic exams.
b. The patient may be experiencing serotonin syndrome, so she needs urgent attention.
c. The patient may in withdrawal from alcohol, so she should be placed on an AWS.
d. The patient should be started on antibiotics for potential surgical site infection.

Answers

1. d

2. e

3. a

4. c

5. b

CHAPTER 8

Nursing Management of the Patient With Encephalitis or Meningitis

Malissa Pynes, MD

Introduction

Encephalitis is defined as "inflammation of the brain."[1] Encephalitis can be caused by different etiologies, including infection, autoimmune reaction, or paraneoplastic processes. Certain etiologies are often associated with specific areas of the brain, whereas others can lead to diffuse or scattered inflammation.[2] The location of inflammation will lead to different patient presentations, symptoms, and physical exam findings.

Investigation of encephalitis starts with central nervous system (CNS) imaging. This can include computerized tomography (CT) scan or magnetic resonance imaging (MRI), and sampling of cerebrospinal fluid (CSF) via lumbar puncture. Different causes of encephalitis are treated differently according to which agents and regimens have proven to be effective in similar cases. The variety of treatments available and their specificity for certain disease pathologies make identification of the underlying cause an important first step in proper management of encephalitis.[3]

Meningitis is inflammation of the meninges, which is the protective membrane that covers the brain and spinal cord. The meninges consist of three layers:

- Delicate inner layer (called the pia mater)
- Middle arachnoid layer
- Tough outermost layer (called the dura mater) (Fig. 8.1)[4]

The term *meningitis* is used colloquially to refer to bacterial meningitis. Untreated bacterial meningitis is associated with high rates of mortality.[5] If bacterial meningitis is suspected, treatment for common pathogens should be rapidly initiated even before the exact cause is determined. It is important to remember, though, that meningitis can be caused by different infectious pathogens, including viruses, fungi, parasites, or amoebas.[6] Meningitis, like encephalitis, can have noninfectious causes, including cancer, autoimmune disorders, trauma, surgical manipulation, or medications.[6]

Evaluation of a Patient Presenting With Meningitis

The meningeal irritation that occurs during meningitis leads to a variety of symptoms, including headache, nausea, vomiting, blurry vision, photophobia, and neck stiffness.[7] If inflammation of the neighboring brain tissues is also present (referred to as meningoencephalitis), the patient may have altered mental status, known as encephalopathy. When evaluating patients, bedside exam maneuvers can be performed to assess for meningeal irritation. For example, asking the patient simply to "touch your chin to your chest" can be painful or impossible due to neck rigidity.

- Neck flexion is utilized when assessing for Brudzinski sign (Table 8.1).[8]
  - When positive, neck flexion triggers a reflexive flexion of the patient's knees and hips.
- Kernig sign is tested with the patient lying supine with the hips in flexed position.
  - If positive, when a provider attempts to extend the knee, the patient will resist the knee extension or experience back or thigh pain.

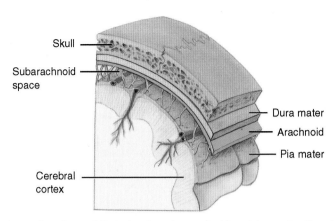

Skull

Subarachnoid space

Dura mater

Arachnoid

Pia mater

Cerebral cortex

Fig. 8.1 Three layers of meninges of the brain: pia mater, arachnoid, and dura mater. (From Corinthian College. *Medical Assistant: Nervous System, Law and Ethics, Psychology and Therapeutic Procedures—Module G*, 2nd ed. Elsevier; 2016.)

TABLE 8.1 ■ Signs of Meningitis

Signs Suggestive of Meningitis	Method	Positive Sign
Kernig sign	With patient lying flat and hips flexed as if sitting in a chair, try to straighten the knees	Inability to straighten or extend the knee or pain in the low back and/or posterior thigh with maneuver
Brudzinski sign	Flex the patient's neck forward as if to touch the chin to the chest	Hips and knees flex or bend
Jolt accentuation of headache	Ask patient to rapidly turn the head from side to side two to three times per second	Worsening of headache

Blood in and around the brain tissues—such as in subarachnoid hemorrhage (SAH)—is irritating to the meninges and can produce similar signs and symptoms as meningitis. As a result, patients who are being evaluated for meningitis should undergo a CT scan of the head to screen for/rule out other problems, such as a SAH.[9] If the CT scan is negative for obvious pathology and does not show signs concerning for significant cerebral (brain) edema (which increases the risk of brain herniation), a lumbar puncture is safe to obtain to evaluate the CSF.

A lumbar puncture can assess for infection, inflammation, cancer, or even a microscopic amount of blood too small to be seen on CT scan. Normal CSF is clear in color. Infection with bacteria can cause the CSF to be cloudy or purulent. Small amounts of subarachnoid blood and its associated red blood cell (RBC) breakdown can lead to xanthochromia, a dark yellow color in the CSF due to the presence of bilirubin.[10] A lumbar puncture with a high opening pressure indicates elevated intracranial pressure and can be seen in cases of cryptococcal (a type of fungus) meningitis.[11] Laboratory studies commonly ordered with a lumbar puncture to evaluate the CSF for meningitis include:

- CSF cell count, which highlights the amount of white blood cells (WBCs) and RBCs
- CSF protein
- CSF glucose

TABLE 8.2 ■ Diagnostic Tests for Meningitis

Test	Bacterial	Viral	Fungal	Tubercular
Opening pressure	Elevated	Usually normal	Variable	Variable
White blood cell count	≥1000/mm³	<100/mm³	Variable	Variable
Cell differential	Predominance of PMNs[a]	Predominance of lymphocytes[b]	Predominance of lymphocytes	Predominance of lymphocytes
Protein	Mild to marked elevation	Normal to elevated	Elevated	Elevated
CSF-to-serum glucose ratio	Normal to marked decrease	Usually normal	Low	Low

[a]Lymphocytosis present 10% of the time.
[b]PMNs may predominate early in the course.
Information from Fishman RA. *Cerebrospinal Fluid in Diseases of the Nervous System*, 2nd ed. Saunders; 1992; Arevalo CE, Barnes PF, Duda M, et al. Cerebrospinal fluid cell counts and chemistries in bacterial meningitis. *South Med J.* 1989;82:1122–1127; Wubbel L, McCracken GH. Management of bacterial meningitis: 1998. *Pediatr Rev.* 1998;19(3):78–84; Zunt JR, Marra CM. Cerebrospinal fluid testing for the diagnosis of central nervous system infection. *Neurol Clin.* 1999;17:675–689; Seehusen DA, Reeves MM, Fomin DA. Cerebrospinal fluid analysis. *Am Fam Physician.* 2003;68(6):1103–1108.

- CSF Gram stain/culture and meningitis/encephalitis panels may also be ordered to further evaluate for CNS infection

Specific infectious etiologies and some neurologic conditions, such as multiple sclerosis, have other specific diagnostic CSF tests. Typical CSF findings in various conditions are shown in Table 8.2.

Bacterial Meningitis

Bacterial meningitis is the deadliest form of meningitis in the acute phase. Patients who are suspected of having bacterial meningitis should always receive treatment as quickly as possible regardless of whether a lumbar puncture is being planned. One study showed that administering antibiotics 6 hours after patient presentation was associated with significantly higher mortality than administering antibiotics 2 hours after presentation.[12] Antibiotic therapy for suspected bacterial meningitis should always be started empirically.

Empiric antibiotic therapy includes multiple medications to cover for the most likely pathogens. If there is a high suspicion for bacterial meningitis, dexamethasone IV should be given either before or at the same time as when antibiotics are started to reduce inflammation and improve outcomes.[13] Antibiotic choice may be adjusted based on each institution's most recent antibiogram, which is a regularly updated database of the common community infections in the area and their susceptibility patterns. Otherwise, empiric antibiotic therapy is determined based on patient age and comorbidities.[14]

- *Streptococcus pneumoniae* is the most common cause of meningitis in adults—particularly in older adults.[15] Most adult patients with bacterial meningitis will be started on vancomycin and a third-generation cephalosporin (ceftriaxone or cefotaxime) to cover common causative bacteria, such as *Neisseria meningitidis* and *S. pneumoniae*.[16]
- Rates of *Neisseria* meningitis have declined over the years due in part to vaccinations, but when outbreaks occur, they are associated with rapid spread and potential for devastating neurologic injury. Historically, many cases of infection with *N. meningitidis* occurred in areas with people living near each other, such as in college dormitories or in military

barracks; thus these institutions now require meningococcus vaccination at intake. *Neisseria* spp. are gram-negative bacteria. Cephalosporins, such as ceftriaxone, are often given to treat *N. meningitidis*. Any patient suspected of having *Neisseria* meningitis should be put on droplet precautions for 24 hours from the start of antibiotics.[17]

- All close contacts of a patient with *Neisseria* meningitis will need antibiotic prophylaxis as soon as possible with rifampin, azithromycin, or ceftriaxone.[6]
- For health care workers, most exposures do not warrant antimicrobial chemoprophylaxis for brief contact unless there was direct exposure to respiratory secretions, such as with suctioning or during intubation.[18]

- Patients age >50 years will also need coverage for *Listeria*, a common bacterial foodborne pathogen, which is found throughout the environment in soil, vegetation, and animals.[19] *Listeria* is more common in older patients and is treated often with ampicillin.
- Immunocompromised patients, such as patients with organ transplants or cancer, and patients who have sustained a penetrating head trauma, or have undergone neurosurgery, will require antibiotic treatment coverage for *Pseudomonas* bacteria. Common antibiotics used include cefepime, ceftazidime, or meropenem.[20]
- In cases of suspected herpes simplex virus (HSV) meningitis, patients may also be treated empirically with IV acyclovir (if renal function is normal).

When the CSF studies start to finalize and diagnoses are ruled in or out, antibiotics, antiviral, and antifungal agents should be tailored to the individualized results. Overall antibiotic duration is dependent upon the specific pathogen. Duration can range from 2 weeks (such as for pneumococcal meningitis) to at least 3 weeks (such as for listerial meningitis[6]).

Viral Encephalitis

Elevated WBC count and lymphocytes in the CSF are indicative of viral encephalitis. Some viruses are included on the standard biofire or meningitis/encephalitis panel, but many others can only be tested with individualized tests. In the case of viral encephalitis, obtaining a thorough exposure history is of high importance. Sexual and travel history can provide insight into diagnosis, including the most common causes of sporadic encephalitis, HSV type 1 (HSV-1), Eastern equine encephalitis, or West Nile virus.[3]

Herpes encephalitis is a deadly viral encephalitis caused by either HSV-1 or HSV-2. Herpes simplex infection is an acute viral disease that spreads from person to person. It is characterized by small, fluid-filled blisters appearing on the lips or genitals. Patients are also often febrile. The herpes virus may become immediately active or remain in the body in an inactive (dormant or latent) state.[21] After being inactive, the virus may then recur (reactivate).

Herpes encephalitis rarely occurs in conjunction with oral or genital lesions. Herpes encephalitis can affect any area of the brain; however, it classically prefers the temporal lobes. Patients with temporal lobe inflammation may present with seizures, express odd feelings (e.g., déjà vu, fear), or express odd sensations (e.g., unusual odor or taste[22]). Brain MRI imaging of an encephalopathic patient that shows temporal lobe hyperintensities may raise suspicion for HSV encephalitis.[3]

Intravenous Immunoglobulin Aseptic Meningitis or Encephalitis

In the correct clinical context, if CSF studies demonstrate elevated protein, increased neutrophils, and negative cultures, a diagnosis of aseptic meningitis or encephalitis may be suspected. Intravenous immunoglobulin (IVIG) therapy poses a very small risk of aseptic meningitis. In these cases, symptoms such as headache or neck stiffness will start to appear within 72 hours of the initiation of IVIG therapy.[23] Aseptic meningitis is estimated to affect 0.6–1% of patients receiving IVIG.[24]

Autoimmune Encephalitis

Several causes of encephalitis are mediated by the immune system. These can occur as a postviral or postinfectious phenomenon. Autoimmune encephalitis can also occur as part of paraneoplastic syndrome due to antibody formation in response to cancer. In many patients the presence of cancer may not be known prior to the onset of neurologic symptoms, and investigation for underlying malignancy may be done with further imaging. However, treatment of autoimmune encephalitis should not be delayed to obtain a formal diagnosis, especially if there is a strong suspicion for autoimmune etiology. Often, in practice, treatment will be started with high-dose steroids, such as IV methylprednisolone 1 g daily.[25] If there is no response to treatment within a few days, or at the end of treatment, the patient may be switched to IVIG or plasmapheresis. Plasmapheresis (also referred to as PLEX) can occasionally be performed via a peripheral IV, but this often requires placement of a central line.

One rare entity to be aware of is NMDA encephalitis. NMDA encephalitis classically affects young females typically ranging from teenagers to those in their 20s (though a patient of any age could be affected). Patients often begin with behavioral changes, which are often diagnosed as primary psychiatric illness, and later develop other neurologic symptoms, such as catatonia, autonomic dysfunction, facial dyskinesias, and seizures.[25] NMDA encephalitis is strongly associated with an underlying ovarian teratoma or mediastinal teratoma.[25] In these cases definitive treatment of encephalitis is only possible with tumor resection, but patients may be left with high residual morbidity.

Many autoantibodies are associated with certain types of cancer. Some important examples are included in the accompanying table, but there are many more.

Name	What Does It Cause?	What Is It Associated With?
Anti-Hu (aka ANNA-1)	Limbic encephalitis	Small cell lung cancer, thymoma, and neuroendocrine tumors[26]
Antiamphiphysin	Encephalomyelitis or stiff-person syndrome	Small cell lung cancer and breast cancer[27]
Anti-AMPAR	Limbic encephalitis or seizures	Lung cancer, thymoma, and breast cancer[26]
Anti-Ma2	Limbic encephalitis or brainstem encephalitis	Testicular cancer, breast cancer, stomach cancer, non-small cell lung cancer, or non-Hodgkin lymphoma[26]
Anti-CASPR2	Usually occurs in patients age >50	Insomnia, dysautonomia, cerebellar dysfunction, encephalopathy, weight loss, and neuropathy[28]
Anti-GAD65	Limbic encephalitis	Small cell lung cancer, thymoma, and neuroendocrine tumor[27]
Anti-LGI1	Limbic encephalitis and faciobrachial dystonic seizures (frequent brief, jerklike movements of the face and ipsilateral arm)	Thymoma, neuroendocrine tumor[26]
Anti- GABA$_B$R	Limbic encephalitis	Small cell lung cancer or neuroendocrine tumor of the lung[28]
Anti-mGLuR5	Encephalitis	Hodgkin lymphoma[29]

Nursing Considerations

Symptoms of a patient with meningitis or encephalitis will vary significantly. Care should be individualized based on many factors especially tailored to the patient's mental status and level of consciousness. A patient with agitation or confusion may be combative, potentially requiring the use of restraints for the safety of the patient and staff. Restraints, lines, and tubes increase the risk of delirium and other complications and should be weaned as soon as it is safe to do so. Patients may also be impulsive or disinhibited. They may try to ambulate unassisted without calling for help, increasing their risk of falling. Such patients might benefit from being in a room close to the nurses' station or having a low bed with floor padding.

Patients with confusion, Glasgow Coma Scale score <15, or slurred speech should be screened for swallowing difficulties, also known as dysphagia. It is often necessary to evaluate the swallowing safety of patients with bedside tests, such as the Yale Swallow Protocol.[30] If a patient's swallowing is determined to be unsafe, the provider caring for the patient will need to be updated, and the patient made NPO (nothing by mouth) accordingly. Speech therapy may be necessary to fully evaluate swallowing safety in difficult cases. In cases where dysphagia is present, alternative enteral access with a nasogastric tube may be required to administer medications and nutrition.

As discussed, certain causes of encephalitis may predispose patients to seizures. Nurses should monitor for abnormal movements or tone in an extremity or intermittent alterations of consciousness and report instances to the provider. Seizure precautions, including padded bed rails, should be initiated.

Conclusion

Meningitis or encephalitis is inflammation of the central nervous system due to various causes. Causes may be infectious, autoimmune, and/or paraneoplastic. Treatment varies depending on etiology, but good bedside care is one of the most critical components of patient management.

References

1. Ellul M, Solomon T. Acute encephalitis: diagnosis and management. *Clin Med (Lond)*. 2018;18(2): 155–159.
2. Hudson SJ, Dix RD, Streilein JW. Induction of encephalitis in SJL mice by intranasal infection with herpes simplex virus type 1: a possible model of herpes simplex encephalitis in humans. *J Infect Dis*. 1991;163(4):720–727.
3. Roos KL, Wilson MR, Tyler KL. Encephalitis. In: Loscalzo J, Fauci A, Kasper D et al, eds. *Harrison's Principles of Internal Medicine*, 21st ed. McGraw Hill; 2022.
4. Weed LH. Meninges and cerebrospinal fluid. *J Anat*. 1938;72(Pt 2):181–215.
5. Bystritsky RJ, Chow FC. Infectious meningitis and encephalitis. *Neurol Clin*. 2022;40(1):77–91.
6. Roos KL, Tyler KL. Acute meningitis. In: Loscalzo J, Fauci A, Kasper D et al, eds. *Harrison's Principles of Internal Medicine*, 21st ed. McGraw Hill; 2022.
7. Roos KL. Encephalitis. *Handbk Clin Neurol*. 2014;121:1377–1381.
8. Thomas KE, Hasbun R, Jekel J, et al. The diagnostic accuracy of Kernig's sign, Brudzinski's sign, and nuchal rigidity in adults with suspected meningitis. *Clin Infect Dis*. 2002;35(1):46–52.
9. Archer BD. Computed tomography before lumbar puncture in acute meningitis: a review of the risks and benefits. *CMAJ*. 1993;148(6):961–965.
10. Carpenter CR, Hussain AM, Ward MJ, et al. Spontaneous subarachnoid hemorrhage: a systematic review and meta-analysis describing the diagnostic accuracy of history, physical examination, imaging, and lumbar puncture with an exploration of test thresholds. *Acad Emerg Med*. 2016;23(9):963–1003.
11. Robertson EJ, Najjuka G, Rolfes MA, et al. Cryptococcus neoformans ex vivo capsule size is associated with intracranial pressure and host immune response in HIV-associated cryptococcal meningitis. *J Infect Dis*. 2014;209(1):74–82.

12. Bodilsen J, Dalager-Pedersen M, Schønheyder HC, et al. Time to antibiotic therapy and outcome in bacterial meningitis: a Danish population-based cohort study. *BMC Infect Dis.* 2016;16:392.
13. van de Beek D, Cabellos C, Dzupova O, et al. ESCMID guideline: diagnosis and treatment of acute bacterial meningitis. *Clin Microbiol Infect.* 2016;22(3):S37–S62.
14. Tunkel AR, Hartman BJ, Kaplan SL, et al. Practice guidelines for the management of bacterial meningitis. *Clin Infect Dis.* 2004;39(9):1267–1284.
15. Centers for Disease Control and Prevention. *Bacterial meningitis.* CDC; 2021.
16. Brouwer MC, Tunkel AR, van de Beek D. Epidemiology, diagnosis, and antimicrobial treatment of acute bacterial meningitis. *Clin Microbiol Rev.* 2010;23(3):467–492.
17. Gardner P. Clinical practice: prevention of meningococcal disease. *N Engl J Med.* 2006;355(14):1466–1473.
18. Gilmore A, Stuart J, Andrews N. Risk of secondary meningococcal disease in health-care workers. *Lancet.* 2000;356(9242):1654–1655.
19. Pagliano P, Ascione T, Boccia G, et al. Listeria monocytogenes meningitis in the elderly: epidemiological, clinical and therapeutic findings. *Infez Med.* 2016;24(2):105–111.
20. Tunkel AR, Hartman BJ, Kaplan SL, et al. Practice guidelines for the management of bacterial meningitis. *Clin Infect Dis.* 2004;39:1267.
21. Whitley RJ. Herpes simplex encephalitis: adolescents and adults. *Antiviral Res.* 2006;71(2-3):141–148.
22. Abou-Khalil B, Misulis KE. Seizure semiology. In: Misulis KE, Abou-Khalil B, Sonmezturk H et al, eds. *Atlas of EEG, Seizure Semiology, and Management.* Oxford University Press; 2022.
23. Jain RS, Kumar S, Aggarwal R, et al. Acute aseptic meningitis due to intravenous immunoglobulin therapy in Guillain-Barré syndrome. *Oxf Med Case Reports.* 2014;2014(7):132–134.
24. Guo Y, Tian X, Wang X, et al. Adverse effects of immunoglobulin therapy. *Front Immunol.* 2018;9:1299.
25. Abboud H, Probasco JC, Irani S, et al. Autoimmune encephalitis: proposed best practice recommendations for diagnosis and acute management. *J Neurol Neurosurg Psychiatry.* 2021;92(7):757–768.
26. Alamowitch S, Graus F, Uchuya M, et al. Limbic encephalitis and small cell lung cancer: clinical and immunological features. *Brain.* 1997;120(Pt 6):923–928.
27. Sarva H, Deik A, Ullah A, et al. Clinical spectrum of stiff person syndrome: a review of recent reports. *Tremor Other Hyperkinet Mov (NY).* 2016;6:340.
28. Dalmau J, Rosenfeld MR, Graus F. Paraneoplastic neurologic syndromes and autoimmune encephalitis. In: Loscalzo J, Fauci A, Kasper D, et al., eds. *Harrison's Principles of Internal Medicine,* 21st ed. McGraw Hill; 2022.
29. Spatola M, Sabater L, Planagumà J, et al. Encephalitis with mGluR5 antibodies: symptoms and antibody effects. *Neurology.* 2018;90(22):e1964–e1972.
30. Ward M, Skelley-Ashford M, Brown K, et al. Validation of the yale swallow protocol in post-acute care: a prospective, double-blind, multirater study. *Am J Speech Lang Pathol.* 2020;29(4):1937–1943.

Questions

Anthony is a 19-year-old previously healthy male who is finishing his third month of college and spending most of his time at his fraternity house. He has been feeling ill for the past 16 hours. His symptoms began with a squeezing, pressurelike headache. The pain gets worse with coughing or sneezing. He reports a "whooshing" sound in both ears. His friends convinced him to go to the student health center for evaluation. Vital signs are 100.6°F, HR 109, BP 109/79, RR 16, O_2 Sat 96%. On examination, he has small purple spots forming a rash on his torso. There are a couple of similar spots in his mouth.

1. What condition are you most concerned about?
   a. *Neisseria meningitis*
   b. Fungal meningitis
   c. Hydrocephalus
   d. Syphilis
   e. Smallpox

2. Once the patient is stabilized, what information obtained in regular intake history is particularly important in this patient's case?
   a. Allergies
   b. Past surgeries
   c. Vaccination history
   d. Birth history
   e. History of recreational drug use

3. What special precautions are required when caring for this patient?
   a. Enteric precautions
   b. N95 respirator with eye shields
   c. Standard precautions
   d. Droplet precautions
   e. No precautions necessary

A 79-year-old female with early-stage dementia who lives with her adult daughter and grandchildren is brought to the emergency department by her family because she has been "acting like a child." She has been disinhibited, and her daughter expresses concern that her rapid movements are going to lead to a fall. When you meet the patient, she is wearing sunglasses and reacts dramatically to the bright lights when sunglasses are removed. She complains of a headache and resists attempts to check her neck movement. She is moving all extremities equally, and her speech is clear. Her vital signs are notable for a temperature of 101.5°F, and lab work notable for WBC 14,000 and Plt 460,000. The patient undergoes a head CT, which is normal.

4. When should antibiotics be started?
   a. If lumbar puncture shows an elevated WBC count
   b. Immediately
   c. After obtaining an MRI brain
   d. Once CSF cultures are obtained
   e. Only if the patient develops signs of sepsis

5. What do you anticipate to occur during the hospital stay?
   a. Start empiric antibiotics immediately and anticipate narrowing of therapy based on culture data.
   b. Since the patient is >50 years, the provider will ensure coverage for *Listeria* and treat appropriately.
   c. The patient will undergo further workup for cancer and autoimmune causes.
   d. Nursing should initiate safety precautions (including 1:1 as needed), monitor for dysphagia, and monitor for seizure activity.
   e. All of the above are anticipated.

Answers

1. a

2. c

3. d

4. b

5. e

CHAPTER 9

Nursing Management of the Patient With Acute Encephalopathy

Victor S. Wang, MD

Introduction

Encephalopathy—often referred to as altered mental status—is a common symptom of various underlying disease states. It can occur in the acute care setting in patients of any age but is particularly prevalent in the elderly population. Encephalopathy itself is a broad term that implies an acute and reversible clinical state of cerebral dysfunction in the absence of structural brain disease. It encompasses aspects of both confusion and delirium.

- Confusion implies an alteration in mentation from the patient's baseline and includes features such as impaired memory, attention, or situational awareness.
- Delirium refers to an acute state of confusion affecting attention and awareness with waxing and waning fluctuations throughout the course of a day.[1-3]

Encephalopathy in the acute care setting requires thorough workup and targeted management of the underlying cause before improvement and resolution will occur. Understanding the etiologies of encephalopathy and how to conduct a proper history and physical exam of an altered patient can improve the interprofessional team's clinical management and equip them to address the family's expectations and concerns.[1-3]

Types of Encephalopathy

Encephalopathy can arise due to a variety of underlying pathologies, including primary/central nervous system dysfunction, metabolic derangements, pharmacologic/toxic stimuli, infections, psychiatric disorders, and other systemic illnesses (Table 9.1). When evaluating a patient, it is important to obtain collateral information regarding their baseline mentation to distinguish acute from chronic neurologic abnormalities and determine the potential for contribution from psychiatric comorbidities (Table 9.2).

Assessment—History and Physical Exam

HISTORY

When evaluating encephalopathy, establishing a clear understanding of the history, progression, associations, and features of symptomatology is critical to assembling an effective plan of care. There are many important questions to ask, and numerous screening tools are available for health care providers to use. Assessments of encephalopathy can be completed by trained nursing staff, and the information obtained should always be communicated to the interprofessional team,

TABLE 9.1 ■ Differential Diagnosis for Encephalopathy by Etiology

Central Nervous System (CNS)	Metabolic	Pharmacologic/ Toxic	Infectious	Psychiatric	Other
Tumor	Sodium (hypo-/ hypernatremia)	Medication (antihypertensives, steroids, sedatives, opiates, sleep aids, anticholinergics, antiepileptics, polypharmacy)	Primary CNS (meningitis, encephalitis, abscess)	Psychosis	Shock (cardiogenic, hypovolemic, hemorrhagic, distributive/ septic)
Stroke (hemorrhagic or ischemic)	Glucose (hypo-/ hyperglycemia)	Alcohol, methanol, ethylene glycol	Urinary tract infection	Depression	Migraine
Edema	Calcium (hypo-/ hypercalcemia)	Illicit drugs	Pneumonia		Delirium (sundowning)
Seizure	Temperature (hypo-/hyper- thermia)	Drug withdrawal (alcohol, benzodiaz- epine, opiate)	Intraabdominal infection		
Dementia	Hypovolemia		Viral (COVID-19)		
	Hypercarbia		Skin/decubitus ulcer/osteo- myelitis/ cellulitis		
	Hypoxemia				

Adapted from Koita J, Riggio S, Jagoda A. The mental status examination in emergency practice. *Emerg Med Clin North Am.* 2010;28(3):439–451.

TABLE 9.2 ■ Characteristics of Delirium vs Dementia vs Psychosis

	Delirium	Dementia	Psychosis
Onset	Acute	Chronic	Variable
Reversibility	Reversible	No	Variable
Clinical Course	Fluctuations throughout the day or daily	Progressive	Variable
Vital Signs	Can be abnormal	Normal	Normal
Level of Consciousness	Altered	Normal	Variable
Hallucinations	Visual	Rare	Auditory
Physical Exam	Can be abnormal	Normal	Normal
Prognosis	Can have rapid decline if not addressed properly	Progressive decline	Variable

emphasizing any elements of the screening protocol that revealed concerning findings.[1-3] Questions that nurses should ask during their evaluation include:

1. When did this change start? When was the patient last known to be at their baseline?
2. What exactly is the change in mentation (e.g., hypoactive vs hyperactive behavior, confusion, forgetfulness, hallucinations)?
3. What is the patient's baseline mental state (e.g., orientation, attention, situational awareness)?
4. How did this change first manifest (e.g., suddenly or gradually)?
5. Is there a discernable pattern to the change (e.g., fluctuations, waxing/waning, continual decline)?

6. Did the onset relate to any other recent changes or events (e.g., medications, toxic ingestion, substance withdrawal, trauma, infection)?

7. Have there been any other symptoms associated with the change (e.g., fever, nausea, vomiting, syncope, shortness of breath, edema)?

DELIRIUM SCREENING TOOLS

Delirium is an acute state of confusion affecting attention and awareness, further characterized by waxing and waning mental status throughout the day. If there is a concern that the patient is experiencing delirium, nurses and physicians should proceed with the Confusion Assessment Method (CAM) diagnostic algorithm (Box 9.1). Using CAM to diagnose delirium requires the presence of features 1 *and* 2 plus *either* 3 or 4.

If there is a concern for substance abuse, nurses should utilize the Clinical Institute Withdrawal Assessment for Alcohol (CIWA), also referred to as the Alcohol Withdrawal Syndrome (AWS) scale (Fig. 9.1), and/or the Clinical Opiate Withdrawal Scale (COWS) (Fig. 9.2). These scoring systems grade the severity of withdrawal and can be used to guide nursing staff through the initiation, monitoring, and management of therapeutic interventions in accordance with their institution's protocols.

PHYSICAL EXAM

When a patient exhibits an acute change in mentation, nurses should always perform a thorough assessment and determine whether the patient is experiencing a medical emergency (see Fig. 9.1). This includes checking a full set of vital signs, determining blood glucose levels (point of care), and

---

BOX 9.1 ■ The Confusion Assessment Method (CAM) Diagnostic Algorithm

Feature 1: Acute onset and fluctuating course
- This feature usually is described by a family member or observed by nursing staff. It is affirmed by positive responses to the following questions:
  - Is there evidence of an acute change in mental status from the patient's baseline?
  - Does the abnormal behavior fluctuate throughout the day (comes and goes), or variably increase and decrease in severity?

Feature 2: Inattention
- This feature is shown by a positive response to the following question:
  - Does the patient have difficulty with focusing attention, being easily distracted, or keeping track of what has been said?

Feature 3: Disorganized thinking
- This feature can be verified by a positive response to the following question:
  - Is the patient's thinking disorganized or incoherent, such as exhibiting rambling or irrelevant conversation, unclear or illogical flow of ideas, or unpredictable switching from subject to subject?

Feature 4: Altered level of consciousness
- This feature is present with any answer other than "alert" to the following question:
  - Overall, how would you rate this patient's level of consciousness?
    - Alert (normal), vigilant (hyperalert), lethargic (drowsy, easily aroused), stupor (difficult to arouse), or coma (unarousable)

Data from Inouye SK, van Dyck CH, Alessi CA, et al. Clarifying confusion: the confusion assessment method. a new method for detection of delirium. *Ann Intern Med.* 1990;113(12):941–948.

Patient_____ Date /__/__/__/ Time____:____
y   m   d (24 hour clock, midnight = 00:00)

Pulse or heart rate, taken for one minute: _____ Blood pressure:____/____

NAUSEA AND VOMITING–Ask "Do you feel sick to your stomach? Have you vomited?" Observation.
0 no nausea and no vomiting
1 mild nausea with no vomiting
2
3
4 intermittent nausea with dry heaves
5
6
7 constant nausea, frequent dry heaves and vomiting

TREMOR–Arms extended and fingers spread apart. Observation.
0 no tremor
1 not visible, but can be felt fingertip to fingertip
2
3
4 moderate, with patient's arms extended
5
6
7 severe, even with arms not extended

PAROXYSMAL SWEATS–Observation.
0 no sweat visible
1 barely perceptible sweating, palms moist
2
3
4 beads of sweat obvious on forehead
5
6
7 drenching sweats

ANXIETY–Ask "Do you feel nervous?" Ovservation.
0 no anxiety, at ease
1 mildly anxious
2
3
4 moderately anxious, or guarded, so anxiety is inferred
5
6
7 equivalent to acute panic states as seen in severe delirium or acute schizophrenic reactions

AGITATION–Observation.
0 normal activity
1 somewhat more than normal activity
2
3
4 moderately fidgety and restless
5
6
7 paces back and forth during most of the interview, or constantly thrashes about

TACTILE DISTURBANCES–Ask "Have you any itching, pins and needles sensations, any burning, any numbness or do you feel bugs crawling on or under your skin?" Observation.
0 none
1 very mild itching, pins and needles, burning or numbness
2 mild itching, pins and needles, burning or numbness
3 moderate itching, pins and needles, burning or numbness
4 moderately severe hallucinations
5 severe hallucinations
6 extremely severe hallucinations
7 continuous hallucinations

AUDITORY DISTURBANCES–Ask "Are you more aware of sounds around you? Are they harsh? Do they frighten you? Are you hearing anything that is disturbing to you? Are you hearing things you know are not there?" Observation.
0 not present
1 very mild harshness or ability to frighten
2 mild harshness or ability to frighten
3 moderate harshness or ability to frighten
4 moderately severe hallucinations
5 severe hallucinations
6 extremely severe hallucinations
7 continuous hallucinations

VISUAL DISTURBANCES–Ask "Does the light appear to be too bright? Is its color different? Does it hurt your eyes? Are you seeing anything that is disturbing to you? Are you seeing things you know are not there?" Observation.
0 not present
1 very mild sensitivity
2 mild sensitivity
3 moderate sensitivity
4 moderately severe hallucinations
5 severe hallucinations
6 extremely severe hallucinations
7 continuous hallucinations

HEADACHE, FULLNESS IN HEAD–Ask "Does your head feel different? Does it feel like there is a band around your head?" Do not rate for dizziness or lightheadedness. Otherwise, rate severity.
0 not present
1 very mild
2 mild
3 moderate
4 moderately severe
5 severe
6 very severe
7 extremely severe

ORIENTATION AND CLOUDING OF SENSORIUM–Ask "What day is this? Where are you? Who am I?"
0 oriented and can do serial additions
1 cannot do serial additions or is uncertain about date
2 disoriented for date by no more than 2 calendar days
3 disoriented for date by more than 2 calendar days
4 disoriented for place and/or person

Total CIWA-A Score_____
Rater's Initials_____
Maximum Possible Score 67

The CIWA-Ar is not copyrighted and may be reproduced freely. This assessment for monitoring withdrawal symptoms requires approximately 5 minutes to administer. The maximum score is 67 (see instrument). Patients scoring less than 10 do not usually need additional medication for withdrawal.

Fig. 9.1 Clinical Institute Withdrawal Assessment for Alcohol (CIWA), also referred to as the Alcohol Withdrawal Syndrome (AWS) Scale. (From Sullivan JT, Sykora K, Schneiderman J, et al. Assessment of alcohol withdrawal: the revised clinical institute withdrawal assessment for alcohol scale (CIWA-ar). *Br J Addict.* 1989;84(11):1353–1357.)

For each item, circle the number that best describes the patient's signs or symptom. Rate on just the apparent relationship to opiate withdrawal. For example, if heart rate is increased because the patient was jogging just prior to assessment, the increase pulse rate would not add to the score.

Patient's Name:_____   **Date and Time:**__/__/__:_____

Reason for this assessment: _____

Resting Pulse Rate:_____beats/minute _Measured after patient is sitting or lying for one minute_ 0 pulse rate 80 or below 1 pulse rate 81-100 2 pulse rate 101-120 4 pulse rate greater than 120	**GI Upset:** _over last 1/2 hour_ 0 no GI symptoms 1 stomach cramps 2 nausca or loose stool 4 vomiting diarrhea 5 multiple episodes of diarrhea or vomiting
Sweating: _over past 1/2 hour not accounted for by room temperature or patient activity._ 0 no report of chills or flushing 1 subjective report of chills or flushing 2 flushed or observable moistness on face 3 beads of sweat on brow or face 4 sweat streaming off face	**Tremor** _observation of outstretched hands_ 0 no tremor 1 tremor can be felt, but not obsrved 2 slight tremor observable 4 gross tremor or muscle twitching
Restlessness: _Observatin during assessment_ 0 able to sit still 1 reports difficulty sitting still, but is able to do so 3 frequent shifting or extraneous movements of legs/arms 5 unable to sit still for more than a few seconds	**Yawning** _Observation during assessment_ 0 no yawning 1 yawning once or twice during assessment 2 yawning three or more times during assessment 4 yawning several times/minute
Pupil size 0 pupils pinned or normal size for room light 1 pupils possibly larger than normal for room light 2 pupils moderately diated 5 pupils so dilated that only the rim of the iris is visible	**Anxiety or Irritability** 0 none 1 patient reports increasing irritability or anxiousness 2 patient obviously irritable or anxious 4 patient so irritable or anxious that participation in the assessment is difficult
Bone or Joint aches _If patient was having pain previously, only the additional component attributed to opiates withdrawal is scored_ 0 not present 1 mild diffuse discomfort 2 patient reports severe diffuse aching of joints/muscles 4 patient is rubbing joints or muscles and is unable to sit still because of discomfort	**Gooseflesh skin** 0 skin is smooth 3 piloerrection of skin can be felt or hairs standing up on arms 5 prominent piloerrection
Runny nose or tearing _Not accounted for by cold symptoms or allergies_ 0 not present 1 nasal stuffiness or unusually moist cycs 2 nose running or tearing 4 nose constantly running or tears streaming down cheeks	Total Sore_____ The total score is the sum of all 11 items Initials of person completing assessment: _____

Score: 5-12 = mild; 13-24 = moderate; 25-36 = moderately; severe; more than 36 = severe withdrawal

This version may be copied used clinically.

Fig. 9.2 Clinical Opiate Withdrawal Scale. (From Wesson DR, Ling W. The clinical opiate withdrawal scale (COWS). _J Psychoactive Drugs._ 2003;35(2):253–259.)

TABLE 9.3 ■ **Glasgow Coma Scale**

Eyes	Verbal	Motor
4 – Spontaneous	5 – Oriented	6 – Follows commands
3 – Loud voice	4 – Confused	5 – Localizes to pain
2 – To pain	3 – Inappropriate words	4 – Withdraws to pain
1 – None	2 – Incomprehensible sounds	3 – Abnormal flexion posturing
	1 – None	2 – Abnormal extension posturing
		1 – None

Think: "GCS ≤8, intubate."
Data from Teasdale G, Jennett B. Assessment of coma and impaired consciousness. A practical scale. *Lancet.* 1974;304(7872):81–84.

calculating the patient's Glasgow Coma Scale (GCS) score (Table 9.3). Nurses should notify the physician team of any alteration from baseline.

- Pay close attention to the patient's level of alertness (e.g., awake, drowsy, lethargic, or unarousable) and what level of stimulation is required to elicit a response.
- Pay attention to the content and characteristics of the patient's thought and speech (e.g., focused, tangential, disoriented, perseverative, or responding to internal stimuli), including any signs of dysarthria (slurred speech) or aphasia (lack of speech).
- Assess the cranial nerves (especially pupils) and look for new signs of nystagmus.
- Assess for focal motor findings (e.g., new weakness or pronator drift).

Common Strategies for the Prevention and Treatment of Delirium[4] (Fig. 9.3)

- Ensure sensory aids are available to the patient (e.g., interpreter, glasses, hearing aids, call bell within reach, phone).
- Ensure patient receives adequate nutrition and hydration.
- Promote normal sleep-wake cycles and appropriate sleep hygiene. At night, turn off lights in the hallways and encourage patients to turn off their own lights. Help patients turn off the TV and other mobile devices before bedtime. Stimulate patients to remain awake with natural sunlight during the day.
- Reorient patients frequently, especially those who are elderly. Review the patient's goals and plan of care for the day. Update the date, care team, and plan of care visibly for patients in their rooms.
- Help patients communicate with their families during the daytime by ensuring that they have a phone nearby and can use it properly.
- Optimize pain control, bowel regimen, urinary retention, and positioning in bed.
- Encourage and facilitate out-of-bed mobilization.
- Notify the physician team if patients develop agitation or hyperactivity; attempt to minimize use of chemical or physical restraints when possible. Provide 1:1 observation when appropriate, or keep patients close to the nursing station for more frequent monitoring.
- In patients with hypoactive delirium, avoid pharmacologic therapy.
- If there is a concern for opiate toxicity, continue to monitor respiratory status and consider naloxone if there is an acute decline in mental status.
- In patients with alcohol or sedative/hypnotic withdrawal, continue AWS/CIWA protocol monitoring and consider the use of as-needed pharmacologic therapy.

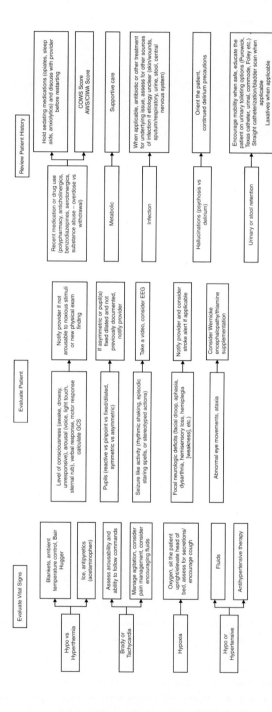

Fig. 9.3 Flow diagram of causes, workup, and management for acute change in mental status (memory, attention/concentration, consciousness). *AWS/CIWA*, Alcohol Withdrawal Scale/Clinical Institute Withdrawal Assessment for Alcohol; *COWS*, Clinical Opiate Withdrawal Scale; *EEG*, electroencephalogram; *GCS*, Glasgow Coma Scale.

TABLE 9.4 ■ Pharmacologic Therapies for Delirium[5]

Medication	Dosage	Adverse Effects/Considerations
Conventional Antipsychotic		
Haloperidol (Haldol)	0.5–1 mg PO, 1–5 mg IV or IM, every 4–6 hours as needed	Extrapyramidal symptoms,[a] prolonged QTc (on ECG), preferred agent of choice
Atypical Antipsychotic		
Quetiapine (Seroquel)	25 mg PO, every 6–8 hours as needed	Extrapyramidal symptoms,[a] prolonged QTc
Olanzapine (Zyprexa)	2.5 mg–5 mg daily	
Risperidone (Risperdal)	0.5 mg daily	
Benzodiazepine		
Lorazepam (Ativan)	0.5–1 mg every 4–6 hours, as needed (PO or IV)	• Paradoxic excitation, respiratory depression, oversedation • Use for alcohol or sedative/benzodiazepine withdrawal

[a]Extrapyramidal symptoms: symptoms typically caused by dopamine blockade or depletion. These include acute dyskinesias (abnormal irregular movements), dystonic reactions (involuntary muscle contractions resulting in abnormal posturing or repetitive movements, including the face, neck, extremities, back, etc.), tardive dyskinesia (involuntary orofacial and tongue movements), parkinsonism (tremor, rigidity, slowed movements), akinesia (lack of movement), akathisia (internal restlessness and a compulsive urge to move), and neuroleptic malignant syndrome (life-threatening condition with high fever, muscle rigidity, stupor, autonomic dysfunction).[6]

■ When indicated, use pharmacologic agents in the treatment of delirium (Table 9.4).
　■ Pharmacologic treatment of delirium should be short term and trialed only after other nonpharmacologic therapies have been attempted and failed. Consult with the primary medical team for questions or concerns regarding efficacy, oversedation, and other adverse events.

Conclusion

Encephalopathy encompasses a broad spectrum of abnormal cognitive states and can be indicative of a significant underlying illness. Nurses should perform routine neurologic exams on their patients, particularly those with prolonged and complicated hospitalizations. Any concerns regarding a patient's mentation should be communicated to the interprofessional team, especially the physicians throughout the day/night and fellow nurses at the change of shifts. Education regarding associated etiologies of encephalopathy and nonpharmacologic interventions to treat potential causes can improve the patient's condition, reduce hospital length of stay, minimize adverse outcomes, and save associated health care costs.[7]

References

1. Miller MO. Evaluation and management of delirium in hospitalized older patients. *Am Fam Physician.* 2008;78(11):1265–1270.
2. Krishnan V, Leung LY, Caplan LR. A neurologist's approach to delirium: diagnosis and management of toxic metabolic encephalopathies. *Eur J Intern Med.* 2014;25(2):112–116.
3. Koita J, Riggio S, Jagoda A. The mental status examination in emergency practice. *Emerg Med Clin North Am.* 2010;28(3):439–451.
4. Inouye SK, Bogardus Jr ST, Charpentier PA, et al. A multicomponent intervention to prevent delirium in hospitalized older patients. *N Engl J Med.* 1999;340(9):669–676.

5. Inouye SK. Delirium in older persons. *N Engl J Med.* 2006;354(11):1157–1165.
6. Blair DT, Dauner A. Extrapyramidal symptoms are serious side-effects of antipsychotic and other drugs. *Nurse Pract.* 1992;17(11):56,62–64,67.
7. Lundstrom M, Edlund A, Karlsson S, et al. A multifactorial intervention program reduces the duration of delirium, length of hospitalization, and mortality in delirious patients. *J Am Geriatr Soc.* 2005;53(4):622–628.

Questions

A 65-year-old male with unknown past medical history is admitted to the hospital with altered mental status, fever, tachycardia, and hypotension. He is admitted to the hospital given concerns for an infection and septic shock of unclear etiology. On workup he is found to have a positive urinalysis, acute kidney injury, and a urine drug screen that is positive for benzodiazepines.

1. The patient is started on antibiotics and fluid resuscitated. After the first day of admission, his mental status improves, but he suddenly becomes agitated, tachycardic, and hypertensive. He is poorly oriented to time or situation and does not engage in proper conversation. At this time, which of the following would be most appropriate for assessing the severity of his condition and guiding further management?
   a. Confusion Assessment Method (CAM) score
   b. Clinical Opiate Withdrawal Scale (COWS) score
   c. Clinical Institute Withdrawal Assessment for Alcohol (CIWA)
   d. Glasgow Coma Scale (GCS) score

2. You correctly identify that the patient is experiencing benzodiazepine withdrawal, which presents similarly to alcohol withdrawal. You administer benzodiazepines according to protocol and note full recovery of the patient's vital signs, mentation, and ability to engage in appropriate conversation. A week later during the same admission, the day nurse signs out to you that the patient is completely oriented and neurologically normal. As the night progresses, you note his mental status begins to fluctuate. He no longer can identify where he is or for what reason. What is the next best course of action after assessing the patient's vital signs and performing a physical examination?
   a. Assess the CAM score.
   b. Assess the CIWA score.
   c. Ask the patient when his last bowel movement occurred.
   d. Call a stroke alert.

3. Based on the CAM score, the patient's new symptoms are consistent with delirium. What intervention is *least* likely to help in this situation?
   a. Reorienting the patient
   b. Turning off the hallway lights
   c. Optimizing pain control
   d. Administering benzodiazepines intermittently

4. The patient becomes physically combative and hyperactive. What intervention is *least* likely to help in this situation?
   a. Notify the provider
   b. 1:1 therapeutic sitter
   c. Benzodiazepines, as needed
   d. Antipsychotics, as needed
   e. Physical restraint if the patient is at risk of harming himself or others

5. After this eventful evening, the patient is calm and completely oriented in the morning. His family arrives and hears about his violent behavior overnight. They worry whether this is something they will have to deal with at home after hospital discharge. Which statement is *least* likely applicable in this situation?
   a. The patient's mentation is likely to improve with family support.
   b. The patient's mentation may have inconsistencies during the day and for up to several days to weeks after hospital discharge.
   c. The patient needs to be kept on a strict day/night schedule to help with reorientation.
   d. The patient is developing permanent neurologic damage and the family should see a neurologist out of concerns for dementia.

Answers

1. c

2. a

3. d

4. c

5. d

Common Procedures and Pathology of the Spine

CHAPTER 10

Nursing Protocol for Elective Spine Surgery

Newton Mei, MD ■ Laura Sweeney, MSN, CRNP, FNP, AGACNP, CNRN

Introduction

Many patients come to the hospital daily for elective spine procedures. Nurses caring for neurosurgical patients should familiarize themselves with the common terminology related to the spine, spinal procedures, and spinal pathology to improve communication in the hospital setting. This chapter will highlight common elective spinal procedures and spinal perioperative pathways developed to aid in the speedy recovery of these patients. By being aware of the protocols and workflows for these patients, nurses can anticipate the plan of care, decrease patients' length of stay in the hospital, and assist with coordinating the best care for the patient postoperatively.

Anatomy and Terminology of the Spine

ANATOMY OF THE SPINE

Knowing the basics of spinal anatomy serves as a foundation for understanding common clinical terminology used in the hospital setting when caring for spine patients.[1] The spine provides structural support for the body and is the protective casing for the spinal cord. The spine is comprised of 33 vertebrae differentiated into five parts from top to bottom as follows (Fig. 10.1)[1,2]:

- Cervical spine: 7 vertebrae
- Thoracic spine: 12 vertebrae
- Lumbar spine: 5 vertebrae
- Sacrum: 5 bones that are fused
- Coccyx: 4 bones that are fused

Between each vertebra are intervertebral discs that act as cartilaginous cushions to absorb vertical compressive stress on the spine. On each side of the vertebra and flanking the spinous process are the lamina. This region of the bone is often cut during spine surgery, and the procedure is referred to as a laminectomy. Nerves exit on the sides of the vertebrae through openings known as the neural foramina. The cylindric tube that houses the spinal cord is known as the vertebral foramen or spinal canal.[1]

COMMON SPINE TERMINOLOGY[3,4]

- Anterior: from the front
- Posterior: from the back
- Lateral: from the side
- Decompression: a spinal decompression is a procedure that alleviates pressure from the spinal cord
- Spinal fusion: a surgical procedure where two or more vertebrae are fused

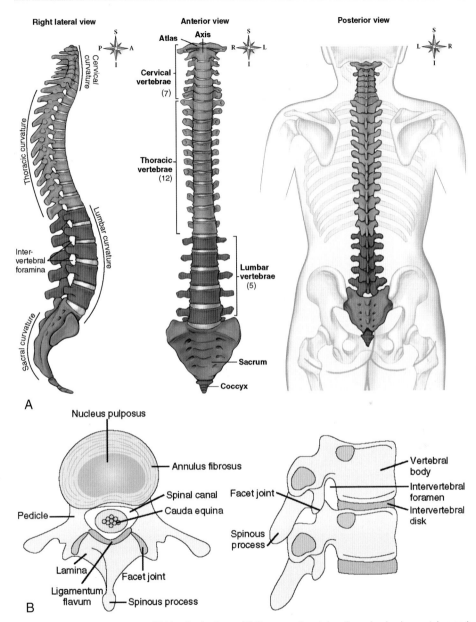

Fig. 10.1 Anatomy of the spine. (A) Vertebral column. (B) Cross-sectional view through a lumbar vertebra and lateral view of the lumbar spine. (A, From Patton K, Bell F, Thompson T, et al. *The Human Body in Health & Disease*, 8th ed. Elsevier; 2023; B, from Firestein G, Budd R, Gabriel SE, et al. *Firestein & Kelley's Textbook of Rheumatology*, 11th ed. Elsevier; 2020.)

- ■ Fusions typically involve metal rods, plates, screws, and cages. At times, patients are fused with bone grafts, using either the patient's own bone (autologous bone) or a synthetic bone graft.
- ■ Laminectomy: cutting and removing the posterior part of the spinal bone by cutting the bilateral laminas

- Foraminotomy: opening of the foramina to release the spinal roots
- Discectomy: partial or total removal of the disc
- Myelopathy: spinal cord lesion/injury that can result from compression and/or inflammation, resulting in progressive neurologic deficits
- Radiculopathy: nerve root injury that can be caused by compression and/or inflammation, resulting in neuropathic pain and associated dermatomal involvement
- Spondylosis: term for degenerative disease in the spine that can result in spinal cord or nerve compression and inflammation
- Spondylolisthesis: term for slippage of vertebrae in relation to each other that can result in spinal cord or nerve compression and inflammation
- Spinal stenosis: narrowing of the spinal canal or vertebral foramina
- Cauda equina syndrome: compression of the nerve roots at the end of the spinal cord (conus medullaris)
  - If this happens acutely, it is a medical emergency, and the patient requires urgent surgical decompression.
  - Associated symptoms include back pain, saddle anesthesia, bowel or bladder dysfunction, and weakness in the lower extremities.[2,4]
- Spine procedures are generally named by their approach, level, and type of surgical intervention, such as:
  - Anterior cervical decompression fusion (ACDF)
  - Posterior lumbar decompression fusion (PLDF)
- Surgeons may also delineate the vertebra involved:
  - Posterior thoracic 1–5 decompression and fusion (PT1–5DF)

Degenerative disk and joint disease occur as part of aging and result from the natural wear-and-tear process of long-term use. Through years of ongoing stress, the spine can develop weakness and tears in its ligaments and discs. The intervertebral discs can lose their height and can herniate into the spinal canal. Osteoarthritis of the spine joints can lead to spondylosis where bony spurs, also known as osteophytes, can form and impinge on nerves or the spinal cord. With the weakness of the ligaments along the spine, vertebrae can slip past each other, resulting in a condition called spondylolisthesis. Stenosis, or narrowing of the spinal canal or neural foramina (the outlet where nerve roots exit the spine), occurs from the abovementioned processes and leads to myelopathy and radiculopathy.[4]

Myelopathy occurs when the spinal cord is compressed and inflamed and can occur at any level of the spinal cord. The higher the level of spinal cord involvement, the more downstream nerves are affected. As such, cervical myelopathy can affect nerves innervating both the upper and lower parts of the body. This can lead to symptoms such as neck stiffness, neck pain, weakness, and paresthesia in the upper extremities, weakness with grip strength, decreased finger dexterity, weakness and paresthesia in the lower extremities, gait imbalance, saddle anesthesia, and bowel and bladder dysfunction. Thoracolumbar myelopathies can lead to back pain, lower extremity weakness, radiculopathy, paresthesia, saddle anesthesia, and bowel or bladder dysfunction.[5]

Surgical treatment for elective spine surgery is usually considered after conservative treatment has failed. Conservative treatment includes outpatient epidural steroid injections (ESI), physical therapy, aqua therapy, and pain medications.[1] Indications for spinal procedures vary and can include worsening myelopathy, persistent pain despite conservative management, significant disability, and decreased functional status. See Fig. 10.2 for common spine procedures and Fig. 10.3 for further indications for surgery.

Elective Spine Surgery Preoperative Pathway

In the preoperative phase, patients intending to undergo elective spine surgery are evaluated by the spine surgery team in the outpatient setting. In addition to the physical examination, patients may undergo imaging (x-rays, computed tomography spine, and/or magnetic resonance imaging [MRI] of the spine) to further evaluate structural deformities and spinal cord pathology.[1] See

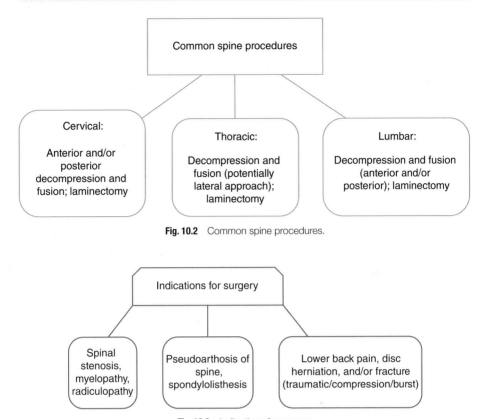

Fig. 10.2 Common spine procedures.

Fig. 10.3 Indications for surgery.

Fig. 10.4 for the preoperative spinal imaging options. The surgeon will then explain to the patient the recommended surgical procedure, describe the associated risks and complications, and obtain the patient's consent. After the evaluation by the surgical team, patients will be requested to present to their primary doctor and/or preadmission testing center for a comprehensive preoperative assessment. During the preoperative assessment, patients will have a cardiovascular risk assessment and receive counseling on their medication management prior to surgery. The patient's other medical problems will also be evaluated and optimized, if possible. Appropriate testing will also be obtained to assist in the patient's assessment and can serve as a baseline for postoperative care.[6]

PERMANENT PACEMAKER AND IMPLANTABLE CARDIOVERTER-DEFIBRILLATORS

MRI with contrast of the spine is the gold-standard imaging modality to evaluate spinal pathology.[1] With the advent of new biotechnology many patients may have implanted devices to manage their chronic medical problems. Permanent pacemakers (PPMs) and implantable cardioverter-defibrillators (ICDs) are especially prevalent in the elderly patient population. It is important to determine whether the patient's PPM/ICD is MRI compatible. The provider should gather information about the patient's PPM/ICD, including company, model, and whether the device is MRI compatible. Some patients may carry cards from the device manufacturer or cardiologists that outline this information. Chest x-rays are sometimes done to determine the positioning of the PPM/ICD leads and wires. If the patient is cleared to undergo MRI imaging, cardiology may be consulted to interrogate and modify the PPM/ICD programming before and after the MRI (Fig. 10.5).[7]

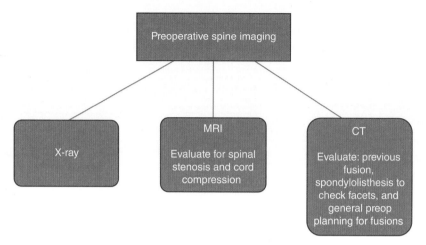

Fig. 10.4   Preoperative Imaging. *CT*, Computed tomography; *MRI*, magnetic resonance imaging.

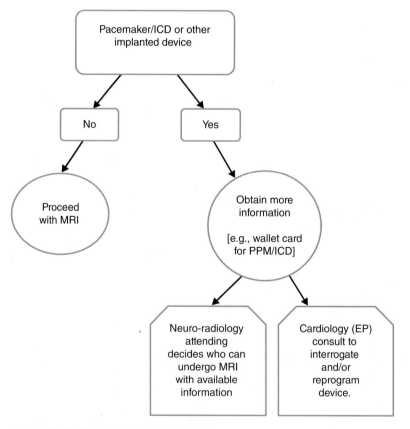

Most older PPM/ICD are not MRI compatible.

Fig. 10.5   Pacemaker and/or implantable cardioverter-defibrillator *(ICD)* for magnetic resonance imaging *(MRI)*. *EP*, Electrophysiology; *PPM*, permanent pacemaker.

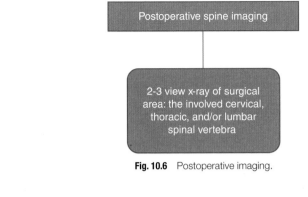

Fig. 10.6   Postoperative imaging.

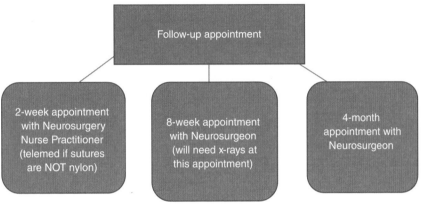

Fig. 10.7   Follow-up pathway.

Postoperative Pathways/Enhanced Recovery After Surgery

Postoperative pathways/protocols were developed to improve outcomes, decrease hospitalization costs, and reduce the length of stay.[8,9] These are commonly referred to as enhanced recovery after surgery.[10] Postoperative spinal pathways are formed from a collection of evidence-based recommendations in postoperative care. The pathways delineated in this chapter can serve as a framework for comprehensive spine units or neurosurgical wards at other institutions (Figs. 10.6, 10.7, 10.8, and 10.9).[11]

NURSING INTERVENTIONS FOR ALL TYPES OF ELECTIVE SPINE PROCEDURES

- Reducing postoperative pulmonary complications using I-COUGH[12]
  - I-COUGH is an acronym that highlights interventions that can be used by nursing in the postoperative setting:
    - *I*ncentive spirometry
    - *C*ough and deep breathing exercises
    - *O*ral hygiene
    - *U*nderstanding: promoting education to patient and family members

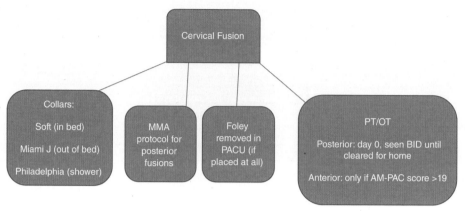

Fig. 10.8 Cervical fusion pathway. *BID,* Twice daily; *MMA,* multimodal analgesia; *PACU,* postanesthesia care unit; *PT/OT,* physical therapy/occupational therapy.

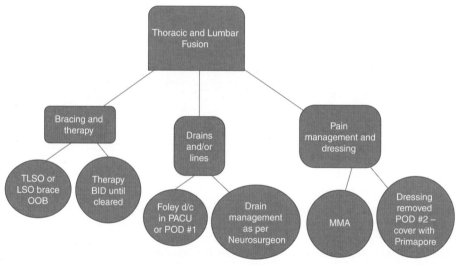

Fig. 10.9 Thoracic and lumbar fusion pathway. *BID,* Twice daily; *MMA,* multimodal analgesia; *OOB,* out of bed; *PACU,* postanesthesia care unit; *POD,* postoperative day.

- Getting out of bed: encouraging patients to get out of bed multiple times in a day and encouraging early mobilization
- Head of bed elevation to reduce the risk of aspiration
- Surgical site monitoring and management
  - Ongoing nursing neurologic assessment and surgical site evaluation[1,13]
  - Surgical drain type, location, and output documentation[13]
  - IV antibiotic prophylaxis per protocol[13]
- Optimizing pain control with multimodal analgesia (MMA)
  - Ongoing pain assessment and review of patient's MMA regimen[10,14]
- Monitor intake and output: optimize nutrition and treat constipation
  - Early postoperative enteral intake[10]
  - Document last bowel movement and bowel regimen
  - Antiemetics PRN for postoperative nausea and vomiting[10,15]

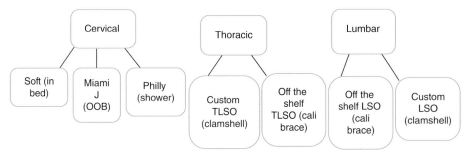

If a patient has a cervical-thoracic fusion they need to wear a CTO brace when out of bed and a Miami J collar when in bed.

Fig. 10.10 Summary of bracing options after spinal fusions. *OOB,* Out of bed.

AFTER CERVICAL SPINE SURGERY[11]

- Patients are often instructed to always wear a cervical collar, both in and out of bed (OOB).
  - The collar provides support to the neck and serves as a reminder to the patient to not turn the neck.[1]
- Typically, patients do not have a Foley catheter placed perioperatively. If the patient does have one placed, the goal should be its removal as early as possible, often in the postanesthesia care unit (PACU)
- ACDF
  - Target length of stay: 1 night
  - AM-PAC score is a validated scoring system that is used to determine discharge disposition to home vs rehab. A score of ≥19 suggests that a patient is functional to return home.[16] Physical therapy and occupational therapy (PT/OT) do not need to be consulted in these patients unless there is an obvious concern for a safe discharge home.
  - Keep head of bed high to reduce swelling in neck
- PCDF
  - Target length of stay: 2 nights
  - PT/OT assessment

AFTER THORACIC OR LUMBAR SURGERY[11]

- Patients are to wear braces when OOB, and braces can be off while in bed,
  - Degree of stability required ultimately depends on the spinal region affected
  - Some braces are standard sizing and others are custom molded to the patient; this may be based on surgeon preference.[1]
    - See Fig. 10.10 for bracing options in spinal stability.
- Indwelling urinary catheters are generally placed perioperatively.
  - Void trials occur on postoperative day 1–2
  - Nursing should monitor for regular voids every 4–8 hours, and use bladder scanners to check for retention.[1]
  - Nursing should check postvoid residuals (PVRs) to ensure adequate bladder emptying.[1]
    - If retaining and unable to void, or having consistently high PVRs, the patient may need intermittent straight catheterization.[1]
- Lumbar laminectomy
  - Target length of stay: 1 night
  - No brace required
  - PT/OT evaluation if there are concerns for a safe discharge to home or the patient has a low AM-PAC score

- A/P TLDF:
  - Target length of stay: 3 nights
  - Patients with underlying scoliosis should get standing x-rays with a brace
  - Brace when OOB per surgeon instructions
  - PT/OT evaluation

Early mobilization is crucial for all spine patients. Early mobilization has been shown to reduce rates of infection and medical complications and quicken the rate of return to function, while serving to emphasize the patient's role in recovery.[10] PT and OT specialists are consulted, and therapy generally is encouraged to start immediately postop unless contraindicated or if the patient is hemodynamically unstable. If comfortable, nursing should feel empowered to get patients OOB prior to formal therapy evaluations. Pain control is also imperative after spinal surgery to allow for improved postoperative mobility and participation in postoperative care.[10,14]

Surgical dressings often remain in place until postoperative day 2. Wounds may be closed either with nylon sutures, dissolvable sutures, staples, surgical skin glue, or adhesive bandages. It is important to know the type of closure material used and to educate patients on follow-up measures for suture/staple removal if appropriate. These wounds should then have an adhesive dressing in place during the hospital stay. At time of discharge, patients are encouraged to shower to reduce the risk of infection. The surgical site may get wet, but after showering, the patient should pat-dry the incision thoroughly. Once discharged home, the patient can either choose to apply a dressing to the surgical site or leave it open to air. Patients should be educated to monitor surgical wounds for any signs/symptoms of infection. Patients should look out for drainage, redness, dehiscence, swelling, tenderness, and any odor and notify the surgeons office for any concerns.[13]

Drains are placed during surgery, and their discontinuation is often dictated by surgeon preference and drainage output. The drainage amount should be recorded by nursing multiple times throughout the day. Sometimes plastic surgery may be consulted for complex surgical site closure. Plastic surgery will often leave surgical drains in place for a prolonged period until drainage reaches a very minimal amount. Because this can take a long time, patients will often be discharged home with these drains. Nursing should be responsible for educating patients on Jackson-Pratt drain management, how to empty the drain, how to measure and record the drainage, and how to apply appropriate suction to the drain.[13] Occasionally patients are discharged home with an incisional wound vacuum to help promote closure of the wound. These vacs are often ordered to be removed on postoperative day 7 unless directed by the surgeon. After removal, these vacs can be discarded in the trash and the incision left open to air afterward.[17,18]

Conclusion

It is important for nurses caring for neurosurgical spine patients to be familiar with the basics of spinal anatomy and the associated terminology to facilitate communication between members of the interprofessional team. With a thorough understanding of the spine pathways, nurses can also assist with patient education and help patients establish achievable goals and expectations. Elective spine surgery protocols are designed to enhance recovery and have been shown to be effective in reducing patient length of stay and accelerating return to function, while reducing complications and readmissions.[10] As a result, many hospitals/institutions are creating their own protocols and pathways. Additionally, nursing interventions are incorporated into the protocol to reduce the risk of postoperative pulmonary complications, catheter-associated urinary tract infections, thromboembolism, postoperative nausea and vomiting, and constipation.

References

1. Ryan D. *Handbook of Neuroscience Nursing: Care of the Adult Neurosurgical Patient.* Thieme; 2019.
2. Gitelman A, Hishmeh S, Morelli BN, et al. Cauda equina syndrome: a comprehensive review. *Am J Orthop (Belle Mead NJ).* 2008;37(11):556–562.

3. Abbasifard S, Abd-El-Barr MM, Ahmadian AA, et al. *Handbook of Spine Surgery*, 2nd ed. Thieme; 2016.

4. Myers CS, Parkinson S. Spinal disorders. In: Ryan D, ed. *Handbook of Neuroscience Nursing: Care of the Adult Neurosurgical Patient*. Thieme; 2019:280.

5. Kern S. *Spine Essentials Handbook: A Bulleted Review of Anatomy, Evaluation, Imaging, Tests, and Procedures*. Thieme; 2019.

6. Wang TY, Price M, Mehta VA, et al. Preoperative optimization for patients undergoing elective spine surgery. *Clin Neurol Neurosurg*. 2021;202:106445.

7. Burke PT, Ghanbari H, Alexander PB, et al. A protocol for patients with cardiovascular implantable devices undergoing magnetic resonance imaging (MRI): should defibrillation threshold testing be performed post-(MRI). *J Interv Card Electrophysiol*. 2010;28(1):59–66.

8. Sivaganesan A, Wick JB, Chotai S, et al. Perioperative protocol for elective spine surgery is associated with reduced length of stay and complications. *J Am Acad Surg*. 2019;27(5):183–189.

9. d'Astorg H, Fière V, Dupasquier M, et al. Enhanced recovery after surgery (ERAS) protocol reduces LOS without additional adverse events in spine surgery. *Orthop Traumatol Surg Res*. 2020;106(6): 1167–1173.

10. Elsarrag M, Soldozy S, Patel P, et al. Enhanced recovery after spine surgery: a systematic review. *Neurosurg Focus*. 2019;46(4):e3.

11. 5 Spine Pathways. Clinical Pathway: Thomas Jefferson University Hospital. p. 5.

12. Cassidy MR, Rosenkranz P, McCabe K, et al. I COUGH: reducing postoperative pulmonary complications with a multidisciplinary patient care program. *JAMA Surg*. 2013;148(8):740–745.

13. Macasieb CO, Mummaneni P. Spine surgery wound and drain management. In: Wang M, Strayer A, Harris O, et al., eds. *Handbook of Neurosurgery, Neurology, and Spinal Medicine for Nurses and Advanced Practice Health Professionals*. Routledge; 2017:183–186.

14. Daniel R, Harrop CM. *Medical Management of Neurosurgical Patients*. Oxford University Press; 2020.

15. Berg S, Bittner EA. *Postoperative Care Handbook of the Massachusetts General Hospital*. Lippincott Williams & Wilkins; 2017.

16. Warren M, Knecht J, Verheijde J, et al. Association of AM-PAC "6-Clicks" basic mobility and daily activity scores with discharge destination. *Phys Ther*. 2021;101(4):pzab043.

17. Dyck BA, Bailey CS, Steyn C, et al. Use of incisional vacuum-assisted closure in the prevention of postoperative infection in high-risk patients who underwent spine surgery: a proof-of-concept study. *J Neurosurg Spine*. 2019;31(3):430–439.

18. Horch RE. Incisional negative pressure wound therapy for high-risk wounds. *J Wound Care*. 2015;24(4): S21–S28.

Questions

A 55-year-old male with neck pain is awaiting spine surgery due to severe myelopathy. He takes rivaroxaban daily due to atrial fibrillation. He also has hypertension, hyperlipidemia, and a pacemaker (placed in 2012). The patient last took rivaroxaban today.

1. He needs an MRI with contrast of the cervical spine. What should the provider or nurse do to ensure patient safety?
   a. Obtain more information regarding the pacemaker.
   b. Ask the patient if he has a card from the pacemaker manufacturer delineating MRI compatibility.
   c. Call cardiology to assist in appropriate programming of the PPM for MRI.
   d. All of the above are correct.

2. The patient needs surgery to alleviate his myelopathic symptoms. What symptoms might he be experiencing? (Select all that apply.)
   a. Decreased with hand dexterity
   b. Gait imbalance
   c. Arm and shoulder pain
   d. Chest palpitations

3. After reviewing all imaging, it was deemed that this patient would be appropriate for ACDF surgery. What does ACDF stand for?
   a. Anterior complete decompression and fusion
   b. Anterior cervical decompression and fusion
   c. Anterior cervical decompression and fixation
   d. Alternative complete decompression and fixation

4. Postoperative protocols after ACDF scenario would include which of the following?
   a. Indwelling urinary catheter removal in PACU (if placed at all)
   b. Out of bed postop day 0, and PT/OT consult if AM-PAC score is <19
   c. Collar at all times
   d. All the above

5. The patient is deemed medically stable for discharge, and his AM-PAC score was 20, so he did not need PT evaluation. Upon discharge, what education is *not* essential for the nurse to provide to the patient?
   a. Assess the wound regularly and notify the provider's office for any drainage, redness, and swelling at the incision site.
   b. Keep the wound dry, always covered, and avoid showering.
   c. Continue to wear your cervical collar as directed and sleep with your head of bed high to reduce swelling.
   d. Keep all follow-up appointments to ensure timely removal of sutures.

Answers

1. d

2. a, b, c

3. b

4. d

5. b

CHAPTER 11

Nursing Management of the Patient With Acute Traumatic Spinal Cord Injury

Renae Fisher, MD ■ Mina Na, DO ■ Kristin Gustafson, DO

Introduction

The spinal cord, which carries motor and sensory signals throughout the body, begins at C1 and terminates around the level of L1. A spinal cord injury (SCI) occurs when there is damage to the neurons that send and receive these signals. This can be caused by direct injury to the spinal cord or from damage to the bones and tissues that surround the spinal cord. There is significant clinical diversity in patients with SCI because the level and completeness of injury can vary widely. Patients with SCI are at risk of developing many complications, especially within the acute care phase.[1] Therefore the role of the neurosurgical nurse is crucial in the direct care and education[2] of these patients to monitor for and prevent complications from arising.

Physical Exam

When a patient presents with a possible SCI, a neuromusculoskeletal physical exam that is accurate, consistent, and reproducible is important in defining neurologic impairments. Having this baseline exam established is important in the event of neurologic change, and in communicating impairment to other providers. The American Spinal Injury Association (ASIA) exam was developed to describe and prognosticate SCI in the acute period and is a universal classification system for grading spinal cord injuries. An ASIA grade includes both the neurologic level of injury and classification letter (e.g., C4 AISA A).[3]

ASIA CLASSIFICATION

- A = Complete injury
    - No motor or sensory function below the level of injury (e.g., C2 ASIA A: ventilator dependent, little to no strength in arms and legs).
- B = Incomplete injury
    - Sensory but not motor function is preserved below the neurologic level of injury, and some sensation is preserved in the lowest sacral segments (S4 and S5).
- C = Incomplete injury
    - Motor function is preserved below the neurologic level of injury (but often weak), and motor and sensory function is preserved at the lowest sacral segments.
- D = Incomplete injury
    - Motor function is preserved below the neurologic level of injury, and at least half of the key muscles below the neurologic level are graded as ≥3 on manual muscle testing (MMT). Motor and sensory function is preserved at the lowest sacral segments (e.g., L4 ASIA D: arms unaffected, may have some mild weakness in legs but can ambulate).
- E = Normal motor and sensory functions

STRENGTH EXAM

MMT is a standardized way to measure muscle strength. It is graded on a scale of 0 (total paralysis) to 5 (normal).

MMT STRENGTH GRADING

- 0 = total paralysis
- 1 = palpable or visual contraction
- 2 = full range of motion with gravity eliminated
- 3 = full range of motion against gravity
- 4 = full range of motion against moderate resistance
- 5 = full range of movement against full resistance (normal strength expected from an unimpaired person)

SENSATION EXAM

The spinal cord carries different sensory signals, including light touch, pressure, pain, and temperature. Checking sensation helps localize spinal cord lesions by elucidating where signals become abnormal. Generally, cervical nerve roots supply the upper limbs, thoracic nerve roots supply the thorax, and lumbar nerve roots supply the lower limbs. Sensation is classified as normal, impaired, or absent.[3]

Common Complications From SCI (Table 11.1)

NEUROGENIC BLADDER

Neurogenic bladder is an inevitable complication after SCI. In neurologically intact individuals, normal voiding depends on a careful synchronization of voluntary control and involuntary reflexes, which are altered with nerve injury. Since bladder dysfunction is expected, it is very important for nurses to time the removal of the indwelling catheter carefully. Subsequently, it is important to monitor bladder volumes after its removal. The bladder overfills at 500 mL. Anything greater than this volume can stretch the bladder and slow the return of bladder function.[4] Some people will not regain volitional bladder function after SCI and will need to use intermittent catheterization to void between four and six times daily.

Before Removing the Foley

- Ensure the patient is hemodynamically stable.
- Check that continuous intravenous (IV) fluids are no longer needed.
- Ensure urine output <2500 mL/day.
- Restrict oral fluids to 2 L daily.

Once Foley Is Removed

- Initiate bladder training protocol (Fig. 11.1)

A Note on External Catheters

- They may be dangerous and inappropriate management options for these patients.
- Place patients at risk of voiding via overflow incontinence.
  - These patients will void small amounts frequently and will be retaining large amounts of urine.
  - Check random bladder scans to ensure volumes are <500 mL.
- Females are at risk of skin breakdown from moisture-associated injury.

TABLE 11.1 ■ **Brief Overview of Common Complications After SCI and Management Options**

Complication	Who Is at Risk?	Management

Neurogenic bladder	All levels of SCI	- Before removing the indwelling catheter ensure:
		  1. hemodynamic stability
		  2. intravenous fluids stopped
		  3. urine output <2500 mL/day
		- When Foley is removed, need bladder training protocol that balances void trials with intermittent catheterizations
		- Goal: always keep bladder volumes <500 mL to avoid overstretching

Neurogenic bowel	All levels of SCI	Start daily, consistently timed, bowel program from day 1 - Give senna about 7 hours before bowel program with suppository (e.g., senna at 12 pm, bowel program at 7 pm) - Insert suppository and perform digital stimulation - To optimize, have patient sit on commode *Do *not* avoid bowel program if patient already had a bowel movement that day
Respiratory failure	SCI: levels C1–T12, higher risk with higher level of injury - Respiratory function can diminish in the first few days	**If not on ventilator:** - Monitor respiratory parameters daily (negative inspiratory force and vital capacity) - Look out for increased work of breathing, higher respiratory rate, signs of fatigue - If mental status diminished or recently returned from cervical surgery, do *not* send patients to MRI without careful monitoring **If using ventilator:** - On ventilator, patients rest on AC mode, not pressure support
Pressure injury	All levels of SCI, especially those with: - Excess moisture - Incontinence - Immobilization - Impaired nutritional status - Impaired sensation	- Avoid use of diapers - Use zinc-based creams - Turn patient every 2 hours while in bed and every 30 minutes while sitting - Avoid shearing forces - Early nutrition consult
Autonomic dysreflexia	SCI: Levels C1–T6, plus patients with: - Sudden, pounding headache - Elevated blood pressure (20 mm Hg above baseline) - Facial flushing	First: Sit up patient Then: Look for noxious stimulus - Most common source is bladder distention, then bowel distension - Recheck blood pressure every 5 minutes until resolution - May use nitro paste if blood pressure is persistently elevated

MRI, Magnetic resonance imaging; *SCI*, spinal cord injury.

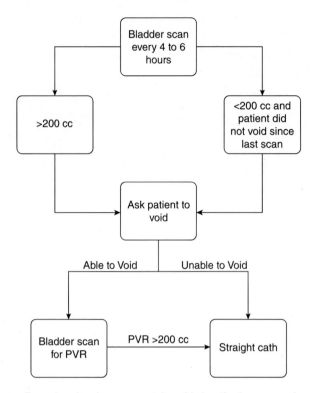

Record each volume separately: voided, cathed or scanned
If patient voids voluntarily and PVR <150cc ×3 notify MD to discontinue order

Fig. 11.1	Bladder training protocol algorithm. *PVR*, Post-void residual.

NEUROGENIC BOWEL

A neurogenic bowel is the loss of normal bowel function caused by a nervous system lesion. There are two main types of neurogenic bowel: upper and lower motor neuron (UMN/LMN) bowel. People with SCI are at risk of UMN bowel, while people with lesions distal to the spinal cord (e.g., cauda equina syndrome) are at risk of LMN bowel. Both types of bowel dysfunction can lead to constipation or fecal incontinence. Poorly managed neurogenic bowel not only leads to a decreased quality of life but can result in autonomic dysreflexia, fecal impaction, or avoidance of social activities[5] (Table 11.2).

Management

Goal: Start a consistently timed bowel program to achieve a formed, soft bowel movement daily without other episodes of fecal incontinence.

Sample UMN Bowel Program
1. Give senna 7 hours before planned bowel routine.
2. Administer suppository followed by digital stimulation, ideally 20–30 minutes after a meal (Box 11.1).

Continue to titrate oral bowel medications: stimulant (senna and/or bisacodyl) and osmotic laxatives (polyethylene glycol) by effect.[5]

TABLE 11.2 ■ Neurogenic Bowel Characteristics Depending on Upper vs Lower Motor Neuron Injury

	Upper Motor Neuron Injury (e.g., spinal cord injury)	Lower Motor Neuron Injury (e.g., cauda equina syndrome)
Hyperreflexic vs areflexic bowel[5]	Hyperreflexic bowel (reflex defecation present)	Areflexic bowel (reflex defecation absent)
Bowel problems	Constipation, diarrhea, and incontinence	Constipation, diarrhea, and incontinence (incontinence is usually the main issue)
Target stool consistency	Soft, formed	Firm, but not hard
Frequency of bowel care	Daily	Daily
Rectal suppository use	Suppositories effective	Suppositories usually *not* effective
Digital stimulation	Digital stimulation is important	Digital stimulation *not* effective; manual removal generally needed

---

BOX 11.1 ■ How to Perform a Digital Stimulation Cycle

Step 1: Explain the procedure of digital stimulation and ensure the patient agrees to it.
Step 2: Insert double-gloved, lubricated finger into the rectum.
Step 3: Slowly rotate the finger in a circular motion giving the rectal mucosal a gentle stretch. Continue until you feel the sphincter relax and flatus/stool passes (typically 20 seconds). Repeat two to three times. Then, wait 5 minutes for any additional stool to descend into the rectal vault. Repeat the cycle until no further stool is present in the rectal vault.

Note: This is ideally performed while on a commode but can be done in bed (with patient lying on their left side).

Important Considerations

- Start bowel program with suppository as early as possible after injury, even on day 1.
- If the patient has been constipated, then has several days of small liquid diarrhea, there may have liquid stool escaping around the impacted area.
- Nurses should continue the bowel routine at the same time every day, even if the patient already had a bowel movement that day.
- If a patient becomes impacted, treatment often involves aggressive laxatives with days of frequent liquid diarrhea. This is bad for the skin and involves frequent bedsheet changes.
- Some patients may experience autonomic dysreflexia (AD) with digital stimulation.
  - Nurses should monitor for sudden, severe headaches, elevated blood pressure, and flushing.
  - If AD occurs, the patient may require pretreatment with antihypertensive medication.
  - If systolic blood pressure is >150 mm Hg, it is recommended that the cycle be discontinued.[6]

PRESSURE INJURY

Pressure injuries (PI) are one of the most feared complications after SCI. They are expensive, common, and can be life threatening. Severe PI may limit seating, which may prevent participation in rehabilitation therapies at critical stages in neurologic recovery. PIs may take months to years to heal. Many PI are preventable but require special care and consideration of the treating team. Factors that contribute to PI formation include unrelieved pressure, shear, friction, moisture, malnutrition, and immobilization.

PI Prevention Strategies for Nurses

- Monitor
  - Do full body skin assessments daily.
  - Address percutaneous endoscopic gastrostomy tube diarrhea, which is very common. Consider decreasing feeding rate, changing formula, changing medication formulation (e.g., sorbitol-containing elixirs, such as liquid acetaminophen often cause diarrhea, while crushed acetaminophen tablets do not), and adding bulking agents, such as guar gum or banana flakes.[7,8]
- Do
  - Use low-air-loss mattress.
  - Turn patient every 2 hours while in bed/every 30 minutes while out of bed.
  - Keep skin dry. If moist, use zinc-based cream.
  - Get the patient out of bed as soon as the spine is stable per the surgeon. Prolonged bedrest is *not* the standard of care after SCI.
  - Encourage protein intake.
- Avoid
  - Raising the head of the bed >30 degrees
  - Diapers
  - External catheters in females

RESPIRATORY COMPLICATIONS

Respiratory complications are common in SCI when patients are injured above the T12 level. The severity of respiratory compromise depends on the level of injury and worsens with higher injuries. The diaphragm is innervated by C3–C5, so injuries at this level or above often require intubation in the acute stage. Injury below these levels also may cause a significant decline in respiratory function due to increased secretions after injury, which is secondary to impaired autonomic balance, decreased strength in the accessory muscles of respiration, and decreased strength in abdominal muscles that are critical for an effective cough. Careful monitoring especially in the initial days after injury is important to monitor for respiratory failure.

Additionally, pneumonia, atelectasis, and mucous plugging are very common respiratory complications.[9] Patients on a ventilator should be optimized to smaller airways by providing higher tidal volumes (10 mL/kg of ideal body weight). This is different from ventilating non-SCI patients.[10] To wean these patients from ventilators, free breathing time off the ventilator is slowly increased to build diaphragm strength.[11]

Management Strategies for Nurses

- Check respiratory parameters daily, including vital capacity and negative inspiratory force.[12]
- Optimize secretion management.
  - Scheduled and as-needed subglottic suctioning
    - Note: Infrequently, suctioning may cause profound bradycardia, which may be treated with atropine.
  - Thin secretions
    - Schedule guaifenesin and/or hypertonic saline nebulizers.
  - Open airways
    - Albuterol (small airways)
    - Ipratropium (larger airways)
  - Schedule cough assist, quad cough, postural drainage, and chest vest.

Important Considerations

- Ventilator-dependent people with SCI rest on assist control, not pressure support.
- People with tracheostomies can eat once they are cleared by speech therapy.
- Always ensure the cuff is fully deflated while patients are on Passy Muir valve (PMV).
  - An inflated cuff while on a PMV can be life threatening.

AUTONOMIC DYSREFLEXIA

Autonomic dysreflexia (AD) is an emergency specific to individuals with SCI at the level of T6 or above. AD is thought to be related to unopposed sympathetic activity below the level of SCI. It is characterized by suddenly elevated blood pressure and can be associated with reflex bradycardia. Often the patient will have a sudden pounding headache and facial flushing.[3] If left untreated, AD may be life threatening due to uncontrolled hypertension with complications such as stroke, cardiac arrhythmias, or seizures. If patients have a chronic SCI, they are often familiar with symptoms and triggers and will state they are "having AD."

If a patient verbally reports AD or has signs and symptoms of AD, it is useful to follow this algorithm:

1. Sit up patient and lower legs (induce orthostasis). Remove the abdominal binder and constrictive clothing.
2. Locate the noxious stimulus. (Hint: Most common source is bladder[6] followed by bowel.)
   a. Check urinary drainage and flush catheter.
   b. Check for bowel impaction or constipation.
   c. Perform a head-to-toe survey for noxious stimuli in areas with poor sensation (foreign objects underneath the patient, ingrown toenails, patient positioning, etc.).
   d. Other possible noxious stimuli include infection, pressure ulcer, venipuncture, and menstruation.
3. Alert the physician if a noxious stimulus cannot be identified. The physician may order a one-time dose of antihypertensive if conservative measures fail.
   a. Keep in mind that if the noxious stimulus is found after an antihypertensive agent is given, the patient may become hypotensive. Therefore it is important to complete a thorough survey.
   b. Topical nitroglycerin paste (applied above the level of injury) is commonly used since it can be wiped off once the noxious stimulus is removed.

Important Considerations

- Individuals with SCI typically have lower blood pressure at baseline, therefore a blood pressure of 120/80 can be considered abnormal and a sign of AD if it is >20 mm Hg over the patient's baseline.

Chronic SCI

Many people with chronic SCI are well versed in their unique needs. They are taught in the rehabilitation stage to direct their own care, especially when it comes to their bowel and bladder needs. It is best to continue their home routine as closely as possible because it may have taken weeks to months of rehabilitation to establish a bowel and bladder routine that works for them. They often hold valuable information about their care, such as what triggers their autonomic dysreflexia or what kind of support they need to safely transfer out of bed. However, unfortunately, some people with chronic SCI may not have received rehabilitation and are not familiar with the concepts of bowel or bladder management. It is especially important to recommend these patients follow up with physical medicine and rehabilitation providers who are specially trained in SCI medicine.

People with chronic SCI are permanently at risk of pressure injury if their sensation is abnormal and their mobility is limited. The same PI prevention guidelines are relevant in the acute and chronic stages. Likewise, respiratory complications and pneumonia remain common years after SCI, so attention to respiratory care is always important postinjury.

Conclusion

After SCI, patients need to learn many new things about their bodies. Nurses who are familiar with SCI medicine can have a tremendously positive impact on these people who are going through a traumatic experience. Teaching the importance and tenets of skin, bowel, and bladder care can reduce the length of hospitalization and prevent life-threatening complications.

Advocating for assistive devices for communication with people with impaired upper limb function is also very important to reduce anxiety and ensure patient safety. Alternative call bells exist that patients can activate with their mouth, such as the Sip & Puff device. If they are ventilator dependent, patients should be asked simple yes or no questions they can answer by closing their eyes or squeezing your hand. Patients on a ventilator who can use their arms can communicate by writing or by using a communication board with simple pictures, letters, or phrases. Consulting speech-language pathology early may be helpful.

References

1. Aito S. Gruppo Italiano Studio Epidemiologico Mielolesioni (GISEM) Group. Complications during the acute phase of traumatic spinal cord lesions. *Spinal Cord.* 2003;41(11):629–635.
2. Rundquist J, Gassaway J, Bailey J, et al. Nursing bedside education and care management time during inpatient spinal cord injury rehabilitation. *J Spinal Cord Med.* 2011;34(2):205–215.
3. Marino R, Maynard FM, Priebe M, et al. Reference Manual for the International Standards for Neurological Classification of SCI. *American Spinal Injury Association.* 2003.
4. Dorsher PT, McIntosh PM. Neurogenic bladder. *Adv Urol.* 2012;2012:816274.
5. Consortium for Spinal Cord Medicine. Clinical practice guidelines: management of neurogenic bowel dysfunction in adults after spinal cord injury. *J Spinal Cord Med.* 2020;21:248–293.
6. Consortium for Spinal Cord Medicine. *Acute Management of Autonomic Dysreflexia: Individuals with Spinal Cord Injury Presenting to Health-Care Facilities.* 2nd ed. Paralyzed Veterans of America; 2001.
7. Edes TE, Walk BE, Austin JL. Diarrhea in tube-fed patients: feeding formula not necessarily the cause. *Am J Med.* 1990;88(2):91–93.
8. Blumenstein I, Shastri YM, Stein J. Gastroenteric tube feeding: techniques, problems and solutions. *World J Gastroenterol.* 2014;20(26):8505–8524.
9. Berlowitz DJ, Wadsworth B, Ross J. Respiratory problems and management in people with spinal cord injury. *Breathe (Sheff).* 2016;12(4):328–340.
10. Fenton JJ, Warner ML, Lammertse D, et al. A comparison of high vs standard tidal volumes in ventilator weaning for individuals with sub-acute spinal cord injuries: a site-specific randomized clinical trial. *Spinal Cord.* 2016;54(3):234–238.
11. Gutierrez CJ, Harrow J, Haines F. Using an evidence-based protocol to guide rehabilitation and weaning of ventilator-dependent cervical spinal cord injury patients. *J Rehabil Res Dev.* 2003;40(5):S99–S110.
12. Consortium for Spinal Cord Medicine. Respiratory management following spinal cord injury: a clinical practice guideline for health-care professionals. *J Spinal Cord Med.* 2005;28(3):259–293.

Questions

A 36-year-old male with no past medical history presents to the emergency department after being restrained as a driver in a motor vehicle accident. Upon arrival, he complains of low back pain and no sensation or movement in his lower extremities. The upper extremities have full strength and sensation. Workup reveals a T4 burst fracture with spinal cord compression. Neurosurgery performed decompression and fusion surgery. Postoperatively, the patient has 0/5 strength in his lower limbs.

1. On day 4, you meet him early in the morning. He is in good spirits. He has not regained any movement in his lower limbs, but he is excited because they removed the Foley catheter. He was started on an external catheter the day previously, and chart review shows he has been producing 4 L urine daily for the past few days. You ask him if he can control when he needs to urinate, and he says, "I have no sensation at all below my chest, so no." What would be a reasonable next step to ensure bladder safety with the external catheter?
   a. Immediately bladder scan the patient and catheterize if retaining >200 mL urine.
   b. Monitor urine output. Alert provider if daily output exceeds 5 L daily.
   c. Wait for patient to void, then check a postvoid residual.
   d. Replace external catheter with diaper.

2. You notice that he voids about 100 cc urine as you are walking into the room with the bladder scanner. Nonetheless, you bladder scan him. The scan volume shows 900 mL urine in his bladder. What is the primary type of urinary incontinence that this patient has?
   a. Overflow incontinence
   b. Urge incontinence
   c. Stress incontinence
   d. He does not have bladder incontinence, since he just voided.

3. You notify the treatment team about his bladder scan volume, and they ask you to reinsert a Foley catheter. When would be an appropriate time to trial removing the Foley again?
   a. Continuous IV fluids are ≤120 mL/hr *and* urine output is <4 L/day.
   b. Continuous IV fluids are stopped *and* urine output is <2500 mL/day.
   c. Continuous IV fluids and urine output do not dictate when to try to remove the Foley.
   d. When his blood pressure is at least 140/90 mm Hg and heart rate ≤130/min.

4. For the first 10 days he did not have any bowel movements. For the last 4 days, he has had four to six liquid stool smears daily. He has become distended and complains of abdominal fullness. What is the most likely cause of the liquid stool smears?
   a. *Clostridium difficile* infection
   b. Fecal impaction with liquid stool leaking around impacted stool
   c. Lactose intolerance
   d. Irritable bowel syndrome with mixed symptoms

5. You speak to the patient about the importance of a daily bowel routine after SCI. You would have preferred to start one immediately after injury, but he was resistant. Now he states, "My stomach really hurts. I'll try anything." You counsel him that the best bowel routine involves eating a good diet, drinking adequate fluids, sitting on a commode if possible, and
   a. drinking prune juice and laxatives daily.
   b. inserting a suppository followed by digital stimulation roughly 7 hours after taking senna.
   c. drinking a bottle of magnesium citrate whenever constipated for >2 days.
   d. inserting a fecal management system.

Answers

1. a

2. a

3. b

4. b

5. b

CHAPTER 12

Spinal Cord Stimulator Management for Nurses

Kevin Hines, MD ▪ Liam P. Hughes, MD ▪ Ellina Hattar, MD
▪ Carol Blyzniuk, BSN, RN ▪ Monét A. Gambrel, BSN, RN
▪ Teresita Devera, MSN, RN, APN-BC ▪ Diane Ferrara Hoffman, MSN, RN, CRNP, ACNP-BC, RNFA ▪ Ashwini Sharan, MD

Introduction

Spinal cord stimulation (SCS) is a rapidly evolving technology with growing indications for the treatment of pain and spinal cord injury (SCI). Indications include neuropathic pain, failed back surgery syndrome, phantom limb pain, and SCI, among others.[1-4] Neuromodulation for chronic pain was developed after Melzack and Wall described the "gate theory" of pain, which proposed a gate in the dorsal horn of the spinal cord allowed transmission of pain to the central nervous system.[5] Pain transmission is regulated by the interplay between different size nerve inputs.[6-8] Peripheral pain transmission is enabled when there is an excess of small fiber activity and suppressed with the activation of large fibers. The first spinal cord stimulator implant was based on this theory that the gate could be electively closed with targeted electrical activation of the large diameter fibers. Currently, spinal cord stimulators are placed within the epidural space and use electrical pulses to suppress neurons within the dorsal horn, effectively neuromodulating the central transmission of pain along the spinothalamic tract of the spinal cord.[9] With a growing number of applications for SCS, it is important for every member of a patient's care team to understand procedural indications, postoperative care, and possible complications. Important aspects include phase of implantation, route of implantation, and treatment modality, as they all influence postoperative care and aim to maximize success of SCS therapy.

Stimulator Implantation

PHASE OF IMPLANTATION

SCS often occurs in two phases: trial and permanent implantation. To determine the eligibility of a patient for permanent implantation, a patient must first have a successful trial of SCS. This is most often achieved by percutaneous lead placement under fluoroscopy.[6,10,11] Patients who undergo this procedure leave the operating room with two external leads exiting the entry site. These leads are anchored to the skin and secured with a sterile dressing for the duration of the trial. The leads are attached to an external battery pack for a trial period of stimulation lasting 7–10 days, during which coverage and efficacy of the stimulation is assessed. At the end of the trial, the dressing and anchor sutures are cut, and the device is removed in the office setting.

Permanent implantation occurs after a successful trial of stimulation is completed and the patient is determined to be an ideal candidate for long-term stimulation.[12,13] After successful lead placement under fluoroscopic guidance, the leads are tunneled to a battery site. This allows for the entire system to be contained under the skin as a completely internal system. The battery, otherwise known as an implantable pulse generator (IPG), may be implanted in a variety of sites. Sites include the flank, buttock, and abdomen, depending on patient preference and maximization of comfort. Patients will leave the operating room with sterile dressings covering the spinal implantation site, the IPG site, and possible additional tunneling sites (Fig. 12.1).[6,12,14]

■ After both trial and permanent implantations, x-rays are obtained to verify correct placement of electrodes and establish a radiographic baseline for future reference.

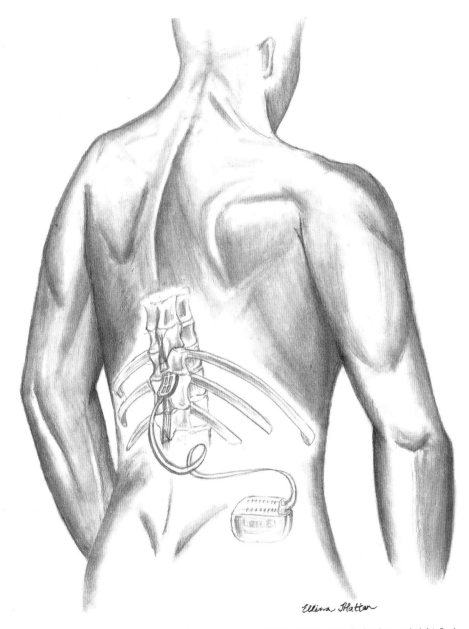

Fig. 12.1 Illustration demonstrating spinal cord stimulator paddle under thoracic lamina and right flank implantable pulse generator placement. (Courtesy Ellina Hattar, MD.)

In certain circumstances a buried trial is performed. During this trial, leads are tunneled beneath the skin to connectors, which are then connected to the external battery. If the trial is successful, the connector leads are removed, and the trial leads only need to be tunneled and connected to an IPG. If the trial is unsuccessful, additional surgery is required to remove the leads.

- Both tunneling of previously buried trial leads and removal of leads after failure are same-day procedures and do not regularly require overnight monitoring of the patient.

ROUTE OF IMPLANTATION

It is important to note that patients may have different routes of implantation of electrodes for SCS. These include:

- Percutaneous access for placement of electrodes
- Laminotomy for placement of a paddle electrode

While differing in technique, both methods allow for access to the epidural space.[15] Spinal cord stimulators may be placed anywhere along the spinal canal but are most often inserted into the thoracic and cervical spine for stimulation. After both percutaneous and laminotomy access procedures, x-rays are obtained to verify correct final placement of electrodes.

Percutaneous Access

In percutaneous access (frequently used for both trial and permanent implantations), fluoroscopy is used to determine an optimal needle entry point. After determining the entry point, the needle is advanced under x-ray guidance until its tip is near the interlaminar opening. At this point a loss of resistance syringe is used to advance the needle closer to the epidural space. This is important because loss of resistance of the syringe indicates entry into the epidural space, which is detected even by small changes in position, thereby minimizing the risk of puncturing the dura and causing a cerebrospinal fluid leak.

After accessing the epidural space, the leads are advanced to the desired level, determined by the modality of therapy and trial results. The leads are then either anchored or tunneled to the IPG site depending on the phase of implantation.[16]

Laminotomy for Paddle Placement

In laminotomy for paddle placement, fluoroscopy is used to localize the desired thoracic level for implantation of the stimulator. An incision is made to expose the spine and create a bony opening that is wide enough for the paddle to slide into the epidural space without resistance. If resistance is encountered, additional laminotomy sites can be created to expose the epidural space at multiple levels. Once adequate access has been achieved, the paddle is implanted and the leads are tunneled to the IPG site. Throughout the procedure, hemostasis is meticulously maintained to prevent hemorrhagic compression of the spinal cord.

- Like percutaneous placement, the patient will have a spinal implantation site, IPG site, and possible tunneling site incisions covered by sterile dressings at the end of the procedure.[17]

Modality of Treatment

Throughout the history of SCS treatment, several modalities have been developed. Initially, treatment was based solely on generating paresthesia in the region of pain. As such, it is normal for some patients undergoing active treatment to experience numbness and tingling in the area targeted by the spinal cord stimulator.[11] In isolation, these symptoms are not necessarily a cause for concern. More recently, nonparesthesia-based treatments have come to the forefront of SCS. Many recent studies have shown improved outcomes with nonparesthesia-based treatments compared to paresthesia-based therapies in the treatment of chronic pain.[18–21] These therapies include:

TABLE 12.1 ■ Summary of Recommendations Regarding Complications of Permanent SCS Implantation

Infection	• Prophylactic antibiotics postoperatively
	• Sterile dressings for 48 hours postoperatively
	• Superficial tissue infection: 7–10 days of gram-positive directed antibiotic therapy
	• Deep tissue infection: culture and susceptibility testing, empiric to targeted antibiotic therapy based on testing, removal of hardware
Hardware	• Postoperative x-ray to verify proper placement
	• Abdominal binder for IPG healing
	• Patient education to avoid lifting, bending, twisting
Perioperative Monitoring	• Blood draw for laboratory studies prior to surgery
	• Stopping antiplatelet and anticoagulation medications prior to and after surgery
	• Inpatient monitoring for laminotomy permanent SCS implantation
	• Blood pressure control postoperatively

IPG, Implantable pulse generator; *SCS*, spinal cord implantation.

- High-frequency stimulation (HF10)
- Burst stimulation
- Differential-target multiplexed stimulation

Understanding the phase, route, and modality of treatment in SCS equips nurses to anticipate the perioperative course in these challenging cases and quickly recognize any complications. Ultimately the management paradigm consists of pain control, infection prevention, hardware complication prevention, and neurologic monitoring. It is important to know if the patient is undergoing active stimulation and what modality of treatment the patient is receiving (paresthesia- or nonparesthesia-based stimulation). This will help ensure that all members of the care team understand what to expect perioperatively in the treatment of these patients. Important measures should be taken to improve outcomes and minimize the risk of complications (Table 12.1).

Perioperative Monitoring and Harm Reduction

INFECTION PREVENTION AND ANTIBIOTICS

Preventing infectious complications is a critical component of SCS management and an important strategy for avoiding additional disability and cost to the patient. Infection rates for SCS implant procedures have steadily declined due to improved quality control and perioperative antibiotic guidelines, with recent reports citing an incidence ranging from 2.4% to 3.1%.[22] SCS infections can be caused by inoculation from skin flora or biofilm development on the implanted device. *Staphylococcus aureus* is the most common organism isolated from cultures, and the most common location of infection is the IPG site.[6] Evaluation begins with determining whether the infection is superficial or involving deep tissues.

- According to recent literature, superficial infections can be treated for 7–10 days with gram-positive directed antibiotic therapy, and the hardware can stay in place.[23]
- If the infection is suspected to involve deeper tissues, the hardware should be removed, and empiric antibiotics should be administered until culture and susceptibility tests return.
  - Studies have reached no consensus on hardware reimplantation timing.[22]

Infection prevention protocols include using careful sterile technique during implantation in the operating room, maintaining sterile dressings for 48 hours after surgery while the dermis is closing, and providing antibiotic prophylaxis perioperatively (Fig. 12.2).

- In permanent implants, the patient may receive 24 hours of oral or intravenous antibiotics, depending on whether the patient remains hospitalized or is discharged immediately following the procedure. Furthermore, there is evidence that supports infection prevention with placement of occlusive dressings for the first 24–48 hours after implantation and patient education on incision care.[24]
  - Current literature strongly recommends not to use perioperative antibiotic prophylaxis for >24 hours.[24]
- In trials, patients are treated with prophylactic oral antibiotics for the 7–10-day duration of the trial due to the presence of a foreign body (the electrode) in continuity with the nonsterile external environment.

PREVENTION OF HARDWARE MIGRATION

Lead migration is a common complication of SCS implantation. Movement of one or both leads occurs in up to 22.6% of patients and causes a sudden recurrence of pain.[9,25–27] Lead malfunction occurs more frequently in the cervical spine due to the greater range of motion of the neck.[28,29] To limit the risk of migration, lead anchors can be utilized to fasten the leads in place during the trial period or permanent fixation.[30-33] To prevent migration, patients are instructed to avoid movements such as lifting, bending, and twisting until scar tissue fastens the leads into place.[6]

IPG migration and internal rotation can be prevented by placement of an abdominal binder. Wearing an abdominal binder for 2 weeks after implantation of the IPG stabilizes the device with external pressure until scar tissue formation secures the IPG in its position. This strategy prevents flipping of the device and complications such as twiddler syndrome, in which the device malfunctions due to malpositioning.[34,35]

- Due to the risk of lead migration during trial lead placement, x-rays should be obtained before permanent implantation to confirm correct positioning for maximal pain relief to the patient.[30]

POSTOPERATIVE HEMATOMA

Spinal epidural hematoma is a rare complication after SCS implantation via laminectomy, with an incidence of ~0.19%.[36] When it does occur, a spinal epidural hematoma is a medical emergency and requires immediate neurosurgical intervention to evacuate the hematoma and relieve compression of the spinal cord. It is imperative for nurses to recognize the signs of cord compression due to a postoperative hematoma, which typically include[37–40]:

- Acute onset of severe back and radicular pain
- Neurologic deficits, such as limb paralysis and new paresthesia
- Loss of bladder and bowel control

Signs of cord compression are sometimes challenging to recognize postoperatively, and patients with a history of chronic pain may experience an exacerbation of pain from implantation itself. Nurses caring for these patients should be suspicious of any acute pain that seems out of proportion to the scale of the procedure, especially when associated with a neurologic deficit, such as new-onset leg weakness. When an issue like this is identified, it is imperative that nursing contact the provider immediately to expedite their care. To mitigate the risk of postoperative hematomas:

- Preoperative labs are obtained to ensure there is no thrombocytopenia or coagulation defect
- Antiplatelet and anticoagulant agents are routinely held before and after the procedure

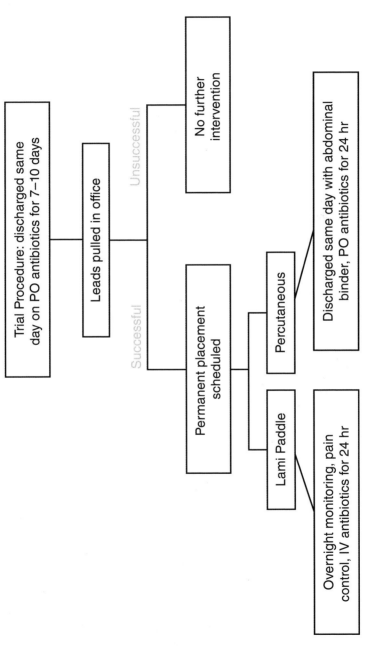

Fig. 12.2 Treatment algorithm for spinal cord stimulation trial, permanent placement, and postoperative course. *IV,* Intravenous; *PO,* by mouth.

- Blood pressure is carefully treated to avoid uncontrolled hypertension postoperatively
- Patients who undergo laminectomy are monitored overnight in the inpatient unit for signs of spinal cord compression

Conclusion

Neuropathic pain is a chronic and debilitating condition with both physiologic and psychosocial impact on the patient. Nursing care of patients receiving SCS requires an understanding of chronic pain, pain generator pathways, and underlying psychosocial factors related to pain. Developing a strong rapport of trust with patients will maximize the chances of success and optimize long-term outcomes of SCS therapy.

A thorough interview and nursing assessment are needed to identify ideal candidates for SCS therapy. The history obtained from patients should include all previously attempted surgeries and medications, noting the extent to which each intervention did or did not alleviate pain. Physical assessment should focus on identifying and documenting the areas of pain and those where pain relief is most desired. Nurses should assess the patient's understanding of the process and ability to adhere to the plan of care to ensure that SCS therapy is a viable treatment option.

Many patients undergoing SCS implantation will experience intense pain at the access sites due to the pathology of their chronic pain, despite the minimally invasive nature of the procedure. Further, nurses should remind patients that the permanent device often is not turned on until 2 weeks postoperatively. This practice simplifies device programming and avoids additional discomfort in the acute postoperative period from holding a charger over the fresh incision to maintain the battery.

Programming device settings for permanent implants may be a challenging and frustrating process for patients, especially until they have recovered from their acute postoperative pain. Extensive patient education is needed to establish reasonable expectations regarding SCS therapy. It is important to convey that the purpose of therapy is to achieve pain reduction and improve overall function rather than cure the pain altogether. Integrating patient beliefs regarding treatment and what they may experience in the future is a critical component of treatment optimization.[41,42] Clear goals, reasonable expectations, comprehensive education, and compassionate care are essential for successfully managing these complex cases.

Patients who undergo SCS procedures should be well established in the health care system prior to considering this therapy. Typically a multidisciplinary team comprised of a chronic pain management physician, primary care physician, and physical therapist should be established prior to surgical consultation. It is important for nurses to help facilitate communication and collaboration with the patient's entire health care team to ensure that their pain is managed effectively during the pre-, peri-, and postoperative periods. Nurses should educate patients in the use of pain medications during each phase of care, ensuring that analgesics are used effectively and responsibly. Despite the many challenges, it is very rewarding to support patients as they learn to manage their pain, regain function, reintegrate into society, and improve the quality of their lives.

References

1. Cameron T. Safety and efficacy of spinal cord stimulation for the treatment of chronic pain: a 20-year literature review. *J Neurosurg Spine*. 2004;100(3):254–267.
2. Harkema SJ, Wang S, Angeli CA, et al. Normalization of blood pressure with spinal cord epidural stimulation after severe spinal cord injury. *Front Hum Neurosci*. 2018;12.
3. Turner JA, Loeser JD, Deyo RA, et al. Spinal cord stimulation for patients with failed back surgery syndrome or complex regional pain syndrome: a systematic review of effectiveness and complications. *Pain*. 2004;108(1):137–147.

4. Kumar K, Taylor RS, Jacques L, et al. Spinal cord stimulation versus conventional medical management for neuropathic pain: a multicentre randomised controlled trial in patients with failed back surgery syndrome. *Pain.* 2007;132(1):179–188.
5. Melzack R, Wall PD. Pain mechanisms: a new theory. *Science.* 1965;150(3699):971–979.
6. Garcia K, Wray JK, Kumar S. *Spinal cord stimulation.* StatPearls Publishing; 2021.
7. Oakley JC, Prager JP. Spinal cord stimulation: mechanisms of action. *Spine.* 2002;27(22):2574–2583.
8. Shealy C, Mortimer J, Reswick J. electrical inhibition of pain by stimulation of the dorsal columns: preliminary clinical report. *Anesth Analg.* 1967;46(4):489–491.
9. Dydyk AM, Tadi P. *Spinal cord stimulator implant.* StatPearls Publishing; 2021.
10. Raff M, Melvill R, Coetzee G, et al. Spinal cord stimulation for the management of pain: recommendations for best clinical practice. *S Afr Med J.* 2013;103(6):423.
11. Jeon YH. Spinal cord stimulation in pain management: a review. *Korean J Pain.* 2012;25(3):143–150.
12. Malige A, Sokunbi G. Spinal cord stimulators: a comparison of the trial period: versus: permanent outcomes. *Spine.* 2019;44(11):e687.
13. Burchiel KJ, Anderson VC, Wilson BJ, et al. Prognostic factors of spinal cord stimulation for chronic back and leg pain. *Neurosurgery.* 1995;36(6):1118–1134.
14. Simopoulos T, Sharma S, Aner M, et al. A temporary vs. permanent anchored percutaneous lead trial of spinal cord stimulation: a comparison of patient outcomes and adverse events. *Neuromodulation.* 2018;21(5):508–512.
15. Zhu J, Gutman G, Collins JG, et al. A review of surgical techniques in spinal cord stimulator implantation to decrease the post-operative infection rate. *J Spine.* 2015;4(1).
16. Kinfe TM, Schu S, Quack FJ, et al. percutaneous implanted paddle lead for spinal cord stimulation: technical considerations and long-term follow-up. *Neuromodulation.* 2012;15(4):402–407.
17. Pahapill PA. Surgical paddle-lead placement for screening trials of spinal cord stimulation. *Neuromodulation.* 2014;17(4):346–348.
18. Kapural L, Yu C, Doust MW, et al. Novel 10-khz high-frequency therapy (hf10 therapy) is superior to traditional low-frequency spinal cord stimulation for the treatment of chronic back and leg pain: the senza-rct randomized controlled trial. *Anesthesiology.* 2015;123(4):851–860.
19. Chakravarthy K, Fishman MA, Zuidema X, et al. Mechanism of action in burst spinal cord stimulation: review and recent advances. *Pain Med.* 2019;20(1):S13–S22.
20. Vallejo R, Kelley CA, Gupta A, et al. Modulation of neuroglial interactions using differential target multiplexed spinal cord stimulation in an animal model of neuropathic pain. *Mol Pain.* 2020;16: 1744806920918057.
21. Deer T, Slavin KV, Amirdelfan K, et al. Success using neuromodulation with BURST (SUNBURST) study: results from a prospective, randomized controlled trial using a novel burst waveform. *Neuromodulation.* 2018;21(1):56–66.
22. Garrigos ZE, Farid S, Bendel MA, et al. Spinal cord stimulator infection: approach to diagnosis, management, and prevention. *Clin Infect Dis.* 2020;70(12):2727–2735.
23. Meglio M, Cioni B, Rossi GF. Spinal cord stimulation in management of chronic pain: a 9-year experience. *J Neurosurg.* 1989;70(4):519–524.
24. Deer TR, Provenzano DA, Hanes M, et al. The neurostimulation appropriateness consensus committee (NACC) recommendations for infection prevention and management. *Neuromodulation.* 2017;20(1):31–50.
25. Kim DD. Rates of lead migration and stimulation loss in spinal cord stimulation: a retrospective comparison of laminotomy versus percutaneous implantation. *Pain Physician.* 2011;14(6):513–524.
26. Rosenow JM, Stanton-Hicks M, Rezai AR, et al. Failure modes of spinal cord stimulation hardware. *J Neurosurg Spine.* 2006;5(3):183–190.
27. Mekhail NA, Mathews M, Nageeb F, et al. Retrospective review of 707 cases of spinal cord stimulation: indications and complications. *Pain Pract.* 2011;11(2):148–153.
28. Vallejo R, Kramer J, Benyamin R. Neuromodulation of the cervical spinal cord in the treatment of chronic intractable neck and upper extremity pain: a case series and review of the literature. *Pain Physician.* 2007(2):305–311.
29. Wolter T, Kieselbach K. Cervical spinal cord stimulation: an analysis of 23 patients with long-term follow-up. *Pain Physician.* 2012;15(3;5):203–212.
30. Osborne MD, Ghazi SM, Palmer SC, et al. Spinal cord stimulator—trial lead migration study. *Pain Med.* 2011;12(2):204–208.

31. Kumar K, Hunter G, Demeria D. Spinal cord stimulation in treatment of chronic benign pain: challenges in treatment planning and present status, a 22-year experience. *Neurosurgery.* 2006;58(3):481–496.
32. Justiz R, Bentley I. A case series review of spinal cord stimulation migration rates with a novel fixation device. *Neuromodulation.* 2014;17(1):37–40.
33. Henderson JM, Schade CM, Sasaki J, et al. Prevention of mechanical failures in implanted spinal cord stimulation systems. *Neuromodulation.* 2006;9(3):183–191.
34. Moens M, Petit F, Goudman L, et al. Twiddler's syndrome and neuromodulation-devices: a troubled marriage. *Neuromodulation.* 2017;20(3):279–283.
35. Son BC, Choi JG, Ha SW. Twiddler's syndrome: a rare hardware complication in spinal cord stimulation. *Asian J Neurosurg.* 2018;13(2):403–406.
36. Levy R, Henderson J, Slavin K, et al. Incidence and avoidance of neurologic complications with paddle type spinal cord stimulation leads. *Neuromodulation.* 2011;14(5):412–422.
37. Kloss BT, Sullivan AM, Rodriguez E. Epidural hematoma following spinal cord stimulator implant. *Int J Emerg Med.* 2010;3(4):483–484.
38. Buvanendran A, Young AC. Spinal epidural hematoma after spinal cord stimulator trial lead placement in a patient taking aspirin. *Reg Anesth Pain Med.* 2014;39(1):70–72.
39. Takawira N, Han RJ, Nguyen TQ, et al. Spinal cord stimulator and epidural haematoma. *Br J Anaesth.* 2012;109(4):649–650.
40. Glotzbecker MP, Bono CM, Wood KB, et al. Postoperative spinal epidural hematoma: a systematic review*Database of Abstracts of Reviews of Effects (DARE): Quality-assessed Reviews [Internet]*: Centre for Reviews and Dissemination; 2010.
41. Bingel U, Wanigasekera V, Wiech K, et al. The effect of treatment expectation on drug efficacy: imaging the analgesic benefit of the opioid remifentanil. *Sci Transl Med.* 2011;3(70):70ra14.
42. Gjesdal K, Furnes B, Dysvik E. Experiences with spinal cord stimulator in patients with chronic neuropathic back pain. *Pain Manag Nurs.* 2014;15(3):e13–e24.

Questions

1. A 55-year-old female patient has just undergone a trial SCS implantation and wants clarification regarding her antibiotic regimen for the trial, specifically how many days she needs to use her prescribed antibiotics. You advise her that antibiotics are required for:
   a. 48 hours
   b. 24 hours
   c. The duration of the trial (7–10 days)
   d. None are required

2. A 47-year-old male patient is admitted following laminotomy for permanent SCS implantation. He is stable with adequate pain management until 3 am when he develops acute-onset severe low back pain, weakness of his left lower extremity, and bladder incontinence. What are the nurse's next steps?
   a. Notify the provider immediately for neurosurgical intervention
   b. Subcutaneous heparin administration
   c. Nothing, this is expected postoperatively after SCS implantation
   d. Increased pain medication dosage

3. Current treatment modalities for SCS include:
   a. High-frequency stimulation
   b. Cross-linked voltage stimulation
   c. Differential-target multiplexed stimulation
   d. a and c
   e. a, b, and c

4. A 73-year-old male patient is preparing to leave the hospital following percutaneous lead placement for permanent SCS implantation. He states that the abdominal binder is uncomfortable and asks why he must wear it. You reply that the binder:
   a. Helps prevents infection
   b. Holds pressure until the IPG pocket scars to keep it in the proper position
   c. Does not really do anything and is unnecessary to wear
   d. Is the primary intervention to stop hematoma formation

5. Recommendations to prevent infection after permanent SCS implantation include:
   a. Intravenous antibiotics for 72 hours
   b. Sterile wound dressing on the implant site for 24–48 hours
   c. No postoperative antibiotics
   d. Removal of sterile wound dressing after 12 hours

Answers

1. c

2. a

3. d

4. b

5. b

CHAPTER 13

Nursing Management of Neoplastic Spinal Cord Compression

Yichao Ethan Zhao, MD, MSc

Introduction

Neoplastic epidural spinal cord compression is a complication of cancer that can cause pain and potentially irreversible loss of neurologic function. Most cases of spinal cord compression occur when cancer metastasizes to the epidural space, often as an epidural extension of vertebral body metastases, and causes secondary compression of the spinal cord. Neurosurgical nurses must be trained to understand the pathogenesis and clinical features of neoplastic epidural spinal cord compression. Early recognition is key to initiating prompt workup and treatment through a multidisciplinary approach alongside physicians and other specialists, and potentially preventing permanent loss of neurologic function. It is important to remember that spinal cord compression may also result from nonneoplastic causes, such as spinal hematoma, abscess, herniated disc, and vertebral fracture. However, moving forward in this chapter, spinal cord compression will refer to any radiologic evidence of thecal sac indentation related to tumor mass effect.

Spinal Cord Anatomy and Pathogenesis

The spinal cord is enclosed within the spinal column. The spinal column is composed of the vertebral body anteriorly, pedicles laterally, and the lamina and spinous process posteriorly. Inside this space lies the thecal sac with the outermost layer comprised of dura mater. Between the bone and dura lies the epidural space, which contains fat and the venous plexus. Spinal cord compression occurs when a tumor extends from the bone and invades the epidural space, causing compression of the thecal sac and obstruction of the venous plexus. This results in vasogenic edema in the white and gray matter of the spinal cord (Fig. 13.1).[1] Metastatic tumors from any primary site can cause spinal cord compression, but lung cancer, breast cancer, prostate cancer, and multiple myeloma are most likely to metastasize to bone.[2]

Clinical Presentation

Patients with spinal cord compression will often complain of pain and tenderness to palpation over the affected area, followed by a progressive loss of neurologic function. The pain typically precedes neurologic symptoms by approximately 6–7 weeks and is often worse at night.[3] Referred pain is common, so it is important to understand that the location of pain is not always the actual location of tumor or injury. Pain that is present only with movement may be indicative of mechanical instability. Common neurologic symptoms include sensory deficits, focal weakness, urinary retention, and bowel and bladder incontinence. Patients may also experience cauda equina syndrome, which is characterized by:

- Back pain
- Unilateral or bilateral sciatica
- Decreased perianal region sensation or saddle anesthesia

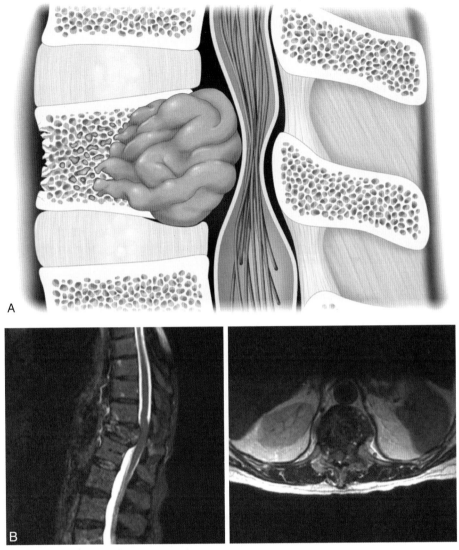

Fig. 13.1 Schematic diagram (A) and midsagittal computed tomography (B) demonstrating spinal cord compression due to metastatic cancer to the vertebral body. (A, From Greenhalgh S, Selfe J. *Red Flags and Blue Lights: Managing Serious Spinal Pathology*, 2nd ed. Elsevier; 2019; B, from Garfin SR, Eismont FJ, Bell GR, et al. *Rothman-Simeone and Herkowitz's The Spine*, 7th ed. Elsevier; 2017.)

- Bowel and bladder dysfunction
- Lower extremity weakness
- Impaired sexual function

Early detection is critical because the patient's neurologic condition prior to definitive treatment (including the overall duration of ambulatory dysfunction) is the most important prognostic indicator for recovery of neurologic function after treatment of spinal cord compression.[4]

Diagnostic Evaluation

A comprehensive neurologic exam is the first step in the evaluation of spinal cord compression. Unless limited by profound weakness or severe pain with movement, examination should include a gait assessment. Imaging studies include magnetic resonance imaging (MRI) and computed tomography (CT) myelogram.

- MRI with and without contrast is the gold standard for diagnosing spinal cord compression.[5]
  - It should be completed and reviewed by a radiologist immediately to facilitate emergent treatment and minimize the risk of permanent neurologic injury.
  - MRI of the entire spine is recommended because one-third of patients have more than one neoplastic lesion, and multiple sites in the spine may be at risk.
- CT myelogram is an alternative imaging procedure to evaluate the spinal cord, nerve roots, and spinal lining.
  - Contrast material is injected into the spinal canal by a spinal needle, then viewed in real time using x-rays and CT imaging.
  - CT myelogram is the recommended imaging modality in cases where MRI is contraindicated—such as for patients with incompatible metallic implants—or when MRI is not feasible due to the patient's body habitus.

Management

Neoplastic spinal cord compression is an oncologic emergency that requires timely diagnosis and prompt surgical evaluation to prevent permanent complications. The treatment approach should focus on pain control, harm reduction, preservation and recovery of neurologic function, and stabilization of mechanical instability. Individualized treatment plans should be formulated through a multidisciplinary approach involving the surgical team, medical oncology, radiation oncology, and the patient's own goals of care. The choice of treatment depends on three important pathologic features:

1. Extent of spinal cord compression
2. Presence or absence of mechanical spinal instability
3. Relative radiosensitivity of the primary tumor

SURGERY AND RADIATION TREATMENT

Surgical stabilization of the spine is indicated for spinal instability regardless of the aggressiveness and radiosensitivity of the primary tumor.[6,7] Patients with high clinical suspicion of mechanical spinal instability should be kept on bed rest, immobilized using spinal bracing, and immediately evaluated by a surgical team. Nurses should clarify with the surgery team whether the patient's injury requires logroll mobility in bed or if the patient should only be moved by the providers in the surgical team. Surgery for rapid decompression of the spinal cord should also be considered in patients with neurologic deficits.

Stabilization of the spine can be achieved by surgical decompression and instrumentation in patients with extensive disease and radioresistant tumors or by minimally invasive interventions, such as vertebroplasty or kyphoplasty in patients who are also suitable candidates for radiation therapy.[8–10] Additional factors that determine surgical candidacy include the patient's comorbidities, functional status, life expectancy, and overall extent of metastatic disease.[11] The combination of surgical decompression and stabilization, followed by radiation therapy to eradicate residual disease, is often done for patients with radioresistant tumors and those with extensive spinal cord compression. This will allow for maximal pain relief, neurologic recovery, and local tumor control.[12,13] Whereas radiosensitive tumors respond well to radiation treatment, tumor response and clinical improvement take time.

- Conventional external beam radiation therapy (cEBRT) can be used to treat patients with radiosensitive tumors who do not meet the criteria for surgery, regardless of the extent of cord compression, and for palliation of pain in patients with very short life expectancy (e.g., ≤3 months).[14]
- With the advent of stereotactic body radiation therapy (SBRT), radioresistant tumors can now be treated with radiation therapy. SBRT allows for high doses of radiation to be delivered to a localized field, thus minimizing toxic doses to the spinal cord and adjacent structures, which previously had been a barrier to treatment with cEBRT.[15]
- Systemic chemotherapy plays a role after definitive treatment for neoplastic spinal cord compression and is occasionally used in place of radiation for select patients with highly chemosensitive tumors.[16–18]

SYSTEMIC STEROIDS

Steroids are often part of the initial treatment regimen and may serve as a bridge to definitive treatment or for palliation of pain.[19] For patients who are poor surgical candidates, steroids and radiation are the mainstay of palliative therapy. Glucocorticoids can temporarily improve neurologic function in patients with spinal cord compression presumably by reducing vasogenic edema and stimulating oncolytic processes in steroid-responsive malignancies (e.g., lymphoma and multiple myeloma).[20,21] For patients with neurologic deficits or pain associated with spinal cord compression, dexamethasone 10 mg intravenously followed by 16 mg orally per day in divided doses is typically recommended.[16]

- Patients receiving steroid therapy should be prescribed stress ulcer prophylaxis to prevent gastrointestinal bleeding.
  - Often this includes either a proton pump inhibitor (e.g., pantoprazole) or H2 blocker (e.g., famotidine).[17]
- Blood glucose levels should be monitored and insulin administered as needed to treat steroid-induced hyperglycemia. Patients with preexisting diabetes are especially at risk for uncontrolled hyperglycemia.
- Sleep disturbance, psychosis, and delirium are common steroid-related adverse effects.[18]

BOWEL AND BLADDER DYSFUNCTION

Patients with spinal cord compression and limited mobility are at risk for developing urinary retention and constipation.[22] Patients should be monitored for urinary retention with postvoid bladder scanning, and Foley catheterization is indicated if urinary retention is present. An aggressive prophylactic bowel regimen is indicated due to the risk of constipation and ileus, which are common complications of autonomic dysfunction, impaired mobility, and opioid analgesics. Conservative use of opioid analgesics is advised to minimize this risk.

VENOUS THROMBOEMBOLISM PROPHYLAXIS

Patients with active malignancy, weakness, deconditioning, and impaired mobility presenting with spinal cord compression are at increased risk for venous thromboembolism (VTE).[23] Although protocols vary across institutions, screening for VTE with lower extremity venous Doppler ultrasound should be considered in this high-risk patient population. Short-term pharmacologic VTE prophylaxis with subcutaneous unfractionated or low-molecular-weight heparin should be prescribed if there is no active bleeding or other contraindications. In addition, patients should be treated with mechanical prophylaxis such as pneumatic venous compression devices or graduated compression stockings. Patients found to have VTE perioperatively may require placement of an inferior vena cava filter to reduce the risk of pulmonary embolism if anticoagulation is contraindicated.[24]

Nursing Interventions

A diagnosis of neoplastic spinal cord compression can generate significant stress and anxiety for patients and their families. Every effort should be made to provide empathetic and supportive care, including collaborative multidisciplinary resources such as social work, spiritual and pastoral care, and psychiatry consultation as needed. Nurses should perform frequent neurologic assessments for close monitoring of the patient's neurologic status and immediately report changes to the provider. Patients with spinal instability should be maintained on flat bedrest, utilizing a logrolling technique to assist with changing position until cleared by the surgical team. Before moving the patient in or out of bed, nurses should clarify mobility/bracing orders with the surgery team, and the patient's mobility should be optimized in collaboration with the physical therapy team. Daily skin inspections should be performed with attention to areas prone to development of pressure ulcers. In patients who cannot move/reposition themselves, specialty mattresses may be utilized to help prevent pressure injuries. An assessment of the patient's nutritional status should also be performed to ensure adequate intake of calories and protein to promote healing. VTE prophylaxis should include mechanical interventions, such as the use of compression stockings and intermittent pneumatic compression devices, and pharmacologic interventions, such as the use of unfractionated or low molecular weight heparin given subcutaneously. Close blood glucose monitoring, dietary control, and delirium precautions should be maintained for patients receiving high-dose steroids.

Conclusion

Patients diagnosed with spinal cord compression are at high risk for clinical deterioration. Neoplastic epidural spinal cord compression can cause irreversible loss of neurologic function if not treated promptly. These patients are also at risk for complications, including prolonged immobility, deconditioning, pressure ulcers, steroid-induced hyperglycemia and behavioral disturbances, and VTE. Diligent nursing management, including frequent neurologic exams, is crucial to the monitoring and prevention of complications.

References

1. Arguello F, Baggs RB, Duerst RE, et al. Pathogenesis of vertebral metastasis and epidural spinal cord compression. *Cancer*. 1990;65(1):98–106.
2. Mak KS, Lee LK, Mak RH, et al. Incidence and treatment patterns in hospitalizations for malignant spinal cord compression in the United States, 1998–2006. *Int J Radiat Oncol Biol Phys*. 2011;80(3):824–831.
3. Kim RY, Spencer SA, Meredith RF, et al. Extradural spinal cord compression: analysis of factors determining functional prognosis–prospective study. *Radiology*. 1990;176(1):279–282.
4. Laufer I, Zuckerman S, Bird JE, et al. Predicting neurologic recovery after surgery in patients with deficits secondary to MESCC: systematic review. *Spine*. 2016;41(20):S224–S230.
5. Li KC, Poon PY. Sensitivity and specificity of MRI in detecting malignant spinal cord compression and in distinguishing malignant from benign compression fractures of vertebrae. *Magn Reson Imaging*. 1988;6(5):547–556.
6. Hussain I, Barzilai O, Reiner AS, et al. Patient-reported outcomes after surgical stabilization of spinal tumors: symptom-based validation of the Spinal Instability Neoplastic Score (SINS) and surgery. *Spine J*. 2018;18(2):261–267.
7. Huisman M, van der Velden JM, van Vulpen M, et al. Spinal instability as defined by the spinal instability neoplastic score is associated with radiotherapy failure in metastatic spinal disease. *Spine J*. 2014;14(12):2835–2840.

8. Mendel E, Bourekas E, Gerszten P, et al. Percutaneous techniques in the treatment of spine tumors: what are the diagnostic and therapeutic indications and outcomes? *Spine*. 2009;34(22):S93–S100.

9. Moussazadeh N, Rubin DG, McLaughlin L, et al. Short-segment percutaneous pedicle screw fixation with cement augmentation for tumor-induced spinal instability. *Spine J*. 2015;15(7):1609–1617.

10. Berenson J, Pflugmacher R, Jarzem P, et al. Balloon kyphoplasty versus non-surgical fracture management for treatment of painful vertebral body compression fractures in patients with cancer: a multicentre, randomised controlled trial. *Lancet Oncol*. 2011;12(3):225–235.

11. Lawton AJ, Lee KA, Cheville AL, et al. Assessment and management of patients with metastatic spinal cord compression: a multidisciplinary review. *J Clin Oncol*. 2019;37(1):61–71.

12. Patchell RA, Tibbs PA, Regine WF, et al. Direct decompressive surgical resection in the treatment of spinal cord compression caused by metastatic cancer: a randomised trial. *Lancet*. 2005;366(9486):643–648.

13. Laufer I, Iorgulescu JB, Chapman T, et al. Local disease control for spinal metastases following "separation surgery" and adjuvant hypofractionated or high-dose single-fraction stereotactic radiosurgery: outcome analysis in 186 patients. *J Neurosurg Spine*. 2013;18(3):207–214.

14. Maranzano E, Latini P. Effectiveness of radiation therapy without surgery in metastatic spinal cord compression: final results from a prospective trial. *Int J Radiat Oncol Biol Phys*. 1995;32(4):959–967.

15. Yamada Y, Bilsky MH, Lovelock DM, et al. High-dose, single-fraction image-guided intensity-modulated radiotherapy for metastatic spinal lesions. *Int J Radiat Oncol Biol Phys*. 2008;71(2):484–490.

16. Vecht CJ, Haaxma-Reiche H, van Putten WL, et al. Initial bolus of conventional versus high-dose dexamethasone in metastatic spinal cord compression. *Neurology*. 1989;39(9):1255–1257.

17. Khan MF, Burks SS, Al-Khayat H, et al. The effect of steroids on the incidence of gastrointestinal hemorrhage after spinal cord injury: a case-controlled study. *Spinal Cord*. 2014;52(1):58–60.

18. Sirois F. Steroid psychosis: a review. *Gen Hosp Psychiatry*. 2003;25(1):27–33.

19. Loblaw DA, Mitera G, Ford M, et al. A 2011 updated systematic review and clinical practice guideline for the management of malignant extradural spinal cord compression. *Int J Radiat Oncol Bio Phys*. 2012;84(2):312–317.

20. Ushio Y, Posner R, Kim JH, et al. Treatment of experimental spinal cord compression caused by extradural neoplasms. *J Neurosurg*. 1977;47(3):380–390.

21. Delattre JY, Arbit E, Rosenblum MK, et al. High dose versus low dose dexamethasone in experimental epidural spinal cord compression. *Neurosurgery*. 1988;22(6 Pt 1):1005–1007.

22. Samson G, Cardenas DD. Neurogenic bladder in spinal cord injury. *Phys Med Rehabil Clin N Am*. 2007;18(2):255–274.

23. Zacharia BE, Kahn S, Bander ED, et al. Incidence and risk factors for preoperative deep venous thrombosis in 314 consecutive patients undergoing surgery for spinal metastasis. *J Neurosurg Spine*. 27(2):189-197.

24. Miyahara T, Miyata T, Shigematsu K, et al. Clinical outcome and complications of temporary inferior vena cava filter placement. *J Vasc Surg*. 2006;44(3):620–624.

Questions

1. What is a favorable prognostic indicator for neurologic recovery following spinal cord compression?
   a. Cancer stage
   b. Ambulatory status at time of presentation
   c. Age
   d. Prior cancer treatment

2. A patient presenting with concern for spinal cord compression is planned for MRI but is found to have an incompatible implantable cardioverter defibrillator (ICD). What is the next appropriate step?
   a. Obtain CT imaging
   b. CT myelogram
   c. ICD reprogramming
   d. Spine x-rays

3. High-dose steroids are started while a patient is awaiting emergent surgical decompression for spinal cord compression. Which of the following should be closely monitored?
   a. Blood glucose
   b. Mood changes
   c. Blood pressure
   d. All of the above

4. A patient is being evaluated for spinal cord compression and is requiring two-person assistance for transfers. The nursing evaluation should include which of the following assessments?
   a. Inspect skin integrity
   b. Frailty assessment
   c. Nutritional status
   d. Pain score
   e. All of the above

5. A patient presenting with spinal cord compression is found to have a T11–L1 osteolytic lesion with vertebral body collapse. The patient is reporting significant back pain with movement of the torso that is relieved when recumbent. What is the most important next step?
   a. Maintain flat bedrest
   b. Assess pain severity
   c. Encourage ambulation
   d. Evaluate need for orthotic brace

Answers

1. b

2. b

3. d

4. e

5. a

CHAPTER 14

Nursing Management of Vertebral Osteomyelitis and Spinal Epidural Abscess

Matthew Brown, MD

Introduction

Vertebral osteomyelitis (VO) is a condition in which a pyogenic (pus-forming) bacterial or fungal infection occurs in one or more bones of the spine. This type of infection typically occurs when a patient develops bacteremia—presence of bacteria in the bloodstream. Bacteria can then travel through the bloodstream and seed one or more vertebral bodies. There are many etiologies of bacteremia, such as intravenous (IV) drug use (contaminated needles can introduce bacteria into the bloodstream) and infections from various alternative sources (e.g., pneumonia, urinary tract infections, foot ulcers). From the vertebrae, infection can spread to the adjacent intervertebral disc, which itself has no direct blood supply. Coinfection of vertebrae and disc is common and referred to as discitis-osteomyelitis, osteodiscitis, or spondylodiscitis.

Direct bacterial or fungal toxicity, combined with the ensuing inflammatory response, lead to tissue damage in the bone and intervertebral disc. This can cause destruction of the disc, loss of vertebral column height, neural foraminal narrowing, and nerve root impingement. If medical management with antibiotics is insufficient or the spine becomes structurally unstable, surgical spine intervention and fixation may be required.[1]

VO may remain a self-contained infection, but often it occurs concurrently with epidural infection. The spinal epidural space contains fat and blood vessels. It is located posterior to the vertebral body and is traversed by nerve roots exiting the spinal cord (Fig. 14.1). Like the vertebral body, the epidural space can be infiltrated by pathogens from the bloodstream. Alternatively, direct inoculation may occur during needle penetration (e.g., epidural anesthesia or glucocorticoid injection) or surgical instrumentation. Due to the lack of an anatomic barrier, such as a compact layer of cortical bone or articular cartilage, there is little to prevent infection in the vertebral body or disc from spreading posteriorly into the spinal epidural space. These infections often begin as a phlegmon (soft tissue infection) and develop over time into an abscess (pus-filled cavity) (Fig. 14.2). A spinal epidural abscess (SEA) carries significant potential for devastating morbidity but is treatable with appropriate medical and surgical intervention.[2]

Initial Management

In most cases, patients with VO present with fever and back pain. SEA should be suspected when there are also neurologic manifestations, such as lower extremity weakness, paresthesias (pins and needles), and urinary or fecal incontinence secondary to spinal cord injury (through direct toxicity and disruption of local blood vessels). Neurologic impairment may localize at or below the affected spinal cord level due to injury of the corticospinal and spinothalamic long tracts. Without prompt treatment, there can be permanent neurologic injury, including paralysis.

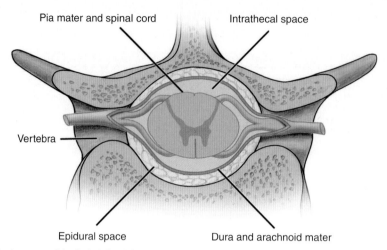

Fig. 14.1   Anatomy of the Spinal Cord. (From Corrin M. In: Baumann MD, Stanwick JC, Donaghue IC, et al., eds., *Biomaterials for Spinal Cord Repair*. Elsevier; 2011.)

When VO or SEA are suspected, blood cultures should be obtained to check for active bacteremia. If positive, these blood cultures help identify the causative bacteria and guide antibiotic management. Antibiotics are typically held prior to obtaining cultures to increase the likelihood of capturing a viable organism that will grow on the culture medium.[3] In the case of hemodynamic instability (such as severe sepsis) or neurologic deficits that are severe or rapidly progressive, antibiotic administration should not be delayed. Always prioritize stabilization of the patient.

Prompt consultation with other specialists should be obtained to guide imaging studies and procedures, to assist in identifying foci of infection elsewhere in the body. If present, these areas of infection could be sources of ongoing bacteremia and may require localized treatment to ensure resolution. For example, many patients with VO have concurrent infective endocarditis, which develops when the infective organism attaches to a heart valve and becomes a potential source of persistent bacteremia[4] (Box 14.1).

Imaging studies are necessary to confirm the diagnosis of VO and SEA. Computed tomography is excellent for detecting abnormalities in bone, but it is inadequate for diagnosing soft tissue abnormalities, such as those seen with an epidural abscess. In these cases, magnetic resonance imaging (MRI) with gadolinium contrast is the study of choice. It is important to remember that patients may need analgesic medications to tolerate lying flat for a prolonged period in the MRI machine, especially if they have severe back pain or spasm of the paraspinal muscles.

Radiographic evidence of VO or SEA plus positive blood cultures are occasionally sufficient data to verify the diagnosis. However, if blood cultures are negative or growing organisms considered to be contaminants (i.e., accidentally sampled from the skin), additional confirmatory tissue sampling may be necessary. Tissue sampling can be accomplished by image-guided needle aspiration biopsy (Table 14.1). In comparison to blood cultures, the culture yield of tissue from a needle aspiration or core biopsy is better preserved despite exposure to antibiotics.[5]

In cases when surgical intervention is needed, deep tissue samples should be obtained intraoperatively (surgical cultures). Indications for surgery include progressive neurologic deficits, epidural or paravertebral abscesses that require drainage, cord compression from vertebral

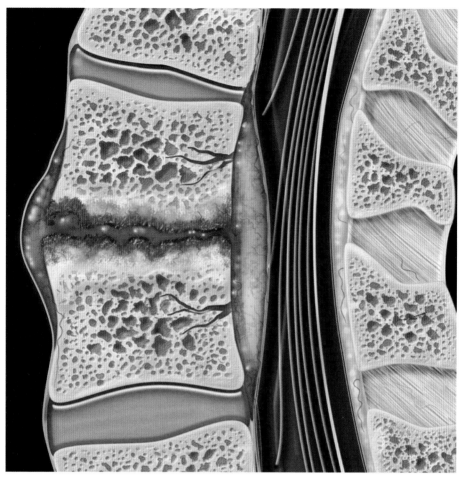

Fig. 14.2 Epidural abscess. (From Ross JS, Bendock BR, McClendon J. *Imaging in Spine Surgery.* Elsevier; 2017.)

BOX 14.1 ■ Recommended Diagnostics

- Bacterial (aerobic and anaerobic) blood cultures (two sets)
- Baseline erythrocyte sedimentation rate and C-reactive protein (both markers of inflammation in the body)
- Spine magnetic resonance imaging
- If epidemiologic or host risk factors are present: Brucella serologies for potential brucellosis, fungal blood cultures, purified protein derivative, or interferon-gamma release assay for extrapulmonary tuberculosis
- Operating room studies: Bacterial (aerobic and anaerobic) and fungal cultures, acid-fast bacilli

---

Data from Berbari EF, Kanj SS, Kowalski TJ, et al. 2015 Infectious Diseases Society of America (IDSA) clinical practice guidelines for the diagnosis and treatment of native vertebral osteomyelitis in adults. *Clin Infect Dis.* 2015;61(6):e26–e46.

TABLE 14.1 ■ Obtaining Image-Guided Aspiration Needle Biopsy

Blood Cultures Data	Recommended Action
• Blood cultures are positive for *Staphylococcus aureus, S. lugdunensis*, or *Brucella*.	• Skip image-guided aspiration biopsy (diagnosis is confirmed by blood cultures alone).
• Blood cultures are negative.	• Obtain a second aspiration biopsy.
• Image-guided aspiration biopsy is positive for a potential skin contaminant (coagulase-negative staphylococci, Propionibacterium species, or diphtheroids). Note: *S. lugdunensis* is the one coagulase-negative staphylococci that acts like *S. aureus* (abscess forming) and must be treated like a pathogen.	
• Blood cultures are negative.	• Perform further testing to exclude difficult-to-grow organisms (e.g., anaerobes, fungi, Brucella species, or mycobacteria).
• Image-guided aspiration biopsy is negative (or indeterminate).	• If further testing is negative, obtain a second aspiration biopsy.[7]

collapse, spinal instability, and persistent or recurrent bloodstream infection despite appropriate antibiotics. Risk factors for severe neurologic deficit include[6]:

- Cervical and thoracic level of involvement
- Presence of epidural abscess
- *Staphylococcus aureus* organism
- C-reactive protein (CRP) >150 mg/L

Antibiotic Selection and Treatment Monitoring

Consultation with an infectious disease specialist is recommended for patients who are diagnosed with VO or SEA. The typical duration of antibiotic treatment is 6 weeks, which underscores the importance of correctly identifying the culprit organism and establishing the most appropriate antibiotic regimen. In the majority of cases, this involves administering antibiotics intravenously. The duration of antibiotic treatment is intended to ensure adequate penetration of the spine, and 6 weeks has been found to be as effective as longer courses.[8]

If the blood cultures and aspiration biopsy are nondiagnostic but there is a high suspicion of infection based on clinical presentation or imaging studies, physicians may resort to prescribing a 6-week course of empiric antibiotic therapy, which covers broadly for the most likely organisms (Box 14.2).

BOX 14.2 ■ Microbes

- The most common organism causing vertebral osteomyelitis is *Staphylococcus aureus*.
- If *S. aureus* is confirmed to be methicillin sensitive, antistaphylococcal penicillin (nafcillin/oxacillin) or cefazolin may be used.
- If the organism is methicillin-resistant *S. aureus*, vancomycin and daptomycin are appropriate alternatives.
  - Vancomycin can be toxic to the kidneys and requires frequent laboratory monitoring and dose adjustments to obtain an ideal and safe trough level.
- Streptococcal species can be treated with ceftriaxone or penicillin class antibiotics, and gram-negative bacilli can be treated with a third- or fourth-generation cephalosporin or a fluoroquinolone.

Once IV antibiotic treatment is initiated and repeat blood cultures are negative for 48–72 hours, long-term IV access, such as a peripherally inserted central catheter (PICC) line, can be inserted at bedside. When stable for discharge, the patient disposition could be home (with home infusion services or daily treatments at an infusion center) or an inpatient rehabilitation facility. Depending on hospital policy, patients with a history of IV drug use often are not candidates for home infusion therapy due to potential risk of the PICC line being used for illegal drug administration.

Regardless, the goal is to facilitate 6 uninterrupted weeks of IV antibiotic treatment. In some instances, under the direction of an infectious disease specialist, antibiotic regimens can be modified to reduce the dosing frequency, thereby enhancing the ease of administration after discharge (e.g., once daily infusion of daptomycin vs three times daily infusion of vancomycin). Blood work should be done weekly while on IV therapy to monitor:

- Kidney and liver function (comprehensive metabolic panel)
- Blood counts (complete blood count with differential)
- Inflammatory markers (erythrocyte sedimentation rate [ESR] and CRP)
- Creatine kinase (if patient is on daptomycin due to its risk of causing rhabdomyolysis [i.e., muscle breakdown])

In addition to completing the full course of IV antibiotics, symptomatic improvement and decreasing inflammatory markers suggest that the treatment has been successful. Both ESR and CRP levels (which have been demonstrated to correlate with clinical response to antibiotics after spinal surgery) should fall, but the CRP level usually falls more rapidly.[9] If the patient is doing well and otherwise showing signs of recovery, repeat imaging of the spine is not necessary and can even generate confusion because radiographic abnormalities sometimes persist despite successful treatment and clinical resolution. Worsening lab values, unresolving symptoms, or persistent neurologic deficits should prompt reevaluation with repeat imaging, blood cultures, or biopsy.

Conclusion

- For patients in whom spinal infection is suspected (i.e., with fever and back pain), draw blood cultures and obtain tissue samples prior to antibiotic administration, if possible. Patients with positive blood cultures should have repeat blood cultures drawn daily to ensure "clearance" (negative blood culture growth at 5 days) of infection.
- While CT is ideal for evaluation of bone, MR imaging with IV gadolinium contrast is required to diagnose epidural abscess.
- Alert the medical team for neurologic changes, especially new or progressive motor weakness, urinary retention, bowel or bladder incontinence. This may prompt initiation of antibiotics or accelerate surgical planning.
- Anticipate the involvement of consultation services and imaging studies to look for other sources of infection. Image-guided bone biopsy or needle aspiration are required unless Staph aureus (or lugdunensis) bacteremia is present, or surgical cultures have already been obtained.
- Patients with VO require 6–8 weeks of uninterrupted IV antibiotic therapy in order to achieve the best likelihood of cure.

References

1. Chen WH, Jiang LS, Dai LY. Surgical treatment of pyogenic vertebral osteomyelitis with spinal instrumentation. *Eur Spine J*. 2007;16(9):1307–1316.
2. Wang TY, Harward II SC, Tsvankin V, et al. Neurological outcomes after surgical or conservative management of spontaneous spinal epidural abscesses: a systematic review and meta-analysis of data from 1980 through 2016. *Clin Spine Surg*. 2019;32(1):18–29.

3. Marschall J, Bhavan KP, Olsen MA, et al. The impact of prebiopsy antibiotics on pathogen recovery in hematogenous vertebral osteomyelitis. *Clin Infect Dis.* 2011;52(7):867–872.
4. Pigrau C, Almirante B, Flores X, et al. Spontaneous pyogenic vertebral osteomyelitis and endocarditis: incidence, risk factors, and outcome. *Am J Med.* 2005;118(11):1287.
5. Saravolatz II LD, Labalo V, Fishbain J, et al. Lack of effect of antibiotics on biopsy culture results in vertebral osteomyelitis. *Diagn Microbiol Infect Dis.* 2018;91(3):273–274.
6. Lemaignen A, Ghout I, Dinh A, et al. Characteristics of and risk factors for severe neurological deficit in patients with pyogenic vertebral osteomyelitis: a case-control study. *Medicine (Baltimore).* 2017;96(21):e6387.
7. Gras G, Buzele R, Parienti JJ, et al. Microbiological diagnosis of vertebral osteomyelitis: relevance of second percutaneous biopsy following initial negative biopsy and limited yield of post-biopsy blood cultures. *Eur J Clin Microbiol Infect Dis.* 2014;33(3):371–375.
8. Bernard L, Dinh A, Ghout I, et al. Antibiotic treatment for 6 weeks versus 12 weeks in patients with pyogenic vertebral osteomyelitis: an open-label, non-inferiority, randomised, controlled trial. *Lancet.* 2015;385(9971):875–882.
9. Khan MH, Smith PN, Rao N, et al. Serum C-reactive protein levels correlate with clinical response in patients treated with antibiotics for wound infections after spinal surgery. *Spine J.* 2006;6(3):311–315.

Questions

1. A 65-year-old male is admitted for lumbar vertebral osteomyelitis. On admission, he is afebrile with stable vital signs, and his leg strength is 5/5 bilaterally. The plan is for image-guided needle aspiration biopsy, scheduled for the next day. Overnight, his lumbar pain acutely worsens, and the nurse notes the lower extremity strength has changed from 5/5 to 3/5. A bladder scan shows urinary retention, which the patient reports is a new problem. How would you care for this patient overnight?
   a. Care team may start antibiotics if surgery is delayed.
   b. Inform the provider of this change immediate, and anticipate surgical consultation.
   c. Order physical therapy evaluation.
   d. Consult urology.
   e. Both a and b.

2. A 33-year-old female who is currently using IV drugs presents with thoracic vertebral osteomyelitis. Blood cultures are positive for *Staphylococcus aureus*, and appropriate antibiotic coverage is initiated. Three days later, she is afebrile, hemodynamically stable, and repeat blood cultures have cleared (negative blood cultures). What is the next step?
   a. Confirm the diagnosis with image-guided aspiration biopsy.
   b. Repeat spine imaging to confirm response to therapy.
   c. Place PICC and send the patient to a skilled nursing facility for IV antibiotics.
   d. Place PICC and consult home infusion therapy.
   e. Convert to oral antibiotics and send the patient home.

3. A 61-year-old female with a history of chronic back pain, prior endocarditis, and diabetes presents with fever. On admission, she is noted to have redness and warmth of the left calf, which is tender to touch. Her urinalysis is suggestive of a urinary tract infection. The patient undergoes transesophageal echocardiogram to evaluate for bacterial vegetations on the heart valves. During the procedure, it is noted that she may have a dental abscess. Subsequently, her back pain becomes acutely worse. Lumbar MRI with contrast is performed and reveals probable T12–L1 vertebral osteomyelitis at the site of an old vertebral compression fracture. Before the final echocardiogram report is available, you are notified by the lab that blood cultures from admission are positive.

Which of the following could be the source of her vertebral osteomyelitis?
a. Urinary tract infection
b. Bacterial cellulitis
c. Endocarditis
d. Dental abscess
e. All the above

4. A patient with recently implanted spinal hardware is admitted for workup of fever. MRI imaging shows a small periprosthetic (next to the hardware) fluid collection, and blood cultures from admission have grown *Staphylococcus epidermidis* in one of the two sets of blood cultures. What is the next best step?
a. Treat with vancomycin for 6 weeks.
b. Repeat blood cultures.
c. Discuss with surgery team regarding possible image-guided needle aspiration biopsy of the fluid collection.
d. Look for other causes of fever.
e. b, c, and d.

5. A 29-year-old female patient with a history of IV heroin abuse was recently diagnosed in the hospital with methicillin-sensitive *S. aureus* spinal epidural abscess and was on IV nafcillin. She left against medical advice 5 days ago and now is readmitted to the hospital as a transfer from an outside hospital with worsening leg weakness. What interventions should the nurse *not* perform?
a. Obtain a full set of vitals and perform a neurologic exam.
b. Draw blood cultures after antibiotics are started.
c. Notify care team of the patient's arrival and prepare the necessary equipment for blood work.
d. Obtain IV access as patient will likely need a prolonged course of IV nafcillin.
e. Counsel the patient that it is important to continue her antibiotic course without interruption.

Answers

1. e

2. c

3. e

4. e

5. b

Medical Management of Common Neurosurgical Issues

CHAPTER 15

Diabetes Management in the Neurosurgical Patient

Swathi Maddula, MD

Introduction

Diabetes mellitus (DM) dates back over 3000 years with the earliest known findings recorded in ancient Egypt, China, and India. At that time, there were documented observations of people who were experiencing polyuria (large volume excretion of urine) and whose urine appeared to be sweet, as it would attract ants.[1–4] The term *diabetes mellitus* stems from the Greek word *diabetes*, meaning "siphon," and the Latin word *mellitus*, meaning "sweet."[3,4] Investigation of pancreatic insulin production and its role in the pathophysiology of diabetes has engaged many researchers over centuries and culminated in the production of the synthetic insulin used today.[5]

DM is a complex metabolic disorder that affects a significant percentage of the American population and the population worldwide. According to the Centers for Disease Control and Prevention and American Diabetes Association (ADA), 11.3% of Americans carried a diagnosis of DM in 2019, and roughly 1.4 million new cases occur each year.[6,7] DM is commonly encountered in the neurosurgical patient population, and acquiring the knowledge and skills needed for management of DM is imperative for providing excellent care to neurosurgical patients during the perioperative period and for the duration of their hospitalization.

Physiology

DM is a metabolic disorder characterized by an imbalance of insulin and glucagon, as a result of an abnormal metabolism of carbohydrates. Ultimately, this leads to an elevated blood glucose level, referred to as hyperglycemia.[4,8] The pancreas contains alpha cells, which are responsible for glucagon production, and beta cells, which are responsible for insulin production. Insulin secretion from the pancreas is triggered by meals and serves to activate cellular uptake of glucose. Consequently, the blood glucose level decreases, and glucose is stored by the cells in the form of glycogen. Glycogen is stored so that it can be used as an energy resource between meals. The conversion of glycogen into usable energy is triggered by glucagon, which is also released by the pancreas. Patients with diabetes experience a disruption of normal glucose processing, which leads to abnormal glucose levels.[3,4,8]

Classification

Understanding the classification of DM is important for guiding therapy.[3,4,8,9] The ADA separates the most common forms of DM into four categories[8]:

- Type 1 is caused by the destruction of beta cells by an autoimmune process. Beta cell destruction results in insulin deficiency.
- Type 2 is related to impaired functionality of beta cells, which leads to decreased insulin secretion and peripheral insulin resistance.

- Gestational diabetes is diagnosed in pregnant individuals who did not have a diagnosis of diabetes prior to pregnancy but who developed diabetes in their second or third trimester.
- Types that are due to other causes:
  - Monogenic diabetes syndromes that pertain to neonatal populations and maturity onset diabetes of the young
  - Exocrine gland dysfunction/diseases, such as cystic fibrosis or pancreatitis
  - Chemical induced, such as by steroids, after organ transplants, and side effects from human immunodeficiency virus treatment

Historically it was believed that type 1 DM occurred mostly in younger patients, and type 2 DM occurred mostly in older patients. While there are certain generalized patterns encountered clinically, after extensive research it was proven that individuals can be diagnosed with either type at any stage of life.[8]

Diagnosis

The ADA uses the following criteria for making a diagnosis of DM[8]:

- Fasting blood glucose ≥126 mg/dL *or*
- Two-hour blood glucose ≥200 mg/dL during an oral glucose tolerance test *or*
- Hemoglobin A1C ≥6.5% *or*
- Random blood glucose ≥200 mg/dL *with* symptoms of hyperglycemia or hyperglycemic crisis

In conjunction with a thorough review of the patient's history and physical exam, these criteria are used to establish the diagnosis of DM. The ADA recommends that all patients with diabetes, a possible history of diabetes, or found to have a blood glucose level >140 mg/dL should have their hemoglobin A1C checked upon admission to the hospital if one has not been checked in the last 3 months.[9]

Inpatient Management

Patients diagnosed with diabetes prior to hospitalization are usually already classified as having one of the types listed earlier, and many are already prescribed a treatment regimen.[4] Documenting the patient's type of diabetes on admission is very important. This information guides management and enables the interprofessional team to prevent adverse outcomes. Nurses play a pivotal role in gathering information about the patient's disease, especially since they are involved in the initial assessment of each patient. Nurses should ask questions related to the patient's history of diabetes, treatment regimen (including any recent changes that have been made), and any complications previously experienced.[8] Possible complications include diabetic ketoacidosis (DKA), often related to insufficient doses of insulin, or hypoglycemia, caused by excessive insulin administration. In addition to insulin, many patients are prescribed oral medications that require adjustment during their hospitalization and the perioperative period.[9,10]

When a patient with diabetes is scheduled for a neurosurgical procedure, it is imperative that the patient's blood glucose be optimally controlled and maintained as close as safely possible to the targets outlined by the ADA[10]:

- In the hospital, treatment for critically ill patients should begin when the blood glucose is >180 mg/dL.
- Therapy should be titrated to maintain the blood glucose level between 140 and 180 mg/dL.
- Glucose levels <110 mg/dL should be avoided.

TYPE 1 DIABETES

Upon admission to the hospital, patients with type 1 diabetes generally should continue or stay close to their home insulin regimen.[9] Because type 1 diabetes is characterized by insulin deficiency

TABLE 15.1 ■ **Pharmacokinetics of Subcutaneous Insulin Preparations**

Insulin	Onset	Peak (hours)	Duration (hours)
Rapid acting			
Aspart with niacinamide	2–4 minutes	1–2	3–5
Aspart	5–15 minutes	1–2	4–6
Lispro	5–15 minutes	1–2	4–6
Glulisine	5–15 minutes	1–2	4–6
Short acting			
Regular insulin	30–60 minutes	2–3	6–10
Intermediate acting			
NPH	2–4 hours	4–10	12–18
Long acting			
Detemir	2 hours	Variable	12–24
Glargine	2 hours	None	20–24
Degludec	2 hours	None	24+

From Furlong K, Villuri S. Blood glucose management in the neurosurgical patient. In: Daniel R, Harrop C, eds. *Medical Management of Neurosurgical Patients*. Oxford University Press; 2019:179.

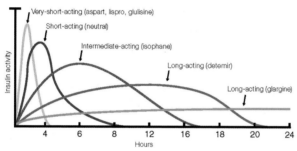

Fig. 15.1 Graphic visualization of the onset time and duration of various insulin types. (From Knights K, Rowland A, Darroch S. *Pharmacology for Health Professionals*, 5th ed. Elsevier; 2019.)

due to the destruction of beta cells, patients with this type are insulin dependent. These patients require a continuous infusion of insulin or a precise and proactive regimen of intermittent subcutaneous insulin injections to avoid DKA even when they are not eating. If a patient is on an insulin pump at home, this typically can be continued during hospitalization to ensure consistent and timely insulin administration. This, however, depends on the anticipated duration of the procedure and if the patient is cognitively and physically able to reliably participate in assisting with managing the pump.[9]

There are many types of insulin and different ways of administering the desired total daily dosage (Table 15.1, Fig. 15.1). The insulin regimen prescribed for each patient may vary according to the patient's medical comorbidities, appetite and nutritional intake, planned surgical procedures and periods of withholding food and fluid, baseline glucose control, and physician preference. Close monitoring of the patient's glucose is essential because the prescribed regimen may need to be modified numerous times before achieving safe and effective glucose control. When calculating an ideal inpatient regimen, nurses and physicians should bear in mind that patients with type 1 diabetes may require a dose reduction of 10–20% of their home long-acting insulin regimen to avoid hypoglycemia. If glucose levels are uncontrolled or too high perioperatively, an insulin drip, which is a continuous infusion of regular insulin, may be considered. This will require more frequent monitoring of blood glucose levels and active titration of the drip rate. Consultation with endocrinology can be pursued in severe or complicated cases.[9,10]

TYPE 2 DIABETES

In comparison to type 1 diabetes, patients with type 2 diabetes may be treated with a greater variety of modalities in the outpatient setting, including lifestyle modifications (such as diet and exercise), oral medications, insulin, or a combination of these options. In general, when a patient is hospitalized, oral diabetes medications are held. This helps patients avoid side effects during the acute stress response that the body experiences while hospitalized. Furthermore, many neurosurgical patients require imaging studies with intravenous contrast during their hospitalization and often one or more surgical interventions. Intravenous contrast (along with other medications) and intraoperative hemodynamic fluctuations can contribute to kidney injury and other deleterious systemic effects, which may be exacerbated if oral antihyperglycemics were continued.[9,10] When a patient is scheduled for elective surgery on a specific day, oral medications, such as metformin and sulfonylureas, should be held within 24 hours before the procedure.[10] They are restarted based on the provider's assessment of the patient's clinical progression and dietary intake postoperatively.

Patients with type 2 diabetes managed with insulin are usually ordered their home regimen (as tolerated) while hospitalized. However, when an order is placed for nothing by mouth (NPO), and patients cannot eat or drink (such as in the hours preceding a surgery), providers will often reduce the long-acting insulin dose by 50%.[9] Whenever an order for NPO is placed, nurses should verify with the physician team that the insulin regimen has been appropriately reduced/adjusted to match the decreased requirement. This dose reduction should be continued until the patient is able to eat and drink normally again. Failure to decrease the insulin dosage when patients cannot eat or drink risks causing severe hypoglycemia. Like patients with type 1 diabetes, insulin dosing is based on the provider's preference, type of insulin the patient is prescribed, duration of procedures, concurrent clinical concerns, and the patient's baseline glucose control (Fig. 15.2).[9]

Steroid-Induced Hyperglycemia

Neurosurgical patients often require steroids perioperatively, which commonly results in steroid-induced hyperglycemia. Depending on the severity of hyperglycemia, patients may need to start antihyperglycemic medications, including oral agents and insulin. Even patients without a formal diagnosis of diabetes tend to develop hyperglycemia while receiving steroids, and patients with preexisting diabetes may need to start insulin therapy even if they did not previously require insulin. Patients who are already prescribed insulin usually need to increase their dose. The dosing and type of insulin selected are dependent on many factors, including the patient's history of diabetes, baseline glycemic control, type and dose of steroid prescribed, anticipated duration of steroid treatment, and whether there will be a steroid taper before discontinuation. Management is relatively provider dependent, but nurses should be prepared to educate patients on the role of glucose checks, proper insulin administration, and guidance related to the next steps especially if an adjustment or assessment is required upon discharge.[9,11]

Hypoglycemia

While it is important to maintain strict blood glucose control, it is also important to be wary of the side effects of insulin administration, especially hypoglycemia. Blood glucose targets for hospitalized patients are generally between 140 and 180 mg/dL.[10,12] This goal is aimed to prevent episodes of hypo- and hyperglycemia and account for higher stress levels in the acute care setting.

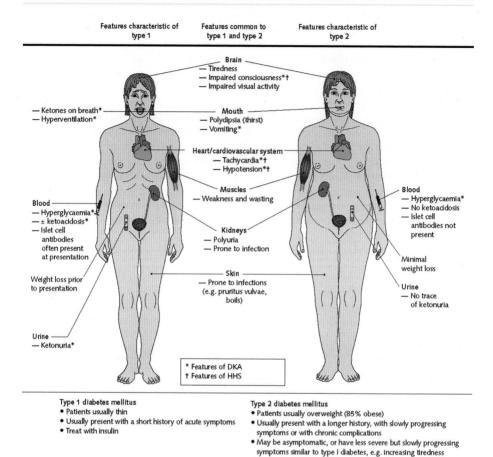

Fig. 15.2   Characteristic ways that type 1 and type 2 diabetes affect the body systems. (From Eiben I, Eiben P, Watson K. *Crash Course: General Medicine*, 5th ed. Elsevier; 2019.)

In the hospital, patients should have their blood glucose checked regularly. In general, patients who are eating should have blood glucose checks before each meal, and those who are NPO or on continuous tube feeding should have blood glucose checks every 4–6 hours.[9,12] Furthermore, patients should have blood glucose assessments ordered "as needed" for nurses to utilize when patients are experiencing symptoms of hypoglycemia.

Symptoms of hypoglycemia include dizziness, confusion, pallor, shakiness, and fast heartbeat. Blood glucose values <70 mg/dL can lead to hypoglycemic coma and even death.[9,12] Management is geared toward bringing glucose levels back up to normal as soon as possible.

- Patients who can eat/drink should be given juice and snacks with sugar and carbohydrates.
- Patients who are NPO, or unable to safely take PO, should receive dextrose injections and/or infusions.

Most health systems have hypoglycemia protocols in place, and orders related to these protocols populate simultaneously with insulin orders. Anyone prescribing or administering insulin should be familiar with these protocols and practices.[9,10] Upon discharge, nurses play a vital role in educating patients and their families on recognizing the signs and symptoms of hypoglycemia and implementing the initial steps in management to prevent complications.

Discharge Planning

Nurses play an important role in diabetes education. Education should be initiated early in the hospital course to ensure complete comprehension. The teaching process should include education on checking glucose levels, drawing up insulin, and administering medications. In some hospitals, reinforcement of these concepts may be supplemented with teaching from a diabetic educator, nutritionist, or registered dietician. Educational materials should be printed out and reviewed with the patient and caregivers. Particular attention should be paid to reviewing any new medications, reviewing potential side effects, and reinforcing how to recognize and manage symptoms of hypo- and hyperglycemia. Upon discharge, nurses should highlight any follow-up appointments, follow-up plans, and provider contact information. Patients will need to know who to reach out to for questions and who to follow up with for medication refills and ongoing monitoring. Providers are a good source of information for further questions or guidance.[4,9]

Conclusion

Patients who are undergoing neurosurgical procedures are susceptible to aberrations in their blood glucoses due to their stressful clinical situation. This can include patients who have preexisting diabetes as well as those who are suffering from steroid-induced hyperglycemia. Recognition and early initiation of interventional measures by nursing for these aberrations and the complications associated with them are imperative. Nurses also play a pivotal role in patient education throughout all phases of the hospitalization and particularly at discharge. Important features of patient education include review of medications along with signs and symptoms of hypoglycemia, hyperglycemia, and other complications. The next steps on how to tackle these complications should also be discussed by nurses and providers.

References

1. Karamanou M, Protogerou A, Tsoucalas G, et al. Milestones in the history of diabetes mellitus: the main contributors. *World J Diabetes.* 2016;7(1):1–7.
2. Lakhtakia R. The history of diabetes mellitus. *Sultan Qaboos Univ Med J.* 2013;13(3):368–370.
3. Sapra A, Bhandari P. *Diabetes mellitus.* StatPearls Publishing; 2022.
4. Sapra A, Bhandari P, Wilhite (Hughes) A. *Diabetes mellitus (nursing).* StatPearls Publishing; 2022.
5. Vecchio I, Tornali C, Bragazzi NL, et al. The discovery of insulin: an important milestone in the history of medicine. *Front Endocrinol (Lausanne).* 2018;9:613.
6. Centers for Disease Control and Prevention. *National and state diabetes trends.* CDC; 2022.
7. American Diabetes Association. *Statistics about diabetes.* ADA; 2022.
8. American Diabetes Association. Classification and diagnosis of diabetes: standards of medical care in diabetes—2021. *Diabetes Care.* 2021;44(1):S15–S33.
9. Furlong K, Villuri S. Blood glucose management in the neurosurgical patient. In: Daniel R, Harrop C, eds. *Medical Management of Neurosurgical Patients.* Oxford University Press; 2019:175–189.
10. Godoy DA, Di Napoli M, Biestro A, et al. Perioperative glucose control in neurosurgical patients. *Anesthesiol Res Pract.* 2012;2012:690362.
11. Hwang JL, Weiss RE. Steroid-induced diabetes: a clinical and molecular approach to understanding and treatment. *Diabetes Metab Res Rev.* 2014;30(2):96–102.
12. American Diabetes Association Professional Practice Committee. Diabetes care in the hospital: standards of medical care in diabetes—2022. *Diabetes Care.* 2022;45(1):S244–S253.

Questions

Cory came to the hospital for back pain and was found to have an epidural abscess. His mother has type 1 diabetes and his father has type 2 diabetes. On admission, Cory had a hemoglobin A1C level of 9%, and he was started on diabetic medications. You learn that Cory will be discharged in the afternoon. You provide him with information on healthy eating, exercise, and medication side effects, and you highlight follow-up information in his discharge paperwork.

1. What should you reinforce as signs and symptoms of hypoglycemia?
   a. Sweating
   b. Altered mental status
   c. Shaking/trembling
   d. All of the above

2. When you are finished going over paperwork, Cory asks you what the difference is between type 1 and type 2 diabetes. What can you tell him?
   a. Type 1 is caused by deficiency in insulin production, and type 2 is caused by insulin resistance.
   b. Type 1 is treated with insulin only, and type 2 is treated with oral medications only.
   c. Type 1 is related to insulin overload, and type 2 is related to insulin deficiency.
   d. Type 1 does not require adherence to a healthy diet and exercise regimen, whereas type 2 does.

Mara was admitted to the hospital after she was found to have cauda equina syndrome. She was evaluated by the neurosurgery team and started on steroids. She is scheduled to undergo surgery. When doing the initial assessment, you find out that she has type 2 diabetes and is currently being treated with both insulin and oral medications.

3. What changes can be anticipated in Mara's diabetic regimen now that she is in the hospital?
   a. If blood glucose is difficult to control with subcutaneous insulin alone, she may require an insulin drip.
   b. Oral diabetic medications may be held due to possible side effects.
   c. Insulin requirements may increase when steroids are administered.
   d. All of the above are correct.

4. It is the night before Mara's surgery, and she is NPO for her procedure. Which of the following changes to her insulin regimen do you anticipate?
   a. Since she is NPO for the procedure, she should be placed on an insulin drip.
   b. She will continue her oral diabetic medications only.
   c. Her home bedtime insulin dosage will be decreased tonight.
   d. All her diabetic medications will be held overnight, since she is NPO, even though none of her blood glucose levels have been low thus far.

Larry is admitted to the hospital for elective surgery for lumbar stenosis. When you perform his initial assessment, you see that he is on two different forms of insulin: glargine before bedtime and lispro before each meal.

5. Which one of the following is considered a long-acting form of insulin?
   a. Lispro
   b. NPH
   c. Glargine
   d. Aspart

Answers

1. d

2. a

3. d

4. c

5. c

CHAPTER 16

Nursing Management of Acute Kidney Injury

Donyell Doram, BS, MD

Introduction

Acute kidney injury (AKI) is not a single disease entity; rather, it is characterized by a sudden decrease in renal function.[1] The kidneys are responsible for maintaining the body's fluid balance and filtering toxins from the body. When the etiology of AKI is reversible, full recovery of renal function is expected. Prompt recognition of changes in renal function, along with adequate treatment, is crucial to prevent new-onset or worsening chronic kidney disease (CKD).[1-3]

The most widely used clinical guidelines and classification system for AKI are from Kidney Disease Improving Global Outcomes (KDIGO). KDIGO assembled their guidelines through large systemic reviews of primarily hospitalized patients, including adults and children, across different countries and clinical settings. According to KDIGO, AKI is defined as[2]:

- Increase in serum creatinine concentration by at least 1.5 times the baseline within 7 days OR
- Increase in serum creatinine concentration by 0.3 mg/dL within 48 hours OR
- Decreased urine output to <0.5 mL/kg/hr for 6 hours

AKI can be divided into stages (Table 16.1).

AKI affects 20% of hospitalized patients, 10% of whom will progress to requiring kidney replacement therapy (KRT).[1] Known colloquially as dialysis, KRT is initiated when medical management alone (such as fluid resuscitation, removing nephrotoxic medications, etc.) is no longer sufficient for preserving or recovering baseline kidney function.

Complications that may result from AKI include CKD, metabolic acidosis, and uremia.[1,4] AKI can occur in patients with or without underlying CKD. Furthermore, incomplete recovery of the initial kidney injury may lead to new-onset or worsening CKD.[1]

Epidemiology and Demographics

Identifying patients who are at risk for AKI will help with early detection of disease and limit adverse outcomes. Elderly patients and those with a history of CKD are the most susceptible.[2,4,5] Furthermore, certain admission diagnoses, such as sepsis, shock, trauma, and hypovolemia from anemia or recent surgery, are risk factors for developing AKI. Lastly, patients with chronic diseases, such as congestive heart failure, cirrhosis, and diabetes, are at a higher risk for AKI when the chronic disease is uncontrolled. Ultimately, proactive monitoring of renal function is essential for patients with any known or suspected risk factors (Table 16.2).

Etiology[1,3-5]

Understanding the patient's reason for admission and the underlying comorbidities can help in the early detection of AKI. Underlying causes for AKI can be broken down into three main categories: prerenal, intrinsic renal, and postrenal (Table 16.3).

TABLE 16.1 ■ KDIGO Acute Kidney Injury Stages

Stage	Serum Creatinine Rise	Urine Output
1	1.5–1.9 times baseline creatinine *or* at least 0.3 mg/dL increase	<0.5 mL/kg/hr for 6–12 hr
2	2–2.9 times baseline creatinine	<0.5 mL/kg/hr for ≥12 hr
3	3 times baseline creatinine *or* increase in creatinine to ≥4 mg/dL *or* initiation of renal replacement therapy	<0.3 mL/kg/hr for ≥24 hr *or* anuria for ≥12 hr

Adapted from Kidney Disease: Improving Global Outcomes (KDIGO) Acute Kidney Injury Work Group. KDIGO clinical practice guideline for acute kidney injury. *Kidney Intl Suppl (2011).* 2012;2(1):8–12.

TABLE 16.2 ■ Risk Factors for Acute Kidney Injury

Exposures	• Sepsis • Critical illness	• Circulatory shock	• Burns/trauma	• Cardiac surgery • Major non-cardiac surgery	• Neph-rotoxic drugs • Poison-ous animals/plants	• Iodin-ated contrast
Susceptibility factors	• Volume depletion • Anemia	• Older age • Female sex • Black race	• Chronic kidney disease • Other chronic cis-eases (liver/heart/lung)	• Diabetes • Hyper-tension	• Cancer	

Adapted from Kidney Disease: Improving Global Outcomes (KDIGO) Acute Kidney Injury Work Group. KDIGO clinical practice guideline for acute kidney injury. *Kidney Intl Suppl (2011).* 2012;2(1):8–12.

PRERENAL

This is the most common cause of community acquired AKI.[1] Kidney injury is triggered by decreased renal perfusion. This can be seen with an elevated blood urea nitrogen:creatinine ratio >20:1.[2,4] Causes within this category include:

- Intravascular volume depletion
  - Overuse of diuretic therapy
  - Osmotic diuresis as seen in diabetic ketoacidosis
  - Extrarenal loss such as vomiting, diarrhea, burns, sweating, and blood loss
  - Hyperthermia
  - Anemia from hemorrhage
  - Cirrhosis
  - Nephrotic syndrome
- Systemic vasodilation
  - Sepsis
  - Cirrhosis
  - Anaphylaxis
- Reduced cardiac output
  - Cardiogenic shock
  - Pericardial disease
  - Valvular heart disease
  - Pulmonary embolism

TABLE 16.3 ■ **Distinguishing Acute Kidney Injury Etiologies**

Prerenal: Decreased Renal Perfusion Without Intrinsic Damage	Intrinsic Renal: Due to Direct Damage to the Kidney Itself	Postrenal: Obstruction of the Urinary Tract
Intravascular Volume Depletion	Tubular	Extrarenal
• Overuse of diuretics	• Medications	• Prostate hypertrophy
• Diabetic ketoacidosis	• Drugs: MDMA/Ecstasy	• Neurogenic bladder
• Gastrointestinal loss: diarrhea/vomiting/hyperthermia	• Synthetic cannabinoids	• Nephrolithiasis
• Nephrotic syndrome	• Pigments: myoglobin/hemoglobin	• Malignancy
• Cirrhosis	• Contrast media	• Retroperitoneal fibrosis
Systemic Vasodilation	• Hypercalcemia	Intrarenal
• Sepsis	• Light chain disease: multiple Myeloma/amyloidosis	• Crystals
• Anaphylaxis	Interstitial	• Clots
• Cirrhosis	• Medications	• Tumor
• Neurogenic shock	• Systemic infections	
Reduced Cardiac Output	• Systemic disease: sarcoidosis, leukemia/lymphoma	
• Sepsis	Glomerular	
• Cardiogenic shock	• Immune-mediated disease due to infection or autoimmune complement disorder	
• Heart failure		
• Pericardial disease	• Thrombotic microangiopathy	
• Pulmonary hypertension	Vascular	
• Pulmonary embolism	• Renal atheroembolic disease	
	• Renal vein thrombosis	
	• Hypertension	
	• Renal infarction	
	Acute phosphate Nephropathy	
	• Oral sodium phosphate for bowel prep colonoscopy	

From Levey AS, James MT. Acute kidney injury. *Ann Intern Med*. 2017;167(9); Rahman M, Shad F, Smith MC. Acute kidney injury: a guide to diagnosis and management. *Am Fam Physician*. 2012;86(7):631–639.

- Normotensive hemodynamic causes
- Due to the use of nonsteroidal antiinflammatory drugs (NSAIDs), which prevent compensatory afferent vasodilation of the kidneys

INTRINSIC RENAL

This is due to direct damage to the kidney itself. AKI due to intrarenal causes has unpredictable outcomes, with mortality ranging from 30% to 80%.[4] Categories include:

- Acute tubular necrosis (ATN), a type of AKI caused by toxic or ischemic damage to the tubular epithelium
  - This is the most common intrinsic cause in hospitalized patients.
  - Sepsis accounts for the majority of ATN etiology in critical care patients.[4]
  - Common causes are toxins/medications or prolonged hypoperfusion/hypotension.
    - Medications: iodinated contrast, aminoglycosides, vancomycin, cisplatin[1]

- Acute interstitial nephritis (AIN), an immune mediated tubulointerstitial injury. Common etiologies include:
  - Infections
  - Autoimmune diseases
  - Medications: sulfonamides, beta lactams, NSAIDs, diuretics, proton pump inhibitors[1]
- Glomerular diseases, a collection of kidney diseases that affect the glomerulus of the nephron, leading to changes such as hematuria, proteinuria, and decreased glomerular filtration
  - This can be due to infections or autoimmune diseases.
- Vascular diseases of the renal arteries or veins caused by atheroembolic disease, hypertension, or renal vein thrombosis

POSTRENAL

Obstruction of the urinary tract
- Extrarenal causes (occurring outside the kidney itself)
  - Prostate hypertrophy
  - Neurogenic bladder
  - Kidney stones
  - Malignancy
- Intrarenal causes (occurring within the kidney)
  - Crystals: Acyclovir and methotrexate can cause crystal nephropathy.[1]
  - Clots
  - Tumors

History

On admission, patients should have a detailed history and physical examination done to help providers identify patients at risk for or actively developing AKI. Patients with AKI are often asymptomatic in the initial stages, but those with urinary tract obstruction may have pain/discomfort from the inability to void.[1,2] Changes in urinary output may be the first objective sign detected.

Asking patients about their past medical history will help pinpoint those patients most susceptible to AKI, especially if they have underlying CKD and other uncontrolled comorbidities. A thorough review of symptoms will also help detect patients at risk for AKI and may help distinguish the type of AKI developing. General questions should include assessment of volume status (oral intake, blood loss, vomiting, diarrhea) and asking about any new medications, both prescribed and over the counter. Distinguishing characteristics/presenting symptoms and signs can be seen within each category of AKI.
- Prerenal: decreased perfusion from bleeding, vomiting, diarrhea, burns/wounds, congestive heart failure
- Intrinsic renal: fever, hypotension, fatigue, rash, weight loss, myalgias, arthritis
- Postrenal: difficulty emptying bladder, bladder fullness, urinary frequency, blood in the urine, flank pain

PHYSICAL FINDINGS

Physical findings to monitor include[3]:
- Vital signs: These will help in detecting sepsis or shock, both major contributors to AKI.
  - Look for low blood pressure, fever or hypothermia, increased heart rate, increased respiratory rate.
- Cardiac exam: Look for jugular venous distension (JVD), listen for murmurs, and note any abnormal rate or rhythm.

- Lung exam: Listen for rales or rhonchi to assess for pulmonary congestion or respiratory infiltrate disease.
- Volume status: Monitor for JVD, leg edema, changes in capillary refill, oral mucosa (dry or moist), and turgor of the skin (e.g. forehead or sternum).
- Skin
  - Palpable purpura: can be an indication of vasculitis
  - Maculopapular rash: can be seen in drug-induced interstitial nephritis
  - Livedo reticularis and ischemic toes: present in atheroembolic disease
- Lower extremities: Monitor for edema, changes in pulse quality, and muscle tenderness (which can be seen in rhabdomyolysis).

Diagnostic Workup[1,3-5]

Initial testing should include general labs:
- Blood urea nitrogen (BUN), serum creatinine (Cr), electrolytes, complete blood count (CBC), urinalysis, and urine electrolytes. These laboratory values can determine the BUN:Cr ratio and fractional excretion of sodium (FeNa).
  - BUN:Cr ratio can help distinguish prerenal from intrinsic causes of AKI.
    - Prerenal causes typically produce a BUN:Cr ratio 20:1.
    - Intrinsic causes typically produce a BUN:Cr ratio 10:1–20:1.
  - Fractional excretion of sodium is calculated based on the concentrations of sodium and creatinine in the blood and urine. It is used to determine if the cause of AKI is pre-, intra-, or postrenal pathology.
    - Fractional excretion of sodium = ([Urine sodium/Plasma sodium] / [Urine creatinine/Plasma creatinine]) × 100
    - FeNa <1% can suggest a prerenal etiology.
    - FeNa >1% can suggest damage to the kidney.
    - This calculation is not useful in patients who are on diuretics due to increased natriuresis and may not be accurate in patients with CKD.[2]
- CBC can also be useful in distinguishing the causes of AKI.
  - Volume depletion from hemorrhage or hemolysis can cause prerenal AKI.
  - Prolonged hypovolemia can cause ATN.
  - Eosinophilia can be seen in AIN.
  - Thrombocytosis can be seen in critically ill patients who develop disseminated intravascular coagulation (DIC).[3]

A renal ultrasound is the first line of diagnostic testing. Evaluation of kidney size can identify underlying CKD. Furthermore, it can also be useful in finding signs of postrenal causes. Hydronephrosis (swelling of the kidney) can be an indicator of either renal or bladder obstruction. Furthermore, a CT without contrast may be considered to decide the level of obstruction or if there is any concern for kidney stones.

When obstruction is suspected, nurses should utilize bladder ultrasound. A normal postvoid residual (PVR) value is ≤50 mL.[4] Nurses should report volumes >100 mL to the provider. An increased PVR can be an initial indicator of obstruction. The provider may begin working up obstructive causes such as benign prostate hyperplasia.

Prevention Strategies

Full recovery of renal function is possible when the cause is reversible and treated swiftly. If not identified and treated, mortality can be as high as 80%.[6] For this purpose, developing prevention strategies and early-stage management is crucial.

Hemodynamic monitoring and management[1]

Nurses play an essential role in the identification, monitoring, and management of patients with AKI. By monitoring vital signs and intake/output, nurses are first to notice significant changes in volume status, which can indicate alteration in kidney function. Nurses are empowered to stop intravenous (IV) fluids in patients who are tolerating an adequate oral diet with stable volume status and request IV fluid initiation in patients who appear dry or are not taking in oral nutrition. They can also request Foley catheter placement in a critically ill patient for close intake and output monitoring or remove the Foley when monitoring is no longer needed. Furthermore, nurses should discuss with the provider about any use of nephrotoxic medication and ensure that antibiotic levels are routinely monitored. Lastly, nurses should ensure that IV fluid resuscitation occurs pre- and postadministration of radiocontrast media especially in high-risk patients.

Pearls and Considerations

- Critically ill patients should have close urinary output monitoring and routine lab monitoring of kidney function.
- Volume status of the patient can be the first clue to the development of AKI.
- Decreased oral intake, vomiting, and diarrhea should prompt the consideration of IV fluid resuscitation
- Patients requiring IV contrast studies or procedures should have a baseline renal function panel checked.
  - IV fluids prior and post can potentially prevent contrast-induced AKI.
  - Diuretics, NSAIDs, angiotensin-converting enzyme inhibitors/angiotensin receptor blockers should also be held prior to contrast administration.
- Antibiotics should be renally dosed and therapeutic drug levels checked.
- Home medication reconciliation is essential because common causes of AKI come from overuse of diuresis or NSAIDs.
- Although a patient may void, there is still potential for incomplete emptying.
  - If urinary output has declined, bladder scanning should be done.

Conclusion

Major risk factors for AKI in the hospitalized setting include patients of older age and those previously diagnosed with CKD. Patients with chronic diseases, such as diabetes, congestive heart failure, and cirrhosis, need close monitoring of renal function due to their increased risk for AKI. Underlying causes for AKI can be broken down into three main categories: prerenal, intrinsic renal, and postrenal. The common cause of prerenal AKI is poor perfusion (sepsis, shock, hypovolemia, diuretics). Intrinsic causes include medications, infections, and prolonged prerenal causes, such as sepsis. Postrenal AKI is due to obstructed urine flow through the urinary tract, such as prostate enlargement and nephrolithiasis. Prerenal AKI is the most common cause of AKI in hospitalized patients. Volume status can be the key in identifying these patients.

References

1. Levey AS, James MT. Acute kidney injury. *Ann Intern Med.* 2017;167(9):ITC66ITC80. doi:10.7326/AITC201711070.
2. Kidney Disease. Improving Global Outcomes (KDIGO) Acute Kidney Injury Work Group. KDIGO clinical practice guideline for acute kidney injury. *Kidney Intl Suppl (2011).* 2012;2(1):8–12. doi:10.1038/kisup.2012.7KDIGO.
3. Rahman M, Shad F, Smith MC. Acute kidney injury: a guide to diagnosis and management. *Am Fam Physician.* 2012;86(7):631–639.

4. Molitoris BA. Acute kidney injury. In: Goldman L, Schafer AI, eds. *Goldman-Cecil Medicine*. 26th ed. Elsevier; 2020:748–753.e2.

5. Bellomo R, Kellum JA, Ronco C. Acute kidney injury. *Lancet*. 2012;380(9843):756–766.

6. Ympa YP, Sakr Y, Reinhart K, et al. Has mortality from acute renal failure decreased? A systematic review of the literature. *Am J Med*. 2005;118(8):827–832.

Questions

1. A 55-year-old male presents with right lower extremity weakness and low back pain. Symptoms started 3 days ago after he was lifting boxes at his job. He has a past medical history of diabetes (DM), hypertension (HTN), and chronic low back pain. On exam his vitals are stable, except his blood pressure (BP) is elevated 170/90. He appears to be in pain, but otherwise he appears nontoxic, awake, and alert. Pertinent positives include lower abdominal discomfort on palpation, strength 2/5 on the right lower extremity in comparison to the left, and decreased rectal tone. Magnetic resonance imaging of his spine is obtained showing concern for cauda equina, and lab results are all stable except for Cr 1.9. A bladder scan was noted to be 800 cc, and he was unable to void on his own. Previous labs from a month ago noted normal renal function. What could be the etiology of AKI and what should be done next?
   a. Uncontrolled HTN; next step: renal ultrasound
   b. Urinary retention; next step: bladder scan
   c. Uncontrolled DM; next step: urinalysis to determine protein:Cr ratio
   d. Spinal cord injury due to cauda equina; next step: urgent surgery

2. An 85-year-old female with past medical history of osteoarthritis and congestive heart failure (CHF) presents with low back pain and lower extremity weakness left greater than right. Her low back pain started 6 months ago and has been progressively getting worse. She has difficulty ambulating due to the pain. She notes some night sweats and unintentional weight loss. On exam she is nontoxic appearing; however, she looks frail. Her vitals are BP 100/70, HR 100, Temp 98.7°F, 98% RA, RR 12. She has a dry mouth, sunken eyes, degenerative changes to her hands, but no jugular vein distention and no lower extremity edema. She is unable to complete the neurologic exam due to pain. On imaging, the patient was found to have multiple spine lesions concerning for metastatic disease. Her labs show elevated BUN and Cr compared to her baseline. What other vital details should be obtained to help determine her etiology of AKI?
   a. Home medications such as NSAIDs for pain, Lasix for CHF
   b. Patterns of her oral intake with her unintentional weight loss
   c. Monitoring of her urine output, including bladder scans, to monitor for urinary retention
   d. All the above

3. A 45-year-old male is admitted for elective cervical spine surgery. Preadmission testing revealed he had no past medical history, no home medications, and normal labs (CBC, basic metabolic panel [BMP], international normalized ratio/partial thromboplastin time). Postop day 2, the patient was noted to have BP 80s/60, HR 90, pulse ox 98% RA, and RR 12. A 1-L fluid bolus was given, and his BP improved to 95/70, and HR remained at 90. He was started on Celebrex for pain. Postop day 3, his BP was again 80s/60, but HR elevated to 110s. He required and additional 2 L fluid boluses. The patient denied any chest pain or shortness of breath but felt lightheaded when standing. Another bolus was given with minimal improvement. This patient is at risk of developing what type of AKI, and what should be done next?
   a. AIN from new start of Celebrex for pain; change pain medication
   b. Prerenal from hypovolemia; check CBC, BMP, lactate, transfuse for hemoglobin <7, and monitor urine output

   c. ATN; continue to give IV fluid resuscitation with normal saline

   d. He has progressed to CKD; consider for urgent dialysis

4. A 60-year-old male with past medical history of diabetes, hypertension, and chronic lower extremity edema is admitted for fever and low back pain. The low back pain started about 2 weeks ago and was causing him to have difficulty ambulating. He reported fevers at home and a relapse in his IV drug abuse. His home medications include Lantus and hydrochlorothiazide. On exam his vitals are temp 101.3°F, BP 90/70, HR 120, RR 18, and 99% RA. Overall, the patient is toxic appearing and diaphoretic, with tachycardia, tenderness to palpation of his lower back, and weakness of bilateral lower extremities with no rectal tone. CT with contrast showed an epidural abscess with cord compression, and the patient was taken emergently to the operating room. Postop, the patient was started on vancomycin and cefepime. What are the patient's risk factors for developing AKI, and what should be done in early-stage management?

   a. Sepsis causing prerenal AKI; volume status should be monitored postoperatively and patient should have daily labs until stabilized

   b. IV contrast causing ATN; fluid resuscitation prior and after administration of contrast

   c. ATN/AIN from antibiotics; therapeutic levels should be routinely monitored and dose adjusted for renal function

   d. All the above

Answers

1. b

2. d

3. b

4. d

CHAPTER 17

Nursing Management of the Patient With Arrhythmias and Acute Coronary Syndrome

Newton Mei, MD ▓ Grace Pae, MSN, CRNP

Introduction

Many older neurosurgical patients have comorbid cardiac disease, such as atrial fibrillation or coronary artery disease (CAD). Some patients with spine infections may have underlying endocarditis or sepsis that require telemetry monitoring. As a result, patients who have undergone neurosurgery are often placed on cardiac monitoring postoperatively to closely monitor for hemodynamic stability and potential cardiac dysfunction that may occur after surgery. Therefore nurses who care for neurosurgical patients should be well versed in interpreting cardiac rhythms on telemetry and understand the principles of advanced cardiac life support (ACLS). Nurses are at the bedside and are usually the first provider to recognize changes in a patient's status and cardiac rhythm on the monitor. By being able to anticipate and prepare for immediate life-threatening cardiac events, nurses can shorten the response time to interventions, potentially reducing the patient's length of stay and reducing mortality. The nurse's knowledge of cardiac rhythm interpretation, dysrhythmia detection, and bedside assessments can significantly minimize patient harm and improve patient outcomes.

Basics of the Heart

Blood is normally pumped through the heart in one direction and traverses through the four heart valves (e.g., tricuspid valve, pulmonic valve, mitral valve, and aortic valve). The blood returns deoxygenated from the body to the right atrium via the superior vena cava and inferior vena cava. From the right atrium, the blood flows through the tricuspid valve and into the right ventricle. It then is pumped through the pulmonary valve into the pulmonary system via the pulmonary arteries. Blood is oxygenated in the lungs and travels back to the left atrium via the pulmonary veins. The oxygenated blood continues down the mitral valve into the left ventricle and then is propelled past the aortic valve into the aorta and to the rest of the body again (Fig. 17.1).[1,2]

The body depends on the heart to pump blood to all vital organs. The heart has specialized pacemaker cells that initiate electrical activity, which is propagated throughout the heart to coordinate the contraction of heart muscle cells, also known as contractile cells (Fig. 17.2)[1]. The heart's natural pacemaker cells are grouped in the sinoatrial (SA) node, which normally has the highest intrinsic rate, sets the heart rate, and suppresses other pacemaker cells located in other parts of the heart, such as those in the atrioventricular (AV) node and Purkinje fibers.[3] The normal heart rate is between 60 and 100 beats per minute (bpm).[1] Normal electrical activity in the heart travels from the SA node to the AV node to the bundle of His, which divides into the right and left bundle

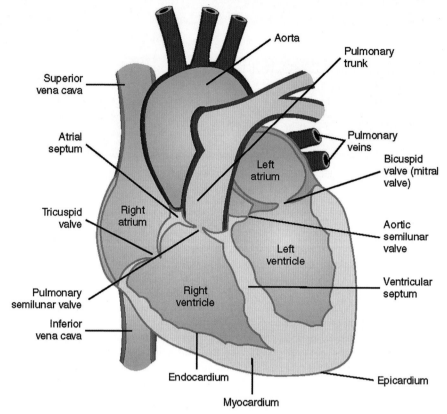

Fig. 17.1   Basic anatomy of the heart. (From Bonewit-West K, *Clinical Procedures for Medical Assistants*, 11th ed. Elsevier; 2022.)

branches, then to the Purkinje fibers.[2] As expected, injury or disturbances along this normal electrical pathway can lead to cardiac arrhythmias and can result in fluctuations in the heart rate.

Telemetry monitoring and electrocardiograms (ECGs) are physical tracings of the electrical activity of the heart. This information can be used to identify cardiac abnormalities, such as conduction delays, myocardial ischemia or infarctions, and electrolyte abnormalities. A normal cardiac cycle begins with the P wave, signifying the firing of the SA node, which leads to atrial depolarization and contraction. The QRS wave follows, signifying depolarization and ventricular contraction. Lastly, the T wave signifies ventricular repolarization and relaxation.[2] There are also four significant intervals: the PR interval, the QRS interval, the QT interval, and the ST segment.

- The PR interval indicates the time it takes from atrial depolarization to ventricular depolarization. Normal PR interval is between 0.12 and 0.2 second. An increased PR interval suggests conduction disease in the AV node.[2]
- The normal QRS interval is <0.10 second.[2] The QRS interval represents the time of ventricular depolarization and contraction. An increase in the QRS interval or a widening of the QRS complex suggests conduction disease such as that seen in bundle branch block (BBB).[2]
- The QT interval represents the time between ventricular depolarization and contraction to repolarization and relaxation. The normal range of the QT interval varies with the patient's heart rate. There are multiple formulas to help calculate the corrected QT (QTc). Many

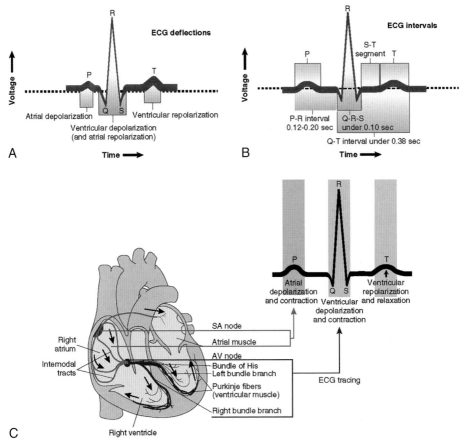

Fig. 17.2 The electrical activity of the heart. (A and B, From Patton KT, Thibodeau G. *Anatomy & Physiology*, 7th ed. Mosby; 2009; C, from Gould BE, Dyer RM. *Pathophysiology for the Health Professions*, 4th ed. Saunders; 2010.)

medications can prolong the QT interval, which can predispose the patient to a dangerous arrhythmia called torsades de pointes, also known as polymorphic ventricular tachycardia (VT).

- When QT prolonging medications are started or doses are adjusted, an ECG will be ordered to monitor their effect on the patient's QTc.[2]

- An elevation of the ST segment from baseline in contiguous leads on the ECG can suggests myocardial infarction, also known as an ST elevation myocardial infarction (STEMI). A depression of the ST segment from baseline can suggest myocardial ischemia or a non-ST elevation myocardial infarction (NSTEMI).[2]

Bradyarrhythmia, Tachyarrhythmia, and Acute Coronary Syndrome

OVERVIEW OF BRADYARRHYTHMIA

Bradycardia is defined as a heart rate <60 bpm.[1] When identified in patients, it is important to fully assess whether the bradycardia is normal versus pathologic. For example, athletes and well-conditioned individuals may have a sinus bradycardia in the 40s, and the bradycardia is considered normal.[4] On the other hand, a different patient who has a heart rate in the 40s but presents with syncope will need further cardiac monitoring and workup.[4] Therefore the clinical manifestation of bradycardia varies between patients. Some patients may be asymptomatic; others may present with syncope, dizziness/presyncope, fatigue, or generalized weakness.[4,5] In general, bradyarrhythmia can be divided into the following categories:

- Sinus node dysfunction (SND)
- Atrioventricular block (AVB)
- Conduction tissue disease

Sinus Node Dysfunction

SND, also known as sick sinus syndrome, is more common in patients age >65 and results from the age-related wear and tear of the sinus node.[6] Other causes of sinus node dysfunction include prior myocardial infarction or ischemia, infiltrating diseases such as sarcoidosis or amyloidosis, and autoimmune diseases.[4] The heart rate is usually <50 bpm and may be associated with sinus pauses >3 seconds.[5] A thorough review of medications that can affect the SA node, such as beta blockers and calcium channel blockers, should be done, and these medications should be adjusted or discontinued if able.[4] Other medical conditions, such as hypothyroidism, hypothermia, and electrolyte imbalances, should also be corrected to prevent exacerbation of the patient's bradycardia.[4] If asymptomatic, the patient can usually be observed without a need for pacemaker placement, but if the patient is symptomatic or has pauses >3 seconds a pacemaker may be indicated.[4]

Atrioventricular Block

The three types of AVB are first, second, and third degree.[2]

- A first-degree heart block is present when the PR interval is >200 milliseconds (ms) (Fig. 17.3).[2]
- A second-degree block can be divided into two types: Mobitz type I and type II (Figs. 17.4 and 17.5).
  - Mobitz type I, also known as Wenckebach, is characterized by the PR interval progressively increasing between heart beats, with an eventual nonconducted P wave.[2]
  - Second-degree AVB Mobitz type II is characterized by a constant PR interval with intermittent nonconducted P waves.[2]
- Third-degree block occurs when electrical activity that originates in the atrium is not conducted to the ventricles. P waves are seen marching on their own, and QRS waves are separately marching at their own rate[2] (Fig. 17.6).

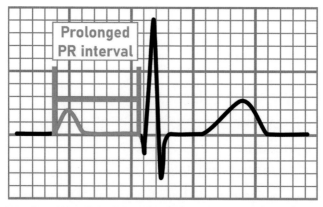

Fig. 17.3 First-degree heart block. (From Al-Hadithi, ABAK, Hobson A, Kirubakaran S. *The Unofficial Guide to ECGs.* Elsevier; 2023.)

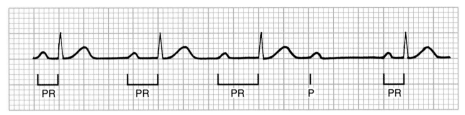

Fig. 17.4   Second-degree atrioventricular block, Mobitz type I. (From Goldberger A, Goldberger Z, Shvilkin A. Atrioventricular (AV) conduction abnormalities, part I: delays, blocks, and dissociation syndromes. In: *Goldberger's Clinical Electrocardiography: A Simplified Approach,* 9th ed. Elsevier; 2018:172–182.)

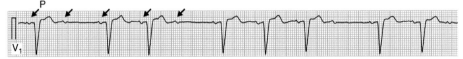

Fig. 17.5   Second-degree atrioventricular block, Mobitz type II. (From Goldberger A, Goldberger Z, Shvilkin A. Atrioventricular (AV) conduction abnormalities, part I: delays, blocks, and dissociation syndromes. In: *Goldberger's Clinical Electrocardiography: A Simplified Approach,* 9th ed. Elsevier; 2018:172–182.)

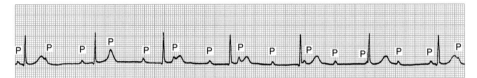

Fig. 17.6   Third-degree atrioventricular block. (From Goldberger A, Goldberger Z, Shvilkin A. Atrioventricular (AV) conduction abnormalities, part I: delays, blocks, and dissociation syndromes. In: *Goldberger's Clinical Electrocardiography: A Simplified Approach,* 9th ed. Elsevier; 2018:172–182.)

A pacemaker is recommended for advanced heart block, such as second-degree AVB Mobitz type II or third-degree AV block.[2,6]

Bundle Branch Block

The heart coordinates ventricular contraction via electrical activity through the bundle branches and Purkinje fibers. A BBB may be a result of injury to the heart muscle. A BBB results in a longer time for electrical activity to move through the heart muscle, resulting in a widening of the QRS interval on ECG. A new left BBB (LBBB) (Fig. 17.7) is more concerning than right BBB (RBBB) (see Fig. 17.7) because it suggests potential acute ischemic heart disease and underlying structural heart disease.[6]

Basic RBBB Criteria[6]
- Wide QRS, ≥120 ms
- RSR' morphology (bunny ears) in V1
- S wave in I and V6 ≥40 ms duration than R wave

Basic LBBB Criteria[6]
- Wide QRS, ≥120 ms
- Broad notched R wave in I, aVL, V5, V6
- No Q waves in I, V5, V6
- Dominant S wave in V1[2]

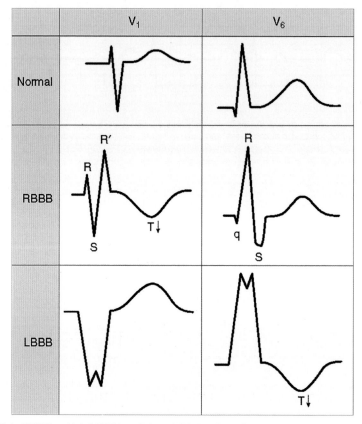

Fig. 17.7   Right *(RBBB)* and left *(LBBB)* bundle branch blocks. (From Goldberger AL, Goldberger ZD, Shvilkin A. *Goldberger's Clinical Electrocardiography: A Simplified Approach,* 9th ed. Elsevier; 2017.)

Overview of Tachyarrhythmia

Tachyarrhythmia can be grouped into two broad categories: supraventricular tachyarrhythmia (SVT) and ventricular tachyarrhythmia (VT). Recognizing the underlying rhythm in the acute hospital setting is key to management and treatment.

Supraventricular Tachycardia

SVT is a collection of rhythms that originate above the ventricles and produce a heart rate >100 bpm (Fig. 17.8). For example, sinus tachycardia, atrial fibrillation with a rapid ventricular rate, and atrial tachycardia are all part of the family of SVT. However, more commonly the term *paroxysmal SVT* is used to refer to regular, narrow-complex tachycardia, such as atrioventricular nodal reentrant tachycardia (AVNRT) and AV reentrant tachycardia (AVRT).[7] A heart rate >100 bpm with electrical activity that originates from the SA node is called sinus tachycardia. Symptoms associated with tachycardia are varied and can include palpitations, chest pain, lightheadedness, syncope, and anxiety.[7]

- Paroxysmal SVT: AVNRT, AVRT[7]
  - Reentrant SVT: most characteristic for its abrupt start and termination
  - Most common type of reentrant SVT: AVNRT

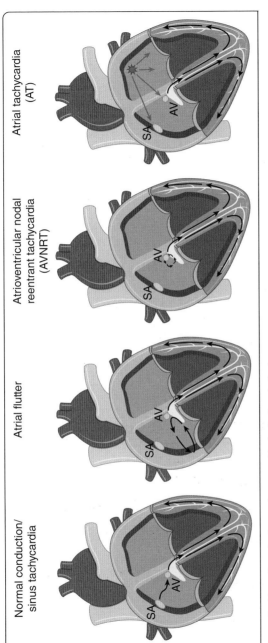

Fig. 17.8A Normal conduction and supraventricular tachyarrhythmias.

- Sinus tachycardia is a physiologic rhythm that is initiated at the sinus node and follows the normal conduction pathway: sinus atrial node → atrioventricular node → His bundle → Purkinje fibers.
- Atrial flutter is a reentrant electrical circuit that can loop around the tricuspid valve.
- Atrial fibrillation is an irregular rhythm that commonly starts from foci in the pulmonary veins and upper atria and results in disorganized electrical activity throughout the atria.
- Atrioventricular nodal reentrant tachycardia is the most common mechanism of what we commonly refer to as supraventricular tachycardia. There is a reentry circuit within or around the AV node.
- Atrial tachycardia occurs when electrical activity is transmitted from a focal site in the atria outside of the sinus node.
- Multifocal atrial tachycardia occurs when there are multiple sites in the atria sending out electrical activity.
- Atrioventricular reentrant tachycardia is a reentry circuit that involves an accessory pathway (white band).
- Orthodromic refers to when electrical activity in the reentrant loop is conducted in the normal direction through the AV node.
- Antidromic refers to when electrical activity in the reentrant loop is conducted in the opposite direction through the AV node.

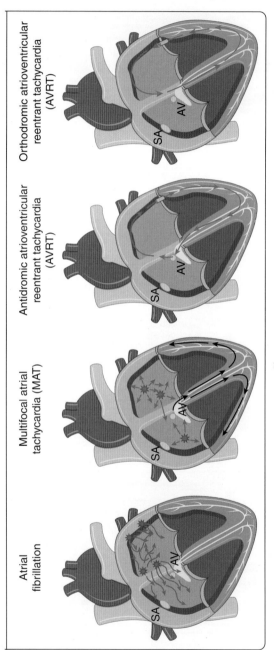

Fig. 17.8A cont'd

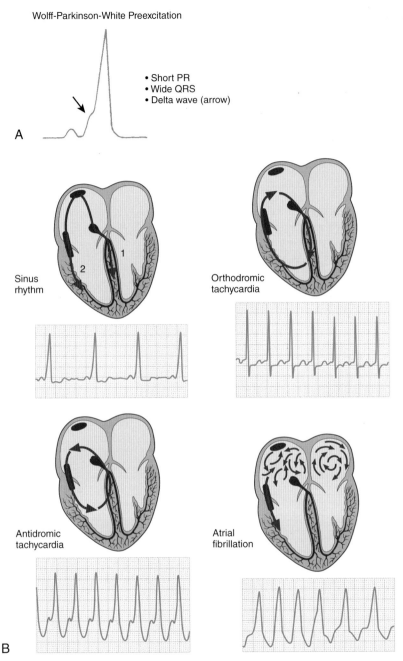

Wolff-Parkinson-White Preexcitation

- Short PR
- Wide QRS
- Delta wave (arrow)

A

Sinus rhythm

Orthodromic tachycardia

Antidromic tachycardia

Atrial fibrillation

B

Fig. 17.8B Wolff-Parkinson-White (WPW) syndrome. (A) Electrocardiogram demonstrating delta waves, where there is an upslope before the QRS complex as a result of premature ventricular depolarization by an early transmission of the action potentials via the accessory pathway (bundle of Kent). (B) Demonstration of the accessory pathway; recall that normally there is no other method for conducting impulses from the atria to the ventricles other than via the AV node. (A, From Goldberger AL, Goldberger ZD, Shvilkin A. *Clinical Electrocardiography: A Simplified Approach,* 8th ed. Saunders; 2012; B, from Colledge NR, Walker BR, Ralston SH. *Davidson's Principles and Practice of Medicine*, 21st ed. Elsevier; 2010.)

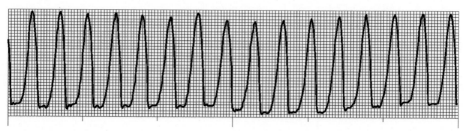

Fig. 17.9 Monomorphic ventricular tachycardia. (From Aehlert, B. (2004). *ECG Study Cards*. St. Louis: Mosby.)

- AVRT seen in Wolff-Parkinson-White (WPW) syndrome, which has a characteristic delta wave on the ECG (Fig. 17.9)
- Atrial tachycardia[7]
  - Electrical activity initiating from an atrial site outside the SA node
  - Focal atrial tachycardia: focal point of origin in the atrium, single P-wave morphology
  - Multifocal atrial tachycardia: multiple points of origin in the atrium, ≥3 distinct P-wave morphologies, irregular rate
- Atrial fibrillation[7]
  - Uncoordinated atrial activity
  - Common cardiac etiology of stroke in neurosurgical patients
  - Associated tachycardia is known as rapid ventricular response
  - ECG: absence of distinct P waves, irregular rate
- Atrial flutter[7]
  - Macroreentrant atrial tachycardia
  - Regular rhythm
  - Sawtooth-like flutter wave on ECG

Ventricular Tachyarrhythmia

Ventricular arrhythmia (VA) can range from premature ventricular complexes (PVC) to ventricular fibrillation (VF), which is deadly. The presence of PVCs is associated with increasing age, and frequent PVCs are associated with increased cardiovascular risk and mortality.[8] Three or more consecutive ventricular complexes that self-resolve are called nonsustained VT, and consecutive complexes lasting >30 seconds are considered sustained VT. VT can also be divided based on its morphology. If the QRS complex has the same shape across beats, it is described as monomorphic. If the QRS complex varies in shape with each beat, it is described as polymorphic[8] (Figs. 17.9, 17.10, and 17.11).

0 Sec.   3 Sec.   6 Sec.

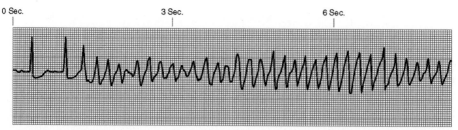

Fig. 17.10 Polymorphic ventricular tachycardia. (From Urden LD, Stacy KM, Lough ME. *Critical Care Nursing*. 9th ed. Elsevier; 2021.)

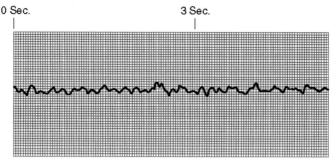

Fig. 17.11 Ventricular fibrillation. (From Urden LD, Stacy KM, Lough ME. *Priorities in Critical Care Nursing.* 9th ed. Elsevier; 2023.)

Patients who have a prolonged QT interval from congenital etiologies, electrolyte abnormalities (hypokalemia or hypomagnesemia), or medications are at higher risk of developing polymorphic VT, also known as torsades de pointes.[1]

VF occurs when there is disordered electrical activity in the ventricles. There is no coordinated ventricular activity, and the heart fails to pump effectively. Both monomorphic and polymorphic VT can degenerate to VF if not promptly treated. VF is not compatible with life and will quickly lead to death if not terminated.[1]

In clinical practice, the term *wide-complex tachycardia* is often used when the QRS on the cardiac monitor or ECG is wide (QRS interval ≥120 ms). All VAs have a wide QRS complex; however, it is important to note that patients with accessory pathways, such as those with WPW or BBB, will also have wide QRS complexes because of conduction aberrancy. Therefore it may be difficult to discern whether the patient is having VT versus SVT with aberrant conduction at first glance. Because VT is the more concerning dysrhythmia, the wide-complex tachycardia should be treated as VT until proven otherwise.[1]

General Management and Treatment of Arrhythmias

When a patient is complaining of cardiac symptoms or if the telemetry is showing a concerning rhythm, the nurse should immediately notify the primary team and feel empowered to initiate the following steps:

1. Assess the patient and ask about symptoms (note any change in mental status or chest discomfort).
2. Evaluate for hemodynamic stability: Measure vital signs and trend any changes (evaluate for hypotension, signs of shock, acute heart failure).
3. Ensure adequate intravenous (IV) access.
4. Print out the concerning cardiac monitoring strips or place the patient on a cardiac monitor if not already on one.[6]
5. Obtain an ECG.[6]

Nurses should alert their institution's rapid response team (RRT) if the patient is hemodynamically unstable, if the patient has a change in mental status, or if the patient's clinical status is deteriorating. Nurses should call a Code Blue and follow ACLS protocol if the patient is pulseless or goes into cardiac arrest.

Bradyarrhythmia Management and Treatment

- Identify and characterize the patient's symptoms associated with bradycardia.[6]
- Identify any factors and reversible causes that may have contributed to the patient's bradycardia[6]:

- Recent medications
- Recent patient activity (e.g., sleeping, eating, physical activity, repositioning, prolonged standing, urinating, defecating, straining, shaving)

The most common treatable causes of acute bradyarrhythmia are acute myocardial infarction, electrolyte abnormalities, hypothyroidism, medications, infection, and metabolic abnormalities.[6] Labs that may be ordered include[6]:

- Thyroid function tests to check for hypothyroidism
- Basic metabolic panel to check for electrolyte abnormalities
- Venous or arterial blood gas to check for metabolic derangements
- Lyme titer if Lyme carditis is suspected especially in a young patient with a new AV block
- Targeted labs to evaluate for infiltrative cardiac diseases, such as sarcoidosis if clinically suspected

If nocturnal bradycardia occurs, patients should undergo screening for sleep apnea. In this case, treatment of the underlying sleep disorder can mitigate bradycardia.[6] Sleep-disordered breathing is common in the United States with an estimated prevalence of >20% in males and close to 10% in females.[6]

Additional cardiac imaging is not recommended for asymptomatic sinus bradycardia or first-degree AV block with no evidence of structural heart disease. In patients with newly identified LBBB, second-degree Mobitz type II AV block, or third-degree AV block, they should undergo transthoracic echocardiography (TTE). For Mobitz type II AV block or third-degree AV block, electrophysiology (EP) cardiology should be consulted to evaluate for potential pacemaker placement.[6]

The following items should be at bedside for emergency situations with bradycardia[9]:

1. Nasal cannula for oxygenation
2. Bag valve mask for mechanical ventilation
3. IV fluids
4. Atropine
5. Transcutaneous pacer

If the patient is symptomatic and hemodynamically unstable, nurses should follow the ACLS adult bradycardia algorithm.[9] Atropine is a parasympatholytic drug that blocks muscarinic acetylcholine receptors at the SA and AV nodes, which results in an increase in heart rate.[5] Atropine, which is part of the ACS bradycardia algorithm, may also be ordered bedside for as-needed administration for cases of symptomatic bradycardia. Of note, atropine is not effective in complete heart block.

Other medications that may be used to increase heart rate include isoproterenol, dopamine, dobutamine, and epinephrine. These medications stimulate the beta receptors at the SA and AV nodes to increase heart rate. IV calcium can be given for calcium channel blocker overdose. Glucagon may be given for beta blocker or calcium channel blocker overdose.[5] For hemodynamically unstable patients who are unresponsive to medications, transcutaneous pacing may be necessary.[5]

Tachyarrhythmia Management and Treatment

- Identify and characterize the patient's symptoms associated with tachycardia.
- Identify any factors and reversible causes that may have contributed to the patient's tachycardia[7]:
  - Recent medications, caffeine intake, other substance ingestion (such as cocaine or stimulants)
  - For sinus tachycardia (presence of P waves followed by QRS on ECG or cardiac monitoring)
  - P waves are upright in leads I, II, aVF and biphasic in V1
  - Evaluate and treat the underlying physiologic causes.
  - Common causes include fever, sepsis, pain, anemia, anxiety, hypovolemia, hyperthyroidism, hypoglycemia, myocardial infarction, congestive heart failure, and pulmonary embolus.
  - Ivabradine can be prescribed for inappropriate sinus tachycardia.[10]

- Look at old ECGs to evaluate for delta waves that would suggest WPW.
- Determine if the rhythm has a wide QRS ≥120 ms, which may suggest VA.
- Ask what the patient was doing at the time of tachycardia (e.g., resting, physical activity, repositioning, wound dressing change).

When a patient is tachycardic, obtaining an ECG and placing a patient on the cardiac monitor will help to diagnose the underlying rhythm. Early recognition of dangerous arrhythmias will lead to improved survival.[7]

Labs that may be ordered include[10]:

- Thyroid function tests to check for hyperthyroidism
- Basic metabolic panel to check for electrolyte abnormalities
- Complete blood count to evaluate for anemia
- Magnesium level to evaluate for hypomagnesemia

The following items should be at bedside in emergency situations with tachycardia[9]:

1. Nasal cannula for oxygenation
2. Bag valve mask for mechanical ventilation
3. IV fluids
4. Adenosine
5. Synchronized cardioversion/defibrillator

Nurses should be aware of the common medications ordered for narrow-complex (QRS <120 ms) tachyarrhythmias:

- Adenosine[7]
  - Recommended in the ACLS protocol for tachycardia
  - Administration can cause chest discomfort, shortness of breath, flushing, and low blood pressure (BP).[7]
  - Sometimes with a fast heart rate it is hard to discern the underlying rhythm. Adenosine causes a temporary AV block, which will slow the heart rate and can potentially terminate paroxysmal SVT if present.[7]
  - If adenosine use reveals the underlying rhythm to be atrial flutter or atrial fibrillation, medications such as beta blockers, calcium channel blockers, or amiodarone may be used to slow the heart rate.
  - Administration must be given through a proximal IV and immediately followed by a saline flush. Continuous ECG should be done during the entire administration.[7]
  - Adenosine use may not be appropriate in patients with advanced AV block, WPW, severe chronic obstructive pulmonary disease/reactive airway disease, or those who are on verapamil/digoxin.[7]
- Beta blockers (atenolol, metoprolol, nadolol, esmolol, propranolol, etc.)[7]
  - Blocks conduction at the AV node
  - Can lead to hypotension, bronchospasm
- Calcium channel blockers (diltiazem or verapamil[7])
  - Blocks conduction at the AV node
  - Can lead to hypotension, liver injury, worsening heart failure
  - Interacts with other medications that are metabolized by the liver
- Digoxin[7]
  - Blocks conduction at the AV node
  - Need to monitor digoxin levels (digoxin toxicity associated with levels >2 ng/mL)
  - Symptoms of digoxin toxicity include anorexia, nausea, vomiting, vision changes
  - Need to be dosed renally
  - Can interact with other medications
- Amiodarone[7]
  - Can cause hypotension; lung, thyroid, corneal, and liver dysfunction

- ■ Interacts with other medications
- ■ Prolongs QT
- ■ Other antiarrhythmics[7]
  - ■ Cardiology/EP may be consulted to assist with medication management to determine if other antiarrhythmics are appropriate and whether an EP study with ablation is appropriate.

Focal Atrial Tachycardia[7,10]

For patients who are hemodynamically stable, the following may be ordered:
- ■ Adenosine, beta blockers, calcium channel blockers
  - ■ If above is ineffective, antiarrhythmics such as ibutilide, flecainide, propafenone, or amiodarone
  - ■ If above is ineffective, synchronized cardioversion may be warranted

For patients who are hemodynamically unstable, the following may be ordered:
- ■ Adenosine if feasible, otherwise synchronized cardioversion will be done

Afterwards, EP may be consulted to determine whether patient is an ablation candidate if the focal atrial tachycardia is recurrent or persistent.

Multifocal Atrial Tachycardia[7,10]

- ■ This is associated with underlying lung and heart disease, low magnesium, or theophylline use.
- ■ Treat underlying disease.
- ■ IV magnesium may be beneficial.
- ■ Beta blockers and calcium channel blockers can be used to slow the heart rate in acute settings.
- ■ If refractory to drug therapy, patient may require EP consultation and potential ablation.

Paroxysmal SVT: AVNRT and Orthodromic AVRT. If the patient is hemodynamically stable with regular SVT, it is reasonable to first attempt vagal maneuvers if clinically feasible. In general, effective vagal maneuvers are done to trigger the vagus nerve to slow the heart rate. Examples of vagal maneuvers include:
- ■ Carotid massage
- ■ Bearing down against a closed glottis for 10–30 seconds
- ■ Inducing the diving reflex by applying an ice-cold towel to the face

If vagal maneuvers are ineffective, the next recommended step along the ACLS pathway is to administer adenosine (if no contraindications) or use beta blockers and calcium channel blockers. If these medications are ineffective or contraindicated, IV amiodarone may be used. If medications are unsuccessful, synchronized cardioversion and EP consultation will be appropriate.[7]

If the patient is hemodynamically unstable with regular SVT, then synchronized cardioversion is recommended per ACLS protocol[7,9] (Fig. 17.12).

Atrial Flutter/Atrial Fibrillation.[7,10,11] For patients who are hemodynamically stable, the following is indicated:
- ■ Beta blockers or calcium channel blockers
- ■ Digoxin
- ■ Amiodarone or other antiarrhythmics
- ■ Discussion with cardiology/EP regarding (pharmacologic vs synchronized) cardioversion vs ablation

For hemodynamically unstable patients, synchronized cardioversion is indicated.

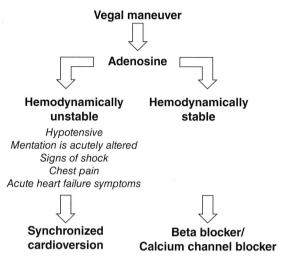

Fig. 17.12 Paroxysmal supraventricular tachycardia management.

Patients with underlying atrial flutter are at a higher risk for stroke. The CHA2DS2-VASc score can be used to risk stratify these patients and determine whether anticoagulation would be beneficial to prevent stroke.[11]

Ventricular Tachyarrhythmia Management and Treatment

Management of VA is challenging and often will require specialist input from cardiology/EP. The nurse's role is primarily to recognize these dangerous rhythms, promptly notify the medical team, activate a RRT/code blue if there are concerns for hemodynamic instability, and follow through with the ACLS protocol. In the acute treatment of a patient with VA, nurses and all providers must first determine if the patient is hemodynamically stable or unstable and assess for a pulse.

- In hemodynamically stable patients with a pulse with monomorphic VT or episodes of nonsustained VT, a 12-lead ECG should be done. Further imaging studies, such as echocardiography, cardiac magnetic resonance imaging, or cardiac computed tomography angiography, may be ordered to further evaluate for underlying structural heart disease. An ischemic workup should be done in all patients with sustained VT, and revascularization should be performed if indicated. Patients may be ordered beta blockers and antiarrhythmics, such as IV procainamide, IV amiodarone, or IV sotalol. Magnesium and potassium should be repleted.[8]
- In hemodynamically unstable patients with a pulse with monomorphic VT, synchronized cardioversion is recommended, and the ACLS protocol should be followed.
- In hemodynamically unstable patients without a pulse with monomorphic VT or VF, defibrillation is recommended, and the ACLS protocol should be followed[8] (Fig. 17.13).
- In patients with polymorphic VT also known as torsades de pointes, the first-line therapy is administration of IV magnesium. Magnesium can help suppress recurrent episodes and prevent degeneration into VF.[1] Medications that prolong the QT interval should be held/discontinued.[1]

Patients with VA should be evaluated by cardiology/EP to optimize medical management and determine if an ablation procedure or an implantable cardioverter defibrillator placement is indicated.[8]

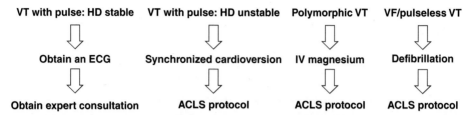

Fig. 17.13 Flowchart for the management of ventricular arrhythmias. The initial intervention for ventricular arrhythmia varies depending on the following: (1) the identified rhythm: monomorphic or polymorphic ventricular tachycardia *(VT)* or ventricular fibrillation *(VF)*, (2) whether the patient has a pulse, and (3) whether the patient is hemodynamically *(HD)* stable. *ACLS,* Advanced Cardiac Life Support; *ECG,* electrocardiogram; *IV,* intravenous.

Overview of Acute Coronary Syndrome

In CAD, atherosclerotic plaques form in the arteries that supply blood flow to the heart musculature. In acute coronary syndrome (ACS), these plaques may rupture or erode, causing thrombus formation, and leading to a sudden partial or complete blockage of blood flow within the coronary arteries and myocardial injury.[12] ACS can be subdivided into three types: STEMI, NSTEMI, and unstable angina (UA).[13]

- STEMI is the result of a complete occlusion by the thrombosis.[1]
  - ECG shows ST elevations in contiguous leads.
  - STEMI has elevated cardiac biomarkers such as troponins.
- UA and NSTEMI are the result of incomplete occlusion by the thrombus.[1]
  - ECG can show ST depressions and/or T wave inversions suggestive of ischemia.[1]
  - UA and NSTEMI are distinguished by the presence of elevated cardiac biomarkers such as troponins.
    - UA does not have elevated biomarkers.
    - NSTEMI has elevated biomarkers.

Symptoms of angina/cardiac chest pain related to ACS include[14]:
- Left-sided substernal chest pain/discomfort
- Descriptions such as pressure, squeezing, tightness, crushing, or heaviness
- Associated symptoms: diaphoresis, nausea, syncope, dyspnea
- Can radiate to the jaw, back arms, or shoulder
- Worsens with activity/emotional stress
- Relieved with rest or sublingual nitroglycerin
- Some patients (e.g., the elderly, patients with diabetes, females) may not have chest pain and will present with atypical symptoms of angina.
  - Patients who have had ACS in the past should be asked about their prior symptoms (anginal equivalent).
  - Some anginal equivalents include epigastric pain, confusion, nausea/vomiting, or shortness of breath.

Acute Coronary Syndrome Management and Treatment

When a patient develops acute chest pain/angina, the nurses should first assess the patient, obtain vital signs to assess for hemodynamic stability, and obtain an ECG.[14] The patient's medical team should also be notified immediately, and nurses should follow the ACLS protocol for ACS. If the patient is hemodynamically unstable, an RRT/code blue should also be activated. If the patient is hemodynamically stable, the nurse can ask the patient questions to better characterize the chest pain.

The newly obtained ECG should be compared with any available prior ECGs to facilitate the detection of any new ischemic changes, such as ST elevations, ST depressions, T-wave inversions, hyperacute T waves, or new LBBB. ECGs that are initially without ischemic changes may be repeated serially to potentially capture ischemic changes that appear later as the patient's ACS evolves.[14]

If ECG indicates a STEMI, the patient will need an emergent cardiac catheterization (also known as invasive coronary angiography) for potential percutaneous coronary intervention (PCI), such as a cardiac stent placement. This should ideally occur within 90 minutes of presentation. In centers where PCI is unavailable or if PCI is delayed, patients without major contraindications (such as prior intracranial hemorrhage, cerebral lesions, stroke in the last 3 months, active bleeding, head or face trauma, recent surgery, uncontrolled hypertension) should receive fibrinolytic therapy, such as alteplase. Afterwards, the patient should then be transferred to a facility where PCI can be done.[13,15]

If the ECG does not show ST elevations but has ST depressions and T-wave inversions concerning for a UA or NSTEMI, cardiac troponins can further assist with diagnosis and management. Elevated troponins that continue to rise are concerning for NSTEMI.[14] Of note, with the development of high-sensitivity troponins, many institutions have laboratory algorithms in place that allow for a rapid rule-out of acute myocardial injury in patients with chest pain or angina but no significant ECG changes. Nurses should be aware of whether high-sensitivity troponins are available at their institution and be familiar with the associated laboratory algorithm used to rule in or out acute myocardial injury.[13]

For patients with a UA/NSTEMI, a TTE may be done at bedside to assess for ventricular dysfunction and wall motion abnormalities. A TTE can also offer insight to other possible cardiopulmonary etiologies for chest pain, such as valvular dysfunction, pulmonary embolus, or pericarditis.[14] For high-risk patients with UA/NSTEMI with persistent chest pain and ECG changes, cardiology will likely recommend cardiac catheterization. If significant obstructive lesions are identified during the angiography, revascularization with PCI or coronary artery bypass graft (CABG) may be done.

For all patients with ACS, optimal medical management is paramount and starts immediately at the time of patient presentation. Nurses should be familiar with the following therapies that may be ordered for the patient and administer the medications accordingly:

- Aspirin (acetylsalicylic acid [ASA]) 162–325 mg[16]
  - When there is a concern for ACS, the patient should first chew a non-enteric-coated aspirin unless there is a contraindication or severe allergy to aspirin.
  - ASA will be continued indefinitely in a patient after a myocardial infarction.[16]
  - Part of dual antiplatelet therapy (DAPT)
    - DAPT is indicated in patients after PCI with cardiac stent placement.
- Nitroglycerin[16]
  - Sublingual nitroglycerin can be given to patients every 5 minutes as needed for chest pain for a total of 3 doses.
  - If chest pain persists despite sublingual nitroglycerin, IV nitroglycerin may be started.
  - Can result in hypotension
  - Contraindicated in patients who recently took a phosphodiesterase inhibitor such as sildenafil and vardenafil within the last 24 hours or tadalafil within the last 48 hours
- Oxygen therapy[16]
  - Apply oxygen therapy for oxygen saturations <90% or in patients with respiratory distress.
- IV morphine[16]
  - Can help with chest pain and dyspnea
- Beta blockers (metoprolol, carvedilol, bisoprolol)[16]
  - Should be started within the first 24 hours of ACS presentation
  - Avoid in patients who have signs of heart failure, shock, or other contraindications to beta blockers.

- High-intensity HMG-CoA reductase inhibitor statins[16]
  - Improves outcomes and decreases mortality after myocardial infarction.
- Angiotensin-converting enzyme inhibitors/angiotensin receptor blockers[16]
  - Recommended for patients with left ventricular ejection fraction <40% on an echo-cardiogram or in patients with hypertension, stable chronic kidney disease, or diabetes mellitus.
- P2Y12 inhibitors (clopidogrel and ticagrelor)[16]
  - May be started in addition to ASA
  - Part of DAPT, which is indicated in patients who had a cardiac stent placed
- Anticoagulation (enoxaparin, unfractionated heparin)[16]
  - Enoxaparin should be avoided in patients with a creatinine clearance <30 mL/min
  - Unfractionated heparin requires partial thromboplastin time monitoring and is continued for 48 hours or until PCI is completed.
  - Monitor for bleeding
- Glycoprotein IIb/IIIa inhibitors (tirofiban, eptifibatide)[16]
  - May be used in patients with planned cardiac catheterization and PCI
  - Monitor for bleeding

Conclusion

Many neurosurgical patients have comorbid conditions that predispose them to potential cardiac dysfunction. Furthermore, in the neurosurgery patient, cardiac rhythm disturbances usually occur within the first 7 days after a brain injury.[17] Therefore nurses caring for neurosurgical patients in the perioperative setting in the hospital need to be comfortable with the diagnosis and management of arrhythmias and ACS. These patients require focused assessments to determine hemodynamic stability, rhythm interpretation, and the use of available resources to guide appropriate management.

Neurosurgical nurses are often the first to identify and assess patients with cardiac complaints and detect arrhythmias on the cardiac monitoring. The nurse should be able to identify concerning assessment findings and rhythm changes before it becomes life threatening. Ultimately, early recognition of cardiac arrest improves mortality, and a delay in defibrillation time was associated with a higher risk of death and decline in neurologic or functional status.[18]

Hospital leadership should facilitate and promote the nurse's ability to interpret cardiac monitoring, set cardiac monitoring alarms appropriately (to reduce false and nonactionable alarms that cause alarm fatigue and sentinel events), correctly document rhythm changes, and respond to emergency and nonemergency cardiac events. This can be achieved through instituting mandatory comprehensive orientation and training programs, assessing staff competency, establishing measures of quality, and conducting periodic competency review evaluations. Such quality measures can increase the identification of life-threatening arrhythmia, improve diagnostic accuracy of rhythm interpretation, and promote adequacy of staffing (in number and quality).[19]

References

1. Lilly LS. *Pathophysiology of Heart Disease: A Collaborative Project of Medical Students and Faculty.* Lippincott Williams & Wilkins; 2012.
2. Green JM, Chiaramida AJ. *12-Lead EKG Confidence: A Step-by-Step Guide.* Springer Publishing Company; 2014.
3. Antzelevitch C, Burashnikov A. Overview of basic mechanisms of cardiac arrhythmia. *Card Electrophysiol Clin.* 2011;3(1):23–45.
4. Mangrum JM, DiMarco JP. The evaluation and management of bradycardia. *N Engl J Med.* 2000;342(10):703–709.
5. Sidhu S, Marine JE. Evaluating and managing bradycardia. *Trends Cardiovasc Med.* 2020;30(5):265–272.

6. Kusumoto FM, Schoenfeld MH, Barrett C, et al. 2018 ACC/AHA/HRS guideline on the evaluation and management of patients with bradycardia and cardiac conduction delay: executive summary: a report of the American College of Cardiology/American Heart Association task force on clinical practice guidelines, and the Heart Rhythm Society. *J Am Coll Cardiol.* 2019;74(7):932–987.
7. Page RL, Joglar JA, Caldwell MA, et al. 2015 ACC/AHA/HRS guideline for the management of adult patients with supraventricular tachycardia: a report of the American College of Cardiology/American Heart Association task force on clinical practice guidelines and the Heart Rhythm Society. *Circulation.* 2016;133(14):e506–e574.
8. Al-Khatib SM, Stevenson WG, Ackerman MJ, et al. 2017 AHA/ACC/HRS guideline for management of patients with ventricular arrhythmias and the prevention of sudden cardiac death: a report of the American College of Cardiology/American Heart Association task force on clinical practice guidelines and the Heart Rhythm Society. *J Am Coll Cardiol.* 2018;72(14):e91–e220.
9. Panchal AR, Bartos JA, Cabañas JG, et al. Part 3: adult basic and advanced life support: 2020 American Heart Association guidelines for cardiopulmonary resuscitation and emergency cardiovascular care. *Circulation.* 2020;142(16/2):S366–S468.
10. Brugada J, Katritsis DG, Arbelo E, et al. 2019 ESC guidelines for the management of patients with supraventricular tachycardia the task force for the management of patients with supraventricular tachycardia of the European Society of Cardiology (ESC) developed in collaboration with the Association for European Paediatric and Congenital Cardiology (AEPC). *Eur Heart J.* 2020;41(5):655–720.
11. January CT, Wann LS, Calkins H, et al. 2019 AHA/ACC/HRS focused update of the 2014 AHA/ACC/HRS guideline for the management of patients with atrial fibrillation: a report of the American College of Cardiology/American Heart Association task force on clinical practice guidelines and the Heart Rhythm Society in collaboration with the Society of Thoracic Surgeons. *Circulation.* 2019;140(2):e125–e151.
12. Libby P. Mechanisms of acute coronary syndromes and their implications for therapy. *N Engl J Med.* 2013;368(21):2004–2013.
13. Bhatt DL, Lopes RD, Harrington RA. Diagnosis and treatment of acute coronary syndromes: a review. *JAMA.* 2022;327(7):662–675.
14. Gulati M, Levy PD, Mukherjee D, et al. 2021 AHA/ACC/ASE/CHEST/SAEM/SCCT/SCMR guideline for the evaluation and diagnosis of chest pain: a report of the American College of Cardiology/American Heart Association joint committee on clinical practice guidelines. *J Am Coll Cardiol.* 2021;78(22):e187–e285.
15. O'gara PT, Kushner FG, Ascheim DD, et al. 2013 ACCF/AHA guideline for the management of ST-elevation myocardial infarction: a report of the American College of Cardiology Foundation/American Heart Association task force on practice guidelines. *J Am Coll Cardiol.* 2013;61(4):e78–e140.
16. Amsterdam EA, Wenger NK, Brindis RG, et al. 2014 AHA/ACC guideline for the management of patients with non–ST-elevation acute coronary syndromes: executive summary: a report of the American College of Cardiology/American Heart Association task force on practice guidelines. *Circulation.* 2014;130(25):2354–2394.
17. Gregory T, Smith M. Cardiovascular complications of brain injury. *Crit Care Pain.* 2012;12(2):67–71.
18. Chen L, Nallamothu B, Spertus J, et al. Association between a hospital's rate of cardiac arrest incidence and cardiac arrest survival. *JAMA Intern Med.* 2013;173(13):1186–1195.
19. Drew BJ, Califf RM, Funk M, et al. Practice standards for electrocardiographic monitoring in hospital settings: an American Heart Association scientific statement from the councils on cardiovascular nursing, clinical cardiology, and cardiovascular disease in the young: endorsed by the International Society of Computerized Electrocardiology and the American Association of Critical-Care Nurses. *Circulation.* 2004;110(17):2721–2746.

Questions

A 65-year-old male patient with a history of diabetes mellitus, congestive heart failure, hyperlipidemia, and hypertension is reporting palpitations on the floor. His vital signs are BP 125/75, respirations 21 breaths/min, and he has an irregular heart rate in the 130s.

1. What are the initial first steps?
    a. Obtain an ECG.
    b. Contact the primary team.
    c. Recheck vital in 4 hours as per protocol.
    d. Both a and b.

2. What medications might be appropriate?
   a. Aspirin
   b. Beta blockers or calcium channel blockers
   c. Ativan for anxiety
   d. Insulin

3. What can the nurse have ready in advance if the patient's condition deteriorates?
   a. IV equipment to ensure access
   b. Bag valve mask, oxygen/nasal cannula
   c. Cardioversion/defibrillator
   d. All of the above

4. What is not a typical sign of acute coronary syndrome?
   a. Often described as "crushing" or "heavy"
   b. Radiates to the jaw, back, arms, or left shoulder
   c. Improves with activity
   d. Associated with diaphoresis, nausea, syncope, dyspnea

5. Why should nursing obtain a troponin and ECG?
   a. To decide if patient should transfer to the cardiology service
   b. To decide if the patient is appropriate for discharge
   c. To evaluate for heart failure exacerbation
   d. To evaluate for cardiac ischemia

Answers

1. d

2. b

3. d

4. c

5. d

CHAPTER 18

Anticoagulation for Venothromboembolism

Lauren Malinowski-Falk, MSN, BA, CRNP, AGACNP-BC
▦ Dina G. Orapallo, MSN, AGACNP-BC ▦ Heather Lynn Yenser, MSN
▦ Anthony Joseph Macchiavelli, MD, SFHM, FACP

Introduction

Neurosurgical patients often experience periods of immobility from the pathology of their spine or brain injuries and from the pain associated with neurologic surgeries. These factors place patients at an increased risk for the development of venous thromboembolism (VTE). According to the Centers for Disease Control and Prevention, a VTE is defined as a blood clot in the venous system and includes both deep vein thrombosis (DVT) and pulmonary embolism (PE).[1]

An untreated DVT can lead to worsening pain and swelling of the affected area. Untreated DVTs can extend and spread and travel to other organs (such as with PE). An untreated PE can lead to potentially serious and life-threatening adverse effects, which include hypoxia, hypotension, and death. Long-term sequelae, such as chronic thromboembolic pulmonary hypertension or postthrombotic syndrome, can also result. In fact, PE is the leading cause of preventable hospital deaths in the United States.[2] To prevent these complications, quick recognition and workup of a DVT is of paramount importance.

Nurses play a critical role in the prevention, detection, and management of VTE. At the bedside, nurses are often the first to recognize the signs and symptoms of VTE and subsequently then are the first to notify the provider to initiate workup. Furthermore, as the treatment for VTE is often anticoagulation (blood thinners), which can cause dangerous bleeding complications, nurses need to feel comfortable providing patients with thorough education to continue self-monitoring after discharge. Overall, having a complete understanding of the pathology, prevention, symptom recognition/diagnosis, and treatment of DVT and PE is essential to providing optimal patient care and improving patient outcomes (Table 18.1).

DEFINITIONS

DVT: A thrombosis occurs when a VTE develops in an area of decreased/diminished blood flow. This commonly occurs in the deep veins of the legs, often near valves. While valves in the veins normally aim to promote blood flow, they can also cause venous stasis and hypoxia.[3]

- Signs and symptoms include asymmetric swelling, redness, warmth, and pain in an extremity.[3]
- If the clot travels through the venous system, it can lodge in the vessels of the lung, leading to PE.[1]

PE: A blockage in the lung's blood vessels due to a blood clot. This disrupts blood flow, causes lung damage, and decreases oxygen levels.

- Signs and symptoms include tachycardia, tachypnea, dyspnea, hypoxia, and pleuritic chest discomfort.[4]

TABLE 18.1 ■ **Epidemiology Facts**

1. There are as many as 900,000 new venous thromboembolism (VTE) events diagnosed annually in the United States.
2. 10–30% of the people diagnosed with VTE will die within 1 month of their diagnosis.
3. There are ~548,000 hospitalizations each year in the United States due to VTE.
4. It is estimated that 100,000 deaths in the United States are directly related to pulmonary embolism.
5. There are $10+ billion associated health care costs due to VTE annually.
6. It is estimated that one-third of the population with a diagnosis of VTE will have a recurrence within the next 10 years.

Data from Centers for Disease Control and Prevention. Data and statistics on venous thromboembolism. February 7, 2020. https://www.cdc.gov/ncbddd/dvt/data.html#:~:text=Estimates%20suggest%20that%20 60%2C000%2D100%2C000,within%20one%20month%20of%20diagnosis.

Diagnostics

The diagnosis of DVT is done through a venous duplex ultrasound.

- An ultrasound probe is used to compress the veins of the extremity, and an inability to compress the vein is diagnostic of DVT.[3]
- Ultrasound imaging can accurately determine the size, chronicity, and degree of occlusion of the thrombus.[3]

The gold standard for diagnosing PE is a computed tomography angiogram (CTA PE).[4] Alternatively, if renal function or contrast dye allergy is a concern, the patient can undergo a ventilation/perfusion scan (VQ scan), and if hemodynamic instability is a concern, the patient can undergo an echocardiogram (ECHO). These alternative studies are considered less accurate.[4]

- **CTA PE**: A CT scan of the chest that uses intravenous (IV) contrast to examine the pulmonary arteries and veins.[4]
- **VQ scan**: A scan that uses radioactive tracer material to examine air flow and blood flow in the lungs.[4]
- **ECHO**: A study that shows findings of right-sided cardiac abnormalities (such as right ventricular [RV] dilation, right heart strain, and increased RV afterload), which suggest the presence of PE.[4]

Causes and Classification of VTE

VTE is classified as either provoked or unprovoked. This classification assists with determining the duration of treatment for VTE.[5] A provoked VTE has a direct underlying cause for the thrombus formation, such as direct trauma or injury to the leg, whereas an unprovoked VTE does not have a clear underlying cause.[6] Factors that place a patient at higher risk for VTE include recent surgery or trauma, malignancy, prolonged immobility, pregnancy, congestive heart failure, varicose veins, obesity, advancing age, and a history of DVT.[3]

Rudolf Virchow, a German physician, discovered three factors that could potentially lead to venous thrombosis formation: venous stasis (when the blood pools in the legs and is unable to be pumped efficiently to the heart), hypercoagulability (altered coagulation pathways in the body), and endothelial injury (damage to the blood vessel wall during trauma or surgery, or vascular inflammation).[6] Today this triad is known as Virchow triad.[6] While venous stasis alone is usually insufficient to cause clot formation, the risk increases when combined with vascular inflammation or hypercoagulability (Fig. 18.1).[3]

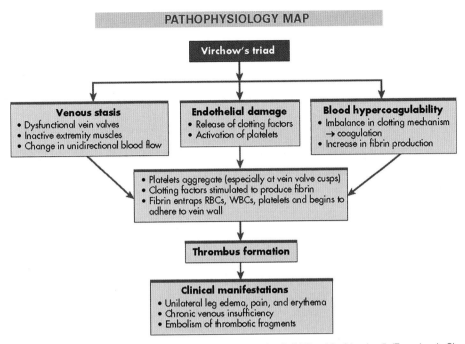

Fig. 18.1 Pathophysiology of Virchow triad. *RBC,* Red blood cell; *WBC,* white blood cell. (From Lewis SL, Dirksen SR, Heitkemper M, et al. *Medical-Surgical Nursing: Assessment and Management of Clinical Problems,* 8th ed. Mosby/Elsevier; 2011.)

DVT Prophylaxis

To decrease the risk of VTE, institutions have implemented DVT prophylaxis protocols. These protocols are designed to combat the risk factors defined in Virchow triad and will often utilize both mechanical/nonpharmacologic and pharmacologic methods. The combination of both methods has been shown to be more effective in VTE prevention (due to an additive effect) than using mechanical/nonpharmacologic or pharmacologic prophylaxis alone.[2]

In the hospital, VTE prophylaxis should be initiated as soon as the risk of immobility begins, often on admission.[3] However, many hospitalized patients will undergo an invasive procedure, and the risk of bleeding during/after the procedure increases with pharmacologic prophylaxis. Therefore nurses must initiate mechanical/nonpharmacologic treatments first (unless contraindicated), then start pharmacologic prophylaxis when cleared by the provider/surgical team.[2]

- Mechanical/nonpharmacologic prophylaxis
  - Early ambulation
    - Used to combat venous stasis while aiding in overall recovery and quicker return to function
  - Intermittent pneumatic compression devices
    - Works by pumping venous blood and reducing stasis
    - Different models available to provide compression to the feet, calf, or up to the thigh
    - Method of choice if unable to use pharmacologic prophylaxis, but only effective if used continuously while patients are nonambulatory[2]
    - Complications: discomfort and skin breakdown, also may not provide enough pressure in obese individuals to compress the deep veins effectively[2]

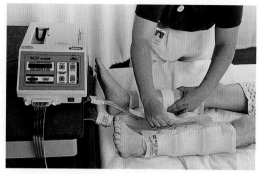

Fig. 18.2 Application of sequential compression stockings, a common form of mechanical venous thrombo-embolism prophylaxis. (From Astle BJ, Duggleby W. *Potter and Perry's Canadian Fundamentals of Nursing*, 7th ed. Elsevier; 2023.)

- Elastic stockings
  - Used to improve venous blood flow and reduce the amount of endothelial injury caused by passive venous dilation that occurs during surgery[2]
  - Complications: improperly fitting stocking may increase venous pressure, which results in delayed venous emptying and an increased risk of VTE (Fig. 18.2)[2]
- Pharmacologic prophylaxis
  - Antiplatelets and low-dose anticoagulation medication
    - Can include low-dose unfractionated heparin, aspirin, warfarin, and low-molecular-weight heparins (LMWH)[2]
    - Complication: bleeding
- Especially risky in the neurosurgical population, as bleeding can cause a hematoma in the brain or spine, leading to devastating neurologic changes
- Initiation of antiplatelet/anticoagulant therapy postoperatively to be discussed with the patient's surgeon

Best Practice in VTE Management

It is imperative to begin treatment once the diagnosis of VTE has been made. With severe, limb-threatening DVTs, providers may consider a more rapid thrombus resolution with mechanical or chemical thrombolysis procedures to rapidly break up the clot.[3] However, more commonly, anticoagulation is prescribed. Anticoagulation interferes with the body's ability to clot, which allows the body to break down existing clots over time.[7] Furthermore, they can aid in symptom resolution, reduce the risk of progression to PE, and prevent new thrombus from forming.[3]

Historically, anticoagulant choices were limited to IV heparin or LMWH for initial therapy, with transition to a vitamin K antagonist (such as warfarin) for treatment duration. The introduction of direct oral anticoagulants (DOACs) created a shift in the first-line treatment choice.[8] DOACs available in the United States for treatment of VTE include apixaban, dabigatran, edoxaban, and rivaroxaban.

DOACs have been shown to have fewer drug interactions, can all be taken orally, and do not require frequent laboratory monitoring to ensure therapeutic levels.[3] They are metabolized in the liver or kidneys, so careful consideration should be taken before prescribing them in patients with altered liver or renal function.[8] Furthermore, they have a long half-life. As a result, patients may require administration of a reversal agent if life-threatening bleeding is a concern or will be required to hold the anticoagulation in advance of any surgical procedure.

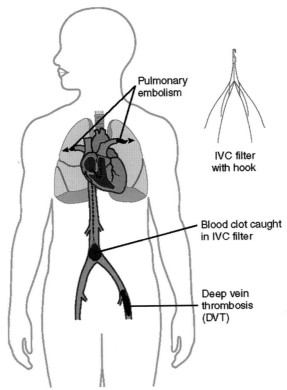

Fig. 18.3   Placement of inferior vena cava *(IVC)* filter to prevent clots from traveling to the lungs. (From Harding MM, Kwong J, Hagler D, et al. *Lewis's Medical-Surgical Nursing: Assessment and Management of Clinical Problems*, 12th ed. Elsevier; 2022.)

Inferior Vena Cava Filter

Sometimes patients who are diagnosed with a VTE cannot safely receive anticoagulation. Often this occurs in patients with recent bleeding (e.g., gastrointestinal bleed), recent surgery (where starting anticoagulation could lead to postop hematoma formation), or a planned upcoming surgery (where anticoagulation can cause life-threatening bleeding). In these cases, consideration should be given for an inferior vena cava (IVC) filter placement. An IVC filter is a mechanical basketlike filtering implanted device that is used to entrap any thrombus from the lower extremities and prevent it from traveling to the lungs and causing a potentially fatal PE.[9] IVC filters do not block normal blood flow to the heart. The filter is inserted through a large vein (often in the groin) and placed ideally below the level of the renal veins (Fig. 18.3).

The IVC filter comes in permanent and retrievable forms. The retrievable form is designed to be removed only once the contraindication to anticoagulation has resolved, and the patient is cleared to start anticoagulation.[2] Complications with IVC filter placement include bleeding/infection at the site, postprocedure thrombosis, and hematoma.[9] Complications once the filter is placed include filter migration/malposition, IVC wall penetration (where part of the filter sticks out from the vessel wall lumen), and IVC filter thrombosis.[9] Complications are more common in filters that are permanent.[9]

In instances where an acute DVT is discovered before a surgical procedure, patients can be started on an IV heparin drip and undergo IVC filter placement. The heparin drip, once started,

---

BOX 18.1 ■ Sample Protocol Used to Titrate Heparin Drip

1. Bolus with heparin at 80 units/kg
2. Begin intravenous (IV) infusion of heparin at 18 units/kg/hr using 25,000 units heparin in 250 mL D5W or a concentration of 100 units/mL
3. Activated partial thromboplastin time (aPTT) 6 hours after rate change and then daily at 7 am
4. Adjust IV heparin daily based on aPTT results
   - aPTT <35 sec, bolus with 80 units/kg and increase rate by 4 units/kg/hr
   - aPTT 35–45 sec, bolus with 40 units/kg and increase rate by 2 units/kg/hr
   - aPTT 46–70 sec, no change
   - aPTT 71–90 sec, decrease rate by 2 units/kg/hr
   - aPTT >90 sec, stop heparin infusion for 1 hour, and decrease rate by 3 units/kg/hr

From Morris DC. *Calculate with Confidence*, 8th ed. Elsevier; 2021.

---

has an immediate effect on blood clotting. It also has a short half-life, and once the drip is stopped, the anticoagulation action clears from the body in ~6 hours.[10] Therefore a heparin drip can be safely stopped 6 hours before any planned surgery, without any adverse bleeding effects.[10] Then, after the procedure, when anticoagulation is contraindicated, the IVC filter will protect the patient against DVT migration. When a patient is placed on a heparin drip, partial thromboplastin times (PTTs) must be monitored.

- Protocols begin with the provider placing an order for weight-based unfractionated heparin infusion and dosing protocol with or without a bolus. The starting rate will also be defined by the provider in the initial order set. A PTT is ordered and drawn 6 hours after initiation of unfractionated heparin infusion.[11] Then the drip rate will be adjusted to meet the overall PTT goal set by the provider.

- As part of the nursing duty, the nurse will verify baseline PTT, platelet level, and actual body weight of the patient for the use of calculations. Once this information is obtained, the nurse will enter it into the pump used to administer the medication. To prevent errors, a second nurse should be required to verify and cosign the initial rate, and any bolus dose ordered.[11]

- Subsequent PTTs will be ordered and drawn by the nurse following the chart algorithm (Box 18.1).

Conclusion

Nursing staff plays a critical role in the prevention of VTE. Nurses should promote early mobilization and ensure proper administration of both mechanical and pharmacologic prevention tools. Nurses should continue to monitor patients for signs and symptoms of DVT and PE while inpatient, and educate patients and their families on warning signs to look out for after discharge. Nurses should be sure to stress signs and symptoms of recurrent VTE, signs and symptoms associated with bleeding, safe medication administration, and drug and alcohol interaction.[1]

Patient education is imperative to ensure an understanding of proper usage of anticoagulation, given the high risk for adverse events. Due to the risks associated with VTE and its treatment options, it may be necessary to engage a family member or friend in the care to ensure full comprehension. Nurses should tailor their teaching to the patient's health literacy (the ability to understand basic health information[12]) and utilize the teach-back method. When using the teach-back method, patients are provided short education by staff, then asked to explain back what they learned in their own words.[13] Ultimately, teach-back has been shown to help patients better manage their disease at home[13] and leads to decreased complications.

References

1. Centers for Disease Control and Prevention. Data and statistics on venous thromboembolism. February 7, 2020. https://www.cdc.gov/ncbddd/dvt/data.html#:~:text=Estimates%20suggest%20that%20 60%2C000%2D100%2C000,within%20one%20month%20of%20diagnosis. Accessed January 22, 2022.
2. Kaboli P, Henderson MC, White RH. DVT prophylaxis and anticoagulation in the surgical patient. *Med Clin North Am.* 2003;87(1):77–110, viii. doi:10.1016/s0025-7125(02)00144-x.
3. Stone J, Hangge P, Albadawi H, et al. Deep vein thrombosis: pathogenesis, diagnosis, and medical management. *Cardiovasc Diagn Ther.* 2017;7(Suppl 3):S276–S284. doi:10.21037/cdt.2017.09.01.
4. Cormican D, Morkos MS, Winter D, et al. Acute perioperative pulmonary embolism: management strategies and outcomes. *J Cardiothorac Vasc Anesth.* 2020;34(7):1972–1984.
5. Ageno W, Farjat A, Haas S, et al. Provoked versus unprovoked venous thromboembolism: findings from GARFIELD-VTE. *Res Pract Thromb Haemost.* 2021;5(2):326–341. doi:10.1002/rth2.12482.
6. Bayer. Thrombus Formation. Thrombosis adviser. https://www.thrombosisadviser.com/en/professionals/knowledge-base/essentials/thrombus-formation. Accessed April 22, 2022.
7. Cleveland Clinic. Anticoagulants. Updated January 10, 2022. Retrieved February 19, 2023. https://my.clevelandclinic.org/health/treatments/22288-anticoagulants.
8. Leentjens J, Peters M, Esselink AC, et al. Initial anticoagulation in patients with pulmonary embolism: thrombolysis, unfractionated heparin, LMWH, fondaparinux, or DOACs? *Br J Clin Pharmacol.* 2017;83(11):2356–2366. doi:10.1111/bcp.
9. Marron RM, Rali P, Hountras P, et al. Inferior vena cava filters: past, present, and future. *Chest.* 2020;158(6):2579–2589. doi:10.1016/j.chest.2020.08.002.
10. Scully C, Wolff A. Oral surgery in patients on anticoagulant therapy. *Oral Surg Oral Med Oral Pathol Oral Radiol Endod.* 2002;94(1):57–64. doi:10.1067/moe.2002.123828.
11. Merli G, Thoma B, Byrne J. *Nurse-Driven Parenteral Anticoagulant Management*: Thomas Jefferson University Hospital; 2021.
12. Schillinger D, Machtinger EL, Wang F, et al. Language, literacy, and communication regarding medication in an anticoagulation clinic: a comparison of verbal vs. visual assessment. *J Health Commun.* 2006;11(7):651–664. doi:10.1080/10810730600934500.
13. Yen PH, Leasure AR. Use and effectiveness of the teach-back method in patient education and health outcomes. *Fed Pract.* 2019;36(6):284–289.

Questions

A 62-year-old male was recently hospitalized for lower extremity weakness and underwent lumbar anterior and posterior decompression and fusion 3 days ago. This morning you do your assessment and find that his left leg is swollen. After notifying the provider, a venous duplex was performed, and he was found to have a right lower extremity femoral vein thrombosis. He does not endorse shortness of breath and his pulse oximetry is 98% on room air. Upon review of his most recent lab values, it was determined that he has normal renal and hepatic function and a stable complete blood count.

1. Can this patient be fully anticoagulated? If so, which anticoagulants should be considered?
   a. Yes, he can be fully anticoagulated with unfractionated heparin.
   b. Yes, he can be fully anticoagulated with apixaban or rivaroxaban.
   c. No, he cannot be fully anticoagulated, and an IVC filter should be considered.
   d. No, he cannot be fully anticoagulated and should follow up outpatient for further workup.

2. Should he receive a CTA given the fact that he has a new diagnosis of a DVT?
   a. Yes, a CTA is indicated—it is the gold standard of diagnosis.
   b. Yes, a CTA is indicated—if he has a DVT it likely went to his lungs.
   c. No, a CTA is not indicated—the contrast will further damage his kidneys.
   d. No, a CTA is not indicated—the patient is stable and has no signs/symptoms of PE.

3. Is this DVT considered provoked or unprovoked?
   a. Provoked from recent surgery
   b. Unprovoked, occurred during the recovery period
   c. Neither
   d. Further investigation studies should be done

4. Where is an ideal location for an IVC filter placement?
   a. Above renal veins
   b. Below renal veins
   c. Iliac vein
   d. Superior vena cava

5. Is there ever a time that this patient could be anticoagulated for treatment of his DVT?
   a. No, because he had recent spine surgery.
   b. Yes, once the risk for bleeding is lower as determined by surgery and vascular medicine.
   c. He should have been started on anticoagulation as soon as the DVT was discovered.
   d. It does not matter because he has an IVC filter.

Answers

1. c

2. d

3. a

4. b

5. b

CHAPTER 19

Nursing Management of the Airway and Shortness of Breath

Lauren Alice Robinson, MSN, AGACNP-BC, CCRN ▪ Lauren Malinowski-Falk, MSN, BA, CRNP, AGACNP-BC

Introduction

Shortness of breath (SOB) or dyspnea is a common complaint among hospitalized neurosurgical patients. The assessment and subsequent treatment of conditions that cause SOB are essential components of bedside nursing. Patients who are short of breath often experience feelings of anxiety and distress. The neurosurgical nurse must understand the common pathophysiology and clinical symptoms of airway compromise and be able to recognize and identify scenarios that need to be brought to the provider's attention urgently/emergently.[1] Furthermore, patients with neurologic compromise may not have the mental faculty to verbally express feelings of SOB. The neurosurgical nurse, as a result, will need to use assessment skills to recognize changes in vital signs that hint at increased respiratory distress, use knowledge to deduce possible causes of the clinical change, and know how to appropriately treat the patient.

The neurosurgical nurse must also have a comprehensive understanding of both pharmacologic and nonpharmacologic treatment options for patients with difficulty breathing. Some of the most effective interventions to improve a patient's respiratory status can be done most efficiently by the bedside nurse, which includes improving physical mobility, teaching breathing and coughing exercises, providing airway maintenance, and applying supplemental oxygen therapy.[2] A thorough understanding of airway management can prevent surgical complications, lead to successful weaning of supplemental oxygen, and allow the nurse to provide the best care possible to this patient population.

Airway and Breathing

Airway management is an essential component of nursing management in the hospital setting and in the neurosurgical patient population. The mnemonic ABCs is a mainstay in new-to-practice training instruction: airway, breathing, circulation. Airway and breathing management are crucial for sustaining life. Patients with an obstructed airway will not be able to breathe properly, leading to decreased oxygen levels in the blood. This hypoxia can lead to confusion, changes in heart rate, increased work of breathing, respiratory distress, SOB, and chest tightness.[3,4] Patients with airway concerns will often experience anxiety related to the feeling of not being able to breathe. They are often hyperaware of the sensation of breathlessness because of the secondary anxiety, distress, and panic that often accompany it. In the hospital, bedside nurses are usually the first to observe any inefficient breathing patterns and increased work of breathing. This is often observed through clinical exam changes such as an increased respiratory rate, accessory muscle use, and shallow breathing.

Common Symptoms of Shortness of Breath: Dyspnea vs Orthopnea

DYSPNEA

Dyspnea is a common symptom that can be a clinical manifestation of multiple disease processes, such as myocardial ischemia or dysfunction, pulmonary disease, anemia, neuromuscular disorders, obesity, or deconditioning.[3] Dyspnea is differentiated as either acute or chronic.[3] The acuity and severity of dyspnea on admission to the hospital predicts increased mortality.[5]

- Acute dyspnea develops over hours to days and is responsible for many hospital admissions.[6]
- Dyspnea is considered chronic when symptoms last for >4–8 weeks.[5]
- On occasion, patients can develop acute on chronic dyspnea, where new symptoms exacerbate underlying pulmonary diseases, such as asthma, chronic obstructive pulmonary disease (COPD), and heart failure (Table 19.1).

ORTHOPNEA

A patient experiences orthopnea when dyspnea develops or worsens in the supine position. It is typically associated with heart failure, but can also be associated with central obesity (obesity

TABLE 19.1 ■ Common Causes of Dyspnea That Frequently Occur in the Hospital

Common Causes of Dyspnea		
	Definition	General Nursing Management
Chronic Obstructive Pulmonary Disease Exacerbation	Acute worsening of chronic bronchitis or emphysema, often caused by inflammation of the bronchial tubes	• Steroid administration (either oral or intravenous [IV]) • Nebulizer treatments • Encourage smoking cessation • Oxygen therapy may worsen hypercapnia in certain patients • Avoid benzodiazepines due to potential respiratory depression • Target SpO2 88–92%
Congestive Heart Failure (CHF) Exacerbation	In CHF, the heart is ineffective as a pump and/or the heart is unable to fill adequately • Often acute on chronic presentation	• Patients will typically examine volume overloaded (increased lower extremity swelling, crackles on lung auscultation, potentially increased oxygen requirement) • Evaluation/interventions typically include ECG, TTE chest imaging, diuresis with IV furosemide, and sodium/fluid restriction • Monitor weight and I&O • OSA and central sleep apnea are commonly associated with heart failure
Aspiration Pneumonitis/ Pneumonia	Inflammation/infection of lung parenchyma • Can be viral, bacterial, or fungal in nature	• May require chest imaging and antibiotic therapy • Monitor and manage fluid status • Prevent the progression of infection • Promote airway secretion clearance • Aspiration precautions • Optimize ventilation and oxygenation

Continued

TABLE 19.1 ■ Common Causes of Dyspnea That Frequently Occur in the Hospital—cont'd

	Common Causes of Dyspnea	
	Definition	**General Nursing Management**
Pulmonary Embolism	Occlusion of pulmonary arteries by a blood clot, fat/air/septic embolus, or tumor tissue	• Chest imaging (typically CT angiogram) • VQ scan • Possible interventional radiology intervention • Anticoagulation for blood clots • Monitor for bleeding and lab monitoring appropriate for the type of anticoagulation (i.e., INR, aPTT, platelets) • Promote adherence to venous thromboembolism prophylaxis measures for prevention
Obstructive Sleep Apnea (OSA)	Partial or complete upper airway obstruction during sleep	• Oxygen monitoring • Continuous positive airway pressure is often used • Avoid medications causing respiratory depression • OSA and central sleep apnea are commonly associated with heart failure
Respiratory Depression From Opioids	Slowing of breathing patterns resulting in failure of oxygen and carbon dioxide exchange due to opioid side effect	• Airway assessment before and after opioid administration • Advocating for patient-controlled analgesia to prevent overdose • Naloxone to treat
Anemia	Deficiency in the quantity of red blood cells (RBCs), hemoglobin, and hematocrit circulating in the body • RBCs transport oxygen, so a deficiency can lead to tissue hypoxia	• Hospital interventions may include blood transfusions, drug therapy, volume replacement, and/or oxygen therapy • Fall prevention

aPTT, Activated partial thromboplastin time; *CT,* computed tomography; *ECG,* electrocardiogram; *I&O,* input and output; *INR,* international normalized ratio; *TTE,* transthoracic echocardiogram.

with significant abdominal fat).[7] Orthopnea occurs due to an increase in capillary pressure and venous return in the supine position. The heart may not be strong enough to pump blood effectively, and the increased intraabdominal pressure impairs the movement of the diaphragm during the inhalation period of breathing. In turn, intrapleural pressure increases, leading to the narrowing or closure of small airways at the base of the lung. This narrowing impairs gas exchange and can result in hypoxemia. Patients with inspiratory muscle weakness may also experience orthopnea due to increased work of breathing when moving the diaphragm against high intraabdominal pressure.

Patients with orthopnea will have trouble breathing when lying flat, and breathing will improve when in a seated or standing position.[7] This may lead to a patient requesting multiple pillows to sleep or the option of sleeping in a recliner chair. Overall, the higher the amount of pillows a patient requires to breathe comfortably, the more severe the orthopnea.[7] Patients may also require supplemental oxygen at night to help ease the SOB when sleeping.

Common Postoperative Respiratory Complications

PULMONARY ATELECTASIS

Atelectasis is a reversible condition that occurs when there is a complete or partial collapse of the lung. It occurs when the lung anatomy is compromised and cannot expand to its standard size with each breath. Patients with atelectasis are commonly asymptomatic. However, if the condition worsens, atelectasis can cause significant breathing issues, and patients with atelectasis might not get enough oxygen in their blood.

Atelectasis can be classified into subtypes[2]:

- Obstructive atelectasis results from the blockage of an airway, preventing effective ventilation.[8]
  - If the atelectasis is caused by an object pressing on the lungs (such as a tumor or cyst), surgical intervention may be required to remove the obstruction itself.
- Nonobstructive atelectasis occurs when there is increased pressure exerted on the lung, causing the alveoli to collapse.[8]
- Postoperative atelectasis is a common postoperative complication of general anesthesia, which is exacerbated by periods of immobility.[8]

Diagnosis is typically done through imaging and a clinical exam. A chest x-ray will show which part of the lung (described by providers as anatomic right upper, middle, and lower lobe, or left upper and lower lobe) is affected and how much of the lung has collapsed. Providers may order serial imaging to monitor for improvement if clinical improvement is not readily apparent. A clinical exam will elicit decreased or absent breath sounds, crackles, and the inability to take a deep breath.[8] Cyanosis (i.e., blue coloring of the skin or lips) is a late sign of compromised oxygenation.[8]

The treatment of atelectasis includes pharmacologic and nonpharmacologic therapies to combat the cause of the atelectasis. Nonpharmacologic nursing intervention options are often preferred to use in patients with SOB because pharmacologic options often have adverse systemic effects.

- Pharmacologic interventions
  - Aimed at breaking up mucus in the lungs and aiding in expectoration if the mucus is impeding air flow or treating any underlying disease causing the atelectasis
  - Commonly administered via oral or nebulized inhaler routes
- Nonpharmacologic interventions[6,9]
  - Airway clearance therapy or chest physiotherapy (chest PT) to help loosen mucus. This is commonly done by manually percussing on a patient's back, using vibrating vests, or using a vibrating bed.
  - Ensure adequate pain control to allow patients to take deep breaths.
- Patients should use a pillow or blanket to split incisions to reduce pain when taking deep breaths.
  - Routinely turning and repositioning immobile patients, and early mobilization and physical therapy for mobile patients[2]
  - Frequent tracheal suctioning in intubated patients or patients with tracheostomies to manually remove mucus out of the airway
  - Educating patients on and encouraging the hourly use of incentive spirometry (IS)
- IS entails a slow, deep inspiration (with the goal being as close as possible to total lung capacity), followed by a pause of 2–5 seconds. Finally, the patient should be instructed to exhale to functional residual capacity slowly.[10]
- In patients with neurologic injury or cognitive impairment, who may have poor compliance with deep breathing or IS use, postoperative continuous positive airway pressure is an effort-independent effective lung expansion maneuver.[11]

Overall, nurses will find they can effectively use a combination of lung expansion maneuvers to increase lung volumes through inspiratory effort, while successfully reducing postoperative pulmonary complications. Lung expansion maneuvers, such as coughing, IS, and voluntary deep breaths, are best taught before surgery, as it is more difficult to emphasize the importance of these strategies to a postoperative patient who may be in pain and sedated from analgesic medication.[4,12]

PULMONARY EDEMA

Pulmonary edema occurs when there is an abnormal accumulation of extravascular fluid in the lung tissue and air space.[13] This buildup will often lead to dyspnea, tachypnea, crackles on exam, and hypoxia. If left untreated it can progress to respiratory failure.[13] Chest imaging will reveal ground-glass opacities, increased congestion/density, and Kerley lines.[14]

- Cardiogenic pulmonary edema occurs due to an inability to remove blood away from the pulmonary circulation.[13] This is most common in patients with cardiac dysfunction and arrhythmias. These patients may have a characteristic cough with pink frothy sputum, as well as peripheral edema, elevated jugular venous pressure, and gallop.[13]
  - This can be brought on during surgery due to overadministration of intravenous fluids and activation of the stress response.[15]
- Noncardiogenic pulmonary edema is caused by lung injury, which causes fluid to move into the alveolar and interstitial spaces in the lung.[13] This type of pulmonary edema can occur in hospitalized patients without any cardiac history and can be a complication of inflammation, infection, general anesthesia, and tracheal intubation.[16]

Treatment is aimed at alleviating symptoms, relieving any airway obstruction, and treating the underlying condition.[13] Identifying the underlying etiology is essential to timely implementation of therapy.[14] Diuretics, used to remove excess intrapulmonary fluid,[15] are the mainstay of treatment, but while higher doses are aimed to improve dyspnea, they can affect the patient's renal function.[13] Invasive and noninvasive ventilatory support are aimed to direct fluid back into the capillaries and reduce overall work of breathing and muscle fatigue.[13,15] Temporizing measures are aimed to help manage symptoms, but ultimately fixing the underlying cause will prevent recurrence.[13] Quick resolution of symptoms can occur if therapy is initiated immediately.[15]

PULMONARY RMBOLISM

A pulmonary embolism (PE) is a blockage in the lung vasculature, which disrupts blood flow, causes ischemic lung damage, and decreases oxygen levels. The signs and symptoms of PE include tachycardia, tachypnea, dyspnea, hypoxia, and pleuritic chest discomfort.[17] Overall, the most frequent risk factor for PE is immobilization, which often occurs when a patient is hospitalized, especially after a surgical procedure.[17] The most common source of PE is from a blood clot that forms in the lower extremity or pelvic veins.[17] A high-risk PE can be classified as either massive or submassive depending on the degree of occlusion of the pulmonary arteries and the patient's hemodynamic compromise.

- Massive PE occurs when either >50% of the pulmonary artery or two or more lobar arteries are occluded.[18] It can result in hypotension, cardiogenic shock, and death if not rapidly treated.[18]
- Patients with submassive PE tend to be hemodynamically stable but will often show signs of right heart strain.[18] These patients will likely have some degree of tachycardia, dyspnea, and hypoxia.[18]

In the case of hemodynamic instability, some institutions have a PE response team that can be activated to assess the patient for possible pulmonary embolectomy or thrombolytic therapy. If the patient is hemodynamically stable, diagnosis can be confirmed with a computed tomography pulmonary angiogram (CTA PE) or VQ scan, and further evaluation can be done with an echocardiogram (ECHO). An ECHO is quick and easy to obtain at the bedside. ECHOs can show findings of right-sided cardiac dysfunction, also known as right heart strain.[17] If the diagnosis of PE is highly suspected or confirmed on imaging, the patient will be evaluated for treatment with anticoagulation (blood thinning medications).

- CTA PE: Uses IV contrast to examine the pulmonary arteries and veins under CT imaging. This study is quick/easy to obtain, with often a high degree of diagnostic accuracy. However, it requires radiation and IV contrast administration, which not every patient can tolerate.[17]
  - Providers should check for contrast allergy, and caution should be taken in those with kidney disease.
- VQ scan: Uses radioactive tracer material to examine air flow and blood flow in the lungs. It requires specialized equipment and trained technicians to administer so it may not be readily available or take a prolonged time to obtain. Furthermore, this test often has high rates of inconclusive results, especially in those with significant underlying lung disease,[17] but it is preferred for those with contraindications to radiation and/or IV contrast.

Treatments should begin as soon as PE is diagnosed to prevent worsening respiratory and hemodynamic compromise,[17] reduce right heart strain, and achieve reperfusion of the pulmonary arteries.[18] The choice of treatment for PE often depends on the size/strain of the blood clot. Options for treatment of PE include thrombolysis (using medications to break down the blood clot), embolectomy (surgical removal of the blood clot), and/or systemic anticoagulation (to prevent extension of blood clot and further formation of clots).[18] However, in the hospital setting, patients who just had surgery are often unable to safely get anticoagulation as it will risk devastating bleeding into surgical sites. Clinicians therefore must strike a balance between the risk of bleeding and the immediate-/long-term benefits of clot dissolution.[17] When surgical and medical treatment is contraindicated, treatment should be aimed at optimizing cardiopulmonary support through supplemental oxygen, inotropic agents, and extracorporeal membrane oxygenation if necessary (Table 19.2).[18]

Tracheostomy Care and Oxygen Therapy

In certain situations, patients may require placement of a tracheostomy to maintain adequate oxygenation and relieve restricted airways. A tracheostomy is a surgically created opening in the anterior wall of the trachea through which a tube can be placed to aid in breathing, airway maintenance, and prolonged mechanical ventilation.[19] Many nurses in the inpatient setting find taking care of patients with chronic or recently placed tracheostomy tubes intimidating. The most common complication in a recently placed tracheostomy is obstruction due to secretions or blood in the postoperative period. To prevent these complications the bedside nurse (in conjunction with the multidisciplinary team) should advocate for regular tracheal suctioning, humidified oxygen, and scheduled daily cleaning or replacement of the inner cannula.[20] When suctioning, pressure should be applied when withdrawing the catheter, not when inserting a suction catheter. Nurses should use caution when applying suction, as excessive pressure can cause mucosal damage, trauma to the trachea, and even lead to atelectasis.[19]

Many patients will require supplemental oxygen therapy during hospitalization. In the patient with a tracheostomy, this is either delivered by mechanical ventilation or via tracheostomy collar. Tracheostomy collars are connected to oxygen via special tubing with humidification and can be titrated according to individual needs. Nurses must ensure that humidification bottles do not empty completely as this can cause dryness, which will thicken secretions and make suctioning and coughing more difficult (Fig. 19.1).

In patients without alternative airways, the choice of oxygen delivery system is decided by the provider, taking into consideration the patient's clinical status, the prescribed dose of oxygen, and patient tolerance of the system. The nurse should monitor the patient via pulse oximetry according

TABLE 19.2 ■ Comparing and Contrasting Management and Characteristics of Pulmonary Atelectasis, Pulmonary Edema, and Pulmonary Embolism

	Pulmonary Atelectasis	Pulmonary Edema	Pulmonary Embolism
Definition	Complete or partial collapse of the lung	Abnormal fluid buildup in lung tissue and air space	Blockage of artery that disrupts blood flow to lung
Postsurgical occurrence	Common postoperative complication exacerbated by immobility and inability to take deep breaths	Complication of intubation and anesthesia, exacerbated in cardiac patients by administration of intravenous (IV) fluids and activation of the stress response	Occurs postop due to immobility, commonly due to a blood clot in the lower extremities that travels to the lungs
Imaging studies	Chest x-ray: used to show how much of the lung has collapsed and monitor for improvement	Chest x-ray: will show ground-glass opacities, increased consolidation, and Kerley lines	Computed tomography pulmonary angiogram: uses IV contrast to examine pulmonary arteries and veins VQ scan: uses radioactive tracer material to examine air and blood flow in the lungs
Symptoms	Commonly asymptomatic	Dyspnea, tachypnea, rales/crackles, and hypoxia	Tachycardia, tachypnea, dyspnea, hypoxia, and pleuritic chest discomfort
Treatment	Aimed at breaking up mucus in the lungs	Diuretics and ventilatory support to direct fluid back into the capillaries and reduce overall work of breathing and muscle fatigue	Thrombolysis: using medications to break down the blood clot Embolectomy: surgical remove of the blood clot Systemic anticoagulation: prevent extension of blood clot and further formation of clots

to parameters dictated by the provider and ensure that the patient remains comfortable. Low-flow nasal cannula typically delivers 25–40% FiO_2 (fraction of inspired oxygen), while high-flow nasal cannula systems have heated and humidified oxygen up to 60 L/min. Patients requiring higher rates of supplemental oxygen will typically require admission to intensive care due to the increased likelihood of needing to be placed on a ventilator.[21]

Conclusion

Nursing care for patients with SOB and respiratory compromise can be challenging for registered nurses. For the patient, respiratory compromise frequently leads to anxiety, panic, thoughts of mortality, and is an overall uncomfortable and frightening experience. Nurses are essential to building rapport and trust in these patients. Appropriate nursing care of these patients requires assessment skills (such as auscultating lung sounds), collecting objective data (such as respiratory

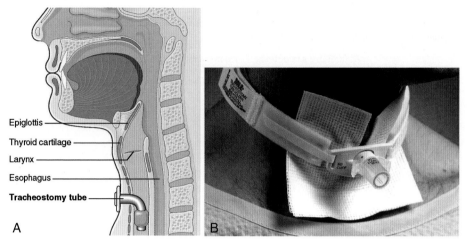

Epiglottis

Thyroid cartilage

Larynx

Esophagus

Tracheostomy tube

A

B

Fig. 19.1 (A) Internal and (B) external visualization of tracheostomy placement. (From Chabner D. *Medical Terminology: A Short Course*, 9th ed. Elsevier; 2022.)

rate and pattern), and intentional interviewing to assess a patient's respiratory status qualitatively.[6] Furthermore, in emergencies, bedside nurses are essential members of the interdisciplinary team as they are often the first to notice a change in a patient's respiratory status and report the change to the provider, while providing oxygen therapy and nonpharmacologic interventions to aid in improvement.

Thankfully, many cases of SOB are caused by simple, short-lived problems. Respiratory tract infections, severe allergic reactions, asthma, mechanical obstruction, pulmonary emboli, heart failure, and pregnancy can all be transient reasons for acute SOB. Chronic breathlessness can be caused by asthma, COPD, interstitial lung disease, cardiomyopathy, deconditioning, obesity, and pulmonary hypertension. Bedside nurses need to understand the pathophysiology behind these conditions to provide the best nursing care for the patient.[6] Literature shows that nursing-based interventions promoting ambulation, chest physiotherapy, and mindful airway maintenance lead to improved patient outcomes.[10]

References

1. Stevens JP, Dechen T, Schwartzstein R, et al. Prevalence of dyspnea among hospitalized patients at the time of admission. *J Pain Symptom Manage*. 2018;56(1):15–22.e2. doi:10.1016/j.jpainsymman.2018.02.013.
2. Woodring JH, Reed JC. Types and mechanisms of pulmonary atelectasis. *J Thorac Imaging*. 1996;11(2): 92–108. doi:10.1097/00005382-199621000-00002.
3. Parshall MB, Schwartzstein RM, Adams L, et al. An official American Thoracic Society statement: update on the mechanisms, assessment, and management of dyspnea. *Am J Respir Crit Care Med*. 2012;185(4):435–452. doi:10.1164/rccm.201111-2042st.
4. Cassidy MR, Rosenkranz P, McCabe K, et al. I COUGH: reducing postoperative pulmonary complications with a multidisciplinary patient care program. *JAMA Surg*. 2013;148(8):740–745. doi:10.1001/jamasurg.2013.358.
5. Stevens JP, Dechen T, Schwartzstein RM, et al. Association of dyspnea, mortality and resource use in hospitalized patients. *Eur Respir J*. 2021;58(3):1902107.
6. Schwartzstein, R. Approach to the patient with dyspnea. *UpToDate*; 2022. Updated April 12, 2023. Accessed May 30, 2022. https://www.uptodate.com/contents/approach-to-the-patient-with-dyspnea.
7. Healthline. *Orthopnea*. Updated September 18, 2018. Accessed October 5, 2022. https://www.healthline.com/health/orthopnea.
8. Grott K, Chauhan S, Dunlap JD. *Atelectasis*: StatPearls Publishing; 2022.

9. Kulur AB, Haleagrahara N, Adhikary P, et al. Effect of diaphragmatic breathing on heart rate variability in ischemic heart disease with diabetes. *Arq Bras Cardiol.* 2009;92(6):423–429, 440–447, 457–463. doi:10.1590/s0066-782 × 2009000600008.
10. Agostini P, Naidu B, Cieslik H, et al. Effectiveness of incentive spirometry in patients following thoracotomy and lung resection including those at high risk for developing pulmonary complications. *Thorax.* 2013;68(6):580–585. doi:10.1136/thoraxjnl-2012-202785.
11. Smetana G, Pfeifer K. Strategies to reduce postoperative pulmonary complications in adults. *UpToDate;* 2022. Updated April 8, 2022. Accessed May 30, 2022. https://www.uptodate.com/contents/strategies-to-reduce-postoperative-pulmonary-complications-in-adults.
12. Moore JA, Conway DH, Thomas N, et al. Impact of a peri-operative quality improvement programme on postoperative pulmonary complications. *Anaesthesia.* 2017;72(3):317–327. doi:10.1111/anae.13763.14.
13. Malek R, Soufi S. *Pulmonary Edema*: StatPearls Publishing; 2022.
14. Barile M. Pulmonary edema: a pictorial review of imaging manifestations and current understanding of mechanisms of disease. *Eur J Radiol Open.* 2020;7:100274. doi:10.1016/j.ejro.2020.100274.
15. Bajwa SS, Kulshrestha A. Diagnosis, prevention and management of postoperative pulmonary edema. *Ann Med Health Sci Res.* 2012;2(2):180–185. doi:10.4103/2141-9248.105668.
16. Liu R, Wang J, Zhao G, et al. Negative pressure pulmonary edema after general anesthesia: a case report and literature review. *Medicine.* 2019;98(17):e15389. doi:10.1097/MD.0000000000015389.18.
17. Cormican D, Morkos MS, Winter D, et al. Acute perioperative pulmonary embolism: management strategies and outcomes. *J Cardiothorac Vasc Anesth.* 2020;34(7):1972–1984. doi:10.1053/j.jvca.2019.11.018.
18. Licha CRM, McCurdy CM, Maldonado SM, et al. Current management of acute pulmonary embolism. *Ann Thorac Cardiovasc Surg.* 2020;26(2):65–71. doi:10.5761/atcs.ra.19-00158.
19. Khanum T, Zia S, Khan T, et al. Assessment of knowledge regarding tracheostomy care and management of early complications among healthcare professionals. *Braz J Otorhinolaryngol.* 2022;88(2):251–256. doi:10.1016/j.bjorl.2021.06.011.
20. Hyzy R, McSparron J. Tracheostomy postoperative care and maintenance and complications in adults. *UpToDate;* 2022. Updated March 14, 2023. Accessed May 30, 2022. https://www.uptodate.com/contents/tracheostomy-postoperative-care-maintenance-and-complications-in-adults.
21. Nagler, J. Continuous oxygen delivery systems for the acute care of infants, children, and adults. *UpToDate.* Updated July 8, 2021. Accessed May 30, 2022. https://www.uptodate.com/contents/continuous-oxygen-delivery-systems-for-the-acute-care-of-infants-children-and-adults.

Questions

Fiona is a 65-year-old female with a past medical history of coronary artery disease, myocardial infarction, hyperlipidemia, hypertension, and chronic pain secondary to degenerative disc disease, who presented to the emergency department with ambulatory dysfunction, coupled with acute onset SOB. The patient's husband is with her and states that her respiratory symptoms began approximately 2 days prior and have progressively worsened, and he brought her to the hospital when she was too weak to get out of bed. The patient and husband deny any aggravating or relieving factors. The patient has a history of COPD and was admitted 10 months ago for acute on chronic respiratory failure. She denies any sick contacts, fever, chills, cough, wheezing, chest pain, palpitations, abdominal pain, nausea, vomiting, or diarrhea. In addition to the SOB and inability to walk, she has been experiencing increased urinary frequency, secondary urinary incontinence, and swelling in her bilateral lower extremities. Her social history includes a 30-pack-year history of smoking cigarettes, but she quit 3 years ago due to increased SOB at home.

1. When initially assessing a patient's respiratory status, it is vital for the nurse to first:
   a. document the husband's description of the patient's SOB; he has been present for previous hospitalizations and knows the patient best.
   b. perform both a subjective and objective assessment and report any immediate concerns to the provider.
   c. place oxygen on the patient, and titrate the FiO_2 based on the patient's presentation.
   d. establish IV access for emergency medication administration.

2. When assessing a patient, which mnemonic is a mainstay for remembering the hierarchy of patient care?
   a. ABC
   b. FIRE
   c. PASS
   d. FAST

3. Fiona calls the nurse to the bedside. She states her SOB has worsened, but the patient's respiratory rate has not changed. What should the nurse do?
   a. Ignore it because it is likely due to anxiety.
   b. Perform a thorough patient assessment and further interview the patient regarding how she feels qualitatively.
   c. Increase the patient's oxygen rate and ask the managing team to put in orders later.
   d. Prepare for intubation.

4. Once Fiona's SOB resolved, imaging revealed lumbar disc herniation, and she is now postoperative day 1 from a lumbar fusion. The following day, the patient develops a low-grade fever with no other apparent signs of infection. What would be the most appropriate nursing intervention?
   a. Wait a few hours and reassess the patient's temperature.
   b. Notify the provider to start antibiotics.
   c. Work with physical therapy to ambulate the patient in the room and perform chest PT.
   d. Patient likely has a surgical site infection, so recommend consulting infectious disease.

5. A few days after surgery, Fiona develops acute tachypnea, dyspnea, and is hypoxic on the monitor. She worsens, despite providing chest PT and pain control with narcotics, and is now on bipap and unable to be weaned. Labs were drawn, which were notable for an increase in creatinine from 0.5 to 2.5. What study do you anticipate being ordered to work up her symptoms?
   a. Chest CTA to assess for PE
   b. Chest x-ray to assess for consolidation
   c. Patient should be started on a heparin drip
   d. VQ scan to assess for PE

Answers

1. b

2. a

3. b

4. c

5. d

CHAPTER 20

Sodium Disorders in Neurosurgical Patients

Jesse Edwards, MD, FHM

Introduction

Sodium abnormalities are frequently encountered among hospitalized patients and are indicative of an increased risk for morbidity and mortality.[1,2] Also known as dysnatremia, abnormal sodium levels represent a problem with water intake, retention, or both. Neurosurgical patients develop dysnatremia at higher rates than the average patient and may be particularly sensitive to its harmful effects.[3-7] It is essential that all staff who care for neurosurgical patients share a common understanding of the clinical significance, symptoms, diagnosis, and treatment of dysnatremia. Learning the fundamentals of sodium and water physiology is a tremendous asset to diagnosing and treating dysnatremia, and it can even help prevent inadvertent medical error.

Physiology and the Consequences of Dysregulation

WATER HOMEOSTASIS: ARGININE VASOPRESSIN AND THIRST

Healthy physiology works to keep blood serum sodium concentration within the range of 135–145 mmol/L and serum osmolality (the overall concentration of solutes in the blood) between 280 and 295 mOsm/kg.[4,5,8–12] Maintaining normal serum sodium and osmolality requires precise regulation of the body's overall water balance, which is achieved by modulating fluid intake and urine output.[10,11] Arginine vasopressin (AVP)—also known as antidiuretic hormone (ADH)—is the hormone responsible for renal retention of free water.[10,11,13]

- AVP is synthesized in the hypothalamus, stored in the posterior pituitary, and released in response to the following conditions[3,4,10,11,14-16]:
  - High serum osmolality
  - High serum sodium concentration
  - Hypovolemia or low arterial blood volume

If any of these conditions develop, AVP and thirst work together to increase water content in the bloodstream by stimulating water retention (reducing urine output) and intake, respectively.[10,14] Conversely, AVP and thirst are inhibited when either serum osmolality or sodium concentration is low, thereby decreasing the water content in the bloodstream.[10,14] Close regulation of water intake and output is very effective at preventing both hyponatremia and hypernatremia from developing.

TONIC STRESS

The initial effect of dysnatremia is an abnormal concentration gradient between the blood serum (extracellular space) and the inside of cells (intracellular space).[3,10] Whether due to a problem with water intake or output, changes in blood serum concentration can exert tonic stress on cells.

- Hypotonic stress[3,10,11,15]
  - Occurs when serum sodium concentration and osmolality are decreasing
  - Water moves from the bloodstream into cells
  - Causes cells to swell
  - Leads to cerebral edema, increased intracranial pressure (ICP), brainstem herniation, and death
- Hypertonic stress[3,9–11,15]
  - Occurs when serum sodium concentration and osmolality are increasing
  - Water moves from inside cells to the bloodstream
  - Causes cells to shrink
  - Leads to cerebral dehydration, vascular injury, intracranial hemorrhage (ICH), cell death, and osmotic demyelinating syndrome (ODS)

CHRONICITY OF DISEASE

Dysnatremia is defined as acute when it has been present <48 hours and chronic when present >48 hours or an unknown duration of time.[4,9,16,17] Acute dysnatremia causes sudden and severe tonic stress, which can dramatically increase the chance that patients will manifest symptoms and sustain one of many potential adverse events.[3,4,18] In cases of chronic dysnatremia, cells have had enough time to implement biochemical adaptations that protect them from immediate harm, but they remain at risk of irreversible damage the longer dysnatremia persists.[4,10,18]

Hyponatremia

CLINICAL SIGNIFICANCE: MORTALITY

Hyponatremia increases the patient's risk of mortality.[3,7,19–22] Even mild hyponatremia is harmful, and studies have shown that patients with any degree of hyponatremia have higher rates of death both in the hospital and after discharge.[22] It is unclear whether the increased risk of mortality is due to hyponatremia itself or to the underlying disease process, but most experts agree that the latter is of greater significance.[21,22]

CLINICAL SIGNIFICANCE: SEVERITY, SYMPTOMS, AND MORBIDITY OF DISEASE

Hyponatremia is most likely to cause symptoms when it is both acute and severe.[3,9,10,15,23,24] The symptoms of hyponatremia are typically neurologic, which reflects the impact of sudden hypotonic stress on brain cells.[15] In contrast, patients with hyponatremia that has developed very slowly may remain asymptomatic for a long time, even until the serum sodium concentration is severely decreased.[3]

Regardless of how quickly it develops, hyponatremia usually does not cause any symptoms as long as sodium remains >125 mmol/L.[10,15] Once the sodium concentration drops below 125 mmol/L, patients may develop malaise, lethargy, confusion, nausea, headache, and restlessness.[3,7,23] Normally, seizures only become a risk when the serum sodium concentration is ≤120 mmol/L.[3,9,10,15] If the sodium level continues to decrease, complications may progress to include vomiting, encephalopathy, respiratory arrest, coma, cerebral edema, increased ICP, brainstem herniation, and death (Box 20.1).[3,7,10,15,24]

DIAGNOSTIC PRINCIPLES OF HYPONATREMIA: VOLUME STATUS

Patients with a sodium level ≤130 mmol/L should be worked up with additional testing.[24] One way to begin is by assessing the patient's extracellular volume (ECV) status.[4,9,16] Accurate assessment of ECV incorporates all information obtained from the patient's history, symptoms, physical

> **BOX 20.1 ■ Hyponatremia: Symptoms and Complications**
>
> Headache, malaise, lethargy, confusion
> Restlessness, muscle weakness
> Nausea, vomiting
> Encephalopathy
> Cerebral edema, increased intracranial pressure
> Pulmonary edema, respiratory arrest
> Coma
> Brainstem herniation
> Death

examination, vital signs, lab results, and imaging studies.[9,13] Hyponatremia is then classified according to the patient's ECV status as either hypovolemic, hypervolemic, or euvolemic.

- Hypovolemic hyponatremia[4,7,9,13,24]
  - History: may include decreased oral intake, vomiting, diarrhea, excessive urination, bleeding, dizziness, fatigue, or syncope
  - Physical exam: dry oral mucous membranes and decreased skin turgor
  - Vital signs: tachycardia, hypotension, and orthostasis
- Hypervolemic hyponatremia[4,9,15,16]
  - History: dyspnea, orthopnea, abdominal distention, weight gain, and swelling; associated with a history of congestive heart failure, cirrhosis, and severe kidney disease
  - Physical exam: ascites, abdominal distention, peripheral edema, pulmonary edema, increased jugular venous distention
  - Vital signs: variable, depending on the causative disease
- Euvolemic hyponatremia[3,4,7,9,24]
  - History, physical exam, and vital signs do not suggest either hypovolemia or hypervolemia
  - Essentially, it is presumed by the exclusion of both hypovolemia and hypervolemia

DIAGNOSIS AND TREATMENT OF COMMON ETIOLOGIES IN NEUROSURGICAL PATIENTS

After the initial assessment of ECV, diagnosis of hyponatremia continues by reviewing the serum osmolality, urine osmolality, and urine sodium level (Fig. 20.1).[3,13,16] Common causes of neurosurgical hyponatremia include hypovolemia, syndrome of inappropriate antidiuretic hormone (SIADH), cerebral salt wasting (CSW), and adrenal insufficiency (AI).[3,5,24]

Hypovolemia

Fluid loss can occur through the kidneys (renal fluid loss) or independently of the kidneys (extrarenal fluid loss). Examples of renal fluid loss include polyuria, CSW, and AI. Extrarenal fluid loss includes problems such as vomiting, diarrhea, bleeding, and decreased oral intake.[7,13,15,24] When there has been a substantial loss of fluid, hypovolemic hyponatremia may develop.[4,5,15,16]

Lab testing in hypovolemic hyponatremia reveals:
- Blood[4,13]
  - Low sodium concentration
  - Low osmolality
  - Elevated creatinine, urea, hemoglobin, protein, and uric acid
- Urine[4,13]
  - High osmolality (often >450 mOsm/kg)
  - Sodium <20 mmol/L, chloride <20 mmol/L

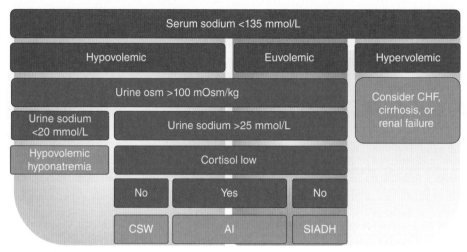

Fig. 20.1   Common etiologies of hyponatremia: diagnostic features. *CHF*, congestive heart failure; *CSW*, cerebral salt wasting; *SIADH*, syndrome of inappropriate antidiuretic hormone.

The treatment of hypovolemic hyponatremia is intravenous fluid (IVF). An isotonic IVF solution such as 0.9% sodium chloride (NaCl) or lactated Ringers (LR) should be used until the patient is hemodynamically stable. Once hemodynamic stability is achieved, providers should change the type and/or rate of IVF infusion to avoid a rapid rebound of the serum sodium level.[5,9,16,23,24]

Syndrome of Inappropriate Antidiuretic Hormone

SIADH is a common source of hyponatremia among neurosurgical patients and can be caused by numerous triggers (Box 20.2).[3,4,10,13,15–23,24] Excessive AVP activity is the hallmark feature of SIADH. As previously stated, low serum osmolality and hyponatremia normally inhibit AVP activity. SIADH, however, is characterized by pathologically persistent AVP activity, which lowers the serum's osmolality and sodium concentration.[3,10,13,15]

BOX 20.2 ■ Common Causes of Syndrome of Inappropriate Antidiuretic Hormone

Intracranial hemorrhage
Traumatic brain injury
Brain tumors
Stroke
Surgery
Respiratory failure, hypoxia, pneumonia
Nausea and vomiting
Severe pain
Physiologic stress
Opioids
Antidepressant and antipsychotic agents

Patients with SIADH are euvolemic, and additional testing reveals the following:

- Blood[3,7,13,15,24]
  - Low sodium concentration
  - Low osmolality
  - Low uric acid, but otherwise normal labs
- Urine[13,15]
  - High osmolality (often extremely elevated, but even as low as >100 mOsm/kg indicates persistent AVP activity)
  - Sodium >40 mmol/L

Restricting both oral and IV fluid is the first-line treatment for SIADH.[3,15,24] Oral fluid restriction to 1 L/day is a reasonable starting point and proves to be effective in many cases. Beyond simple fluid restriction, urea packets and sodium chloride tablets are a good next step in the treatment of SIADH. These salt supplements work by increasing the body's overall solute load and by triggering renal excretion of free water, which concentrates the blood serum by eliminating excess water content.[4,10,16] Loop diuretics (e.g., furosemide) similarly increase renal excretion of free water; they are also used to raise sodium levels by concentrating the blood serum.[4,10,16,24]

Note: Fluid restriction is contraindicated in patients with subarachnoid hemorrhage (SAH) even if they have SIADH due to an increased risk for cerebral vasospasm from low intravascular volume.[16,24,25]

Cerebral Salt Wasting

CSW is a controversial topic, as the true prevalence, pathophysiology, and clinical significance remain subjects of debate.[3,9,15,24] In the neurosurgical patient, CSW occurs most frequently following SAH, traumatic brain injury (TBI), and intracranial aneurysm clipping.[3,4,7,15] The key physiologic feature of CSW is salt wasting via the urine; high salt content excreted in the urine leads to hypovolemia.[3,13,15,24]

Typical lab findings include:

- Blood[3-5,7,13,15]
  - Low sodium concentration
  - Low osmolality
  - Elevated creatinine, urea, hemoglobin, and protein
  - Low uric acid
- Urine[3-5,7,13,15]
  - Osmolality >100 mOsm/kg
  - Sodium >25 mmol/L (often much higher)

Treatment of CSW focuses on volume and solute repletion.[4,15] Hypertonic IVF such as 3% NaCl solution is recommended and can be given as intermittent boluses or as very slow, weight-based continuous infusions.[3,4,16,24] When using hypertonic IVF, sodium levels should be checked frequently, and nurses should review their institutional policies to verify the rate and duration of hypertonic IVF infusion that is permitted via a peripheral line (due to the risk of causing phlebitis or extravasation of the solution). In addition to hypertonic IVF, patients with CSW should be treated with intermittent boluses of isotonic IVF (e.g., 0.9% NaCl solution or LR) to restore and maintain euvolemia.[4,9,10,15,24] Lastly, fludrocortisone is a steroid that decreases renal excretion of sodium, and it can be a helpful addition to the treatment regimen in some cases of CSW.[5,7,24]

Adrenal Insufficiency

Prescribed steroids are the most common cause of AI in neurosurgical patients.[26] In addition, numerous neurosurgical conditions can lead to AI, including SAH, TBI, pituitary tumors, and surgical manipulation of the pituitary and its stalk (such as in the case of a transsphenoidal resection of a pituitary adenoma).[3,24] Neurosurgical AI due to pituitary dysfunction frequently is transient, and recovery is expected over time.[24] Symptoms of AI include fever, hypothermia, orthostasis, hypotension, and tachycardia.[9,26] Patients may present with abdominal pain, nausea, vomiting, decreased appetite, lethargy, and confusion.[9,26]

Cortisol testing is key to making a diagnosis of AI.[3,26]

- Morning cortisol ≥15 μg/dL: excludes the diagnosis of AI
- Morning cortisol <3 μg/dL: confirms the diagnosis of AI[3,27-29]
- Nondiagnostic cortisol level: consider a cosyntropin stimulation test[3,26,29,30]:
  - Check a baseline cortisol level
  - Administer one dose of cosyntropin 250 μg IV
  - Check a repeat cortisol level 30–60 minutes later
- Diagnosis depends on the cortisol level achieved in response to cosyntropin stimulation[3,9,26,29,30]

AI may coincide with either hypovolemia or euvolemia, along with the following findings[3,7,15]:

- Blood[3,26]
  - Low sodium concentration
  - Low osmolality
  - Low glucose, high potassium
  - Low cortisol
- Urine[13,24]
  - Osmolality >200 mOsm/kg
  - Sodium >25 mmol/L

If there is hypotension or the risk of clinical decompensation, treatment for AI should be started without delay, even while cortisol test results are pending.[3,26] Hydrocortisone IV is preferred for the treatment of acute AI, including perioperatively and when patients are at risk for hemodynamic instability.[3,9,23,24] Fludrocortisone may also be used in patients who need targeted inhibition of renal sodium excretion to help restore intravascular volume.[7,24]

TREATMENT PRINCIPLES AND PRECAUTIONS

Acute Hyponatremia

Acute and severe hyponatremia risks causing immediate and devastating harm—it should be corrected quickly, without strictly limiting the rate of sodium improvement.[3,4,8,10,16,23,24] Raising serum sodium by just 3–5 mmol/L in the first 2–4 hours of treatment is effective at preventing seizures and reducing cerebral edema.[3,4] Nurses play a critical role in treatment by obtaining frequent blood draws, monitoring the patient's symptoms, and communicating closely with physicians regarding the plan of care.

Chronic Hyponatremia

In contrast, chronic hyponatremia should not be corrected by more than 6–8 mmol/L in the first 24 hours of treatment.[3,4,10] Asymptomatic patients with chronic hyponatremia can be treated with conservative modalities first (e.g., fluid restriction, urea packets, furosemide). Hypertonic IVF (e.g., 3% NaCl solution) is indicated for symptomatic patients and those at risk of immediate harm due to severe hyponatremia.[4,10]

Osmotic Demyelinating Syndrome

Serum sodium should be closely monitored during treatment because overcorrection of chronic hyponatremia exerts hypertonic stress on brain cells, causing their sudden dehydration and potentially ODS.[8,10,15,16] Symptoms of ODS may not develop until 2–6 days after the overcorrection of hyponatremia occurs.[4,9,15] Nurses should monitor for strokelike symptoms, spastic paresis, movement disorders, altered cognition, and unexplained behavioral changes.[3–5,10] Magnetic resonance imaging (MRI) is the study of choice when establishing the diagnosis.[3]

Factors that increase the risk of ODS include[3,4,9,10,16,23,24]:

- Hyponatremia present >48 hours
- Initial serum sodium <110 mmol/L
- Sodium level increased >12 mmol/L in 24 hours
- Patients with liver disease, malnutrition, hypokalemia, or excess alcohol consumption

If sodium is corrected too quickly in a patient who is at risk for ODS, immediate relowering of the sodium concentration with hypotonic IVF (e.g., dextrose 5% in water solution) or desmopressin (synthetic AVP) can reduce hypertonic stress and lower the risk of developing ODS.[3–5,24]

Hypernatremia

CLINICAL SIGNIFICANCE: MORTALITY

Hypernatremia usually develops as a symptom of disease rather than as a stand-alone pathology.[4,5,18] The presence of hypernatremia often signals that there is an increased risk of mortality, but it is difficult to know how much of that risk is due to the elevated sodium itself versus the underlying disease process.[5,6,18]

CLINICAL SIGNIFICANCE: SEVERITY, SYMPTOMS, AND MORBIDITY OF DISEASE

Like hyponatremia, symptoms of hypernatremia typically are neurologic, and they are most likely to manifest when the rise in sodium level is both acute and severe.[4,10,18] Hypernatremia causes headache, malaise, nausea, vomiting, restlessness, myoclonus, seizures, and coma.[4,18] In extreme cases hypertonic stress and cellular dehydration caused by a rapidly rising sodium concentration leads to vascular injury, ICH, or even ODS.[4,10,18] Most patients are asymptomatic as long as the sodium concentration remains <160 mmol/L.[4,10,18]

DIAGNOSTIC PRINCIPLES OF HYPERNATREMIA: WATER DEFICIT

Normal physiology closely guards against hypernatremia by stimulating thirst (water intake) and AVP secretion (water retention).[4,10,18,31] Hypernatremia can only develop when at least one of these safeguards has been disrupted.[4,10,11,18,31] In fact, patients who can sense thirst and quench thirst are almost always protected against hypernatremia.[11] Hypernatremia always indicates an overall water deficit; it is always hyperosmolar and almost always associated with hypovolemia.[5,10,18]

Evaluation of hypernatremia begins by identifying potential sources of water loss. Common causes of water loss in neurosurgical patients include vomiting, diarrhea, profuse sweating, persistent fever (i.e., insensible losses), osmotic diuresis (e.g., patients with hyperglycemia), loop diuretics, and central diabetes insipidus (CDI).[4,5,10,18,31] Physical exam findings, vital signs, and lab results typically reflect a state of hypovolemia.[18]

The workup of hypernatremia includes testing urine osmolality.[5,10,11,31] If urine osmolality is appropriately high—indicating that the kidneys are retaining as much free water as possible in response to increased AVP secretion—then inadequate water intake must be contributing to the hypernatremia.[4,5,18] Loss of the thirst stimulus (hypodipsia) due to hypothalamic dysfunction is very rare, but neurosurgical patients frequently sustain impaired access to water as a cause of their inadequate intake.[4,5,11]

DIAGNOSIS AND TREATMENT OF COMMON ETIOLOGIES IN NEUROSURGICAL PATIENTS

Impaired Access to Water

Impaired access to water simply means that the patient is unable to drink fluid independently. Patients who are very young, very old, frail, cognitively impaired, critically ill, or otherwise dependent on assistance for self-care (including many hospitalized patients and nursing home residents) are at risk for impaired access to water.[5,10,11,18] Physical or cognitive functional limitations may themselves be enough to cause dehydration and hypernatremia, but nurses should be diligent to identify coexisting disorders that may worsen the water deficit (e.g., fever and sweating, diarrhea, or polyuria). Neurosurgical patients and those with neurologic injury are especially prone to inadequate water intake from paresis or paralysis, immobility, deconditioning, change in consciousness, and dysphagia.[4,5,10,11,18]

When AVP activity is normal, impaired access to water leads to the following:
- Blood[4,10,11]
  - High sodium concentration
  - High osmolality
- Urine[4,10,11]
  - High osmolality (normally >600 mOsm/kg)

Correcting hypernatremia from impaired access to water relies on two basic principles[4,5,11]:
- Treatment and resolution of coexisting disorders, if applicable
- Increased water intake

Oral water intake always is preferred over hypotonic IVF, but often it requires constant caretaker assistance. In some cases (e.g., dysphagia, neurologic injury) even continuous bedside support is not enough to keep the patient hydrated. When the cause of impaired access to water is not likely to resolve quickly, sustainable hydration can be achieved by placement of a gastric feeding tube.[4,5,15,18]

Central Diabetes Insipidus

CDI is caused by decreased pituitary secretion of AVP and the kidneys' subsequent inability to retain water. Common triggers for CDI in neurosurgical patients include pituitary surgery, TBI, SAH, tumors, meningitis, and encephalitis.[4,18,31] The severity and duration of CDI depend on the cause, location, and extent of injury to the hypothalamic-pituitary complex.[4,5,15,31] CDI after pituitary surgery is relatively common and may be transient, phasic, or permanent.[3-5,15,31]

Classic findings of CDI include[31]:
- Blood[5,31]
  - High sodium concentration
  - High osmolality
- Urine[5,31]
  - Low osmolality (lower than blood osmolality)
  - High volume urine output (polyuria)

Treating CDI involves increasing water intake, retention, or both.[15] Oral hydration should always be attempted first; patients should be encouraged to drink enough water to compensate for their high urine output.[4,5,18] If patients cannot drink enough fluid to lower their serum sodium concentration, then desmopressin can be used to increase water retention by the kidneys.[4,5] Desmopressin can be administered orally, intravenously, subcutaneously, or intranasally.[4,5,31]

Nurses should be aware that AVP secretion and urinary excretion of free water can vary considerably after pituitary surgery. As a result, patients may unexpectedly alternate between hypernatremia and hyponatremia, potentially manifesting what are known as biphasic and triple phase responses (Fig. 20.2).[3,4,11,15,31] Although phasic responses are not very common, providers should

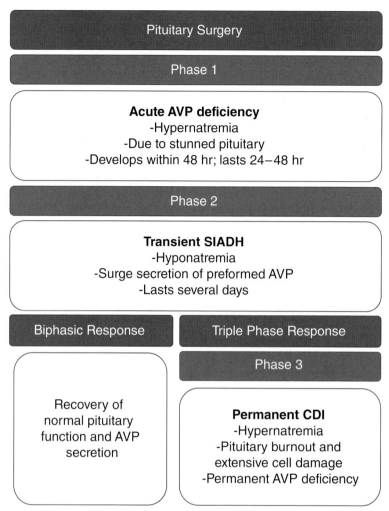

Fig. 20.2 Biphasic and triple phase response after pituitary surgery. *AVP*, arginine vasopressin; *CDI*, central diabetes insipidus; *SIADH*, syndrome of inappropriate antidiuretic hormone

be cautious when managing patients after pituitary surgery to avoid inadvertently worsening dysnatremia in patients with fluctuating AVP activity.[3,4,15,31]

TREATMENT PRINCIPLES AND PRECAUTIONS

Proper management of hypernatremia requires proactive hydration (correcting the free water deficit) and simultaneous treatment of the underlying cause.[4,5,11] Although each underlying disorder may require a different treatment regimen, hydration protocols typically follow common principles pertaining to the acuity and severity of hypernatremia.

Acute Hypernatremia

The hypertonic stress generated by acute and severe hypernatremia poses a significant risk for sudden-onset morbidity (e.g., encephalopathy, seizures, vascular injury, ICH).[10] Generally speaking, oral/enteric hydration with free water is preferred for the correction of hypernatremia, but acutely severe hypernatremia initially requires treatment with hypotonic IVF to quickly reduce the risk of harm.[5,18]

In its acute phase, hypernatremia can be corrected rapidly without concern for causing cerebral edema.[4,5,11,17,18] If the underlying disease process persists, ongoing water loss will counteract treatment efforts, and providers must frequently reassess serum sodium levels, volume status, and the effectiveness of their interventions.[11,18]

Chronic Hypernatremia

Chronic hypernatremia should also be treated by oral/enteric hydration with free water whenever safe and feasible. Nevertheless, hypotonic IVF may be necessary when caring for critically ill patients or those with severely elevated serum sodium levels.[4,5,18]

Hypotonic stress from rapidly lowering chronic hypernatremia is believed to risk causing cerebral edema and seizures.[18] In reality, cerebral edema due to overcorrection of chronic hypernatremia has been reported only in infants and animal models; there have been no substantiated reports of harmful consequences in adults.[4,5,10,11,32] Unfortunately, adult patients often are undertreated, allowed to remain hypernatremic for too long, and may even sustain worse outcomes due to excessively slow rates of correction.[4,11,17,32,33]

Treatment guidelines have traditionally recommended that serum sodium be reduced by ≤0.5 mmol/L/hr and no more than 10 mmol/L/day, though strict adherence to rate-limiting guidelines for the correction of chronic hypernatremia may not be necessary in all cases.[10,11,18,32] Nevertheless, caution remains prudent, especially in neurosurgical patients who may be uniquely sensitive to the devastating consequences of cerebral edema.[32]

Conclusion

Neurosurgical patients frequently develop dysnatremia, and nurses who care for this niche patient population must be prepared to treat sodium disorders daily. When managing sodium disorders, nurses must remain attentive to their patient's ECV status, fluid intake, urine output, and sources of water loss. In all cases it is important to identify the cause and chronicity of the dysnatremia, because these factors determine the management strategies and optimal rates of sodium correction. Coupled with clinical experience, understanding the pathophysiology, diagnosis, and treatment of dysnatremia will equip nurses for their critical role in managing sodium disorders and protecting their patients from harm.

References

1. Holland-Bill L, Christiansen CF, Heide-Jorgensen U, et al. Hyponatremia and mortality risk: a Danish cohort study of 279 508 acutely hospitalized patients. *Eur J Endocrinol.* 2015;173(1):71–81.
2. Al Mawed S, Pankratz VS, Chong K, et al. Low serum sodium levels at hospital admission: outcomes among 2.3 million hospitalized patients. *PLoS One.* 2018;13(3):e0194379.
3. Hannon MJ, Thompson CJ. Neurosurgical hyponatremia. *J Clin Med.* 2014;3(4):1084–1104.
4. Castle-Kirszbaum M, Kyi M, Wright C, et al. Hyponatraemia and hypernatraemia: disorders of water balance in neurosurgery. *Neurosurg Rev.* 2021;44(5):2433–2458.
5. Tisdall M, Crocker M, Watkiss J, et al. Disturbances of sodium in critically ill adult neurologic patients: a clinical review. *J Neurosurg Anesthesiol.* 2006;18(1):57–63.
6. Aiyagari V, Deibert E, Diringer MN. Hypernatremia in the neurologic intensive care unit: how high is too high? *J Crit Care.* 2006;21(2):163–172.
7. Fraser JF, Stieg PE. Hyponatremia in the neurosurgical patient: epidemiology, pathophysiology, diagnosis, and management. *Neurosurgery.* 2006;59(2):222–229.
8. Adrogue HJ, Tucker BM, Madias NE. Diagnosis and management of hyponatremia: a review. *JAMA.* 2022;328(3):280–291.

9. Edwards J, Sharma S, Gulati R. Diagnosis and management of sodium disorders in the neurosurgical patient. In: Daniel R, Harrop C, eds. *Medical Management of Neurosurgical Patients*: Oxford Academic; 2019:156–C9.P75.

10. Sterns RH. Disorders of plasma sodium—causes, consequences, and correction. *N Engl J Med.* 2015;372(1):55–65.

11. Seay NW, Lehrich RW, Greenberg A. Diagnosis and management of disorders of body tonicity—hyponatremia and hypernatremia: core curriculum 2020. *Am J Kidney Dis.* 2020;75(2):272–286.

12. Verbalis JG, Goldsmith SR, Greenberg A, et al. Diagnosis, evaluation, and treatment of hyponatremia: expert panel recommendations. *Am J Med.* 2013;126(10 Suppl 1):S1–S42.

13. Milionis HJ, Liamis GL, Elisaf MS. The hyponatremic patient: a systematic approach to laboratory diagnosis. *CMAJ.* 2002;166(8):1056–1062.

14. Cuzzo B, Padala SA, Lappin SL. *Physiology, Vasopressin*: StatPearls Publishing; 2022.

15. Cole CD, Gottfried ON, Liu JK, et al. Hyponatremia in the neurosurgical patient: diagnosis and management. *Neurosurg Focus.* 2004;16(4):e9.

16. Hoorn EJ, Zietse R. Diagnosis and treatment of hyponatremia: compilation of the guidelines. *J Am Soc Nephrol.* 2017;28(5):1340–1349.

17. Qian Q. Hypernatremia. *Clin J Am Soc Nephrol.* 2019;14(3):432–434.

18. Adrogue HJ, Madias NE. Hypernatremia. *N Engl J Med.* 2000;342(20):1493–1499.

19. Gill G, Huda B, Boyd A, et al. Characteristics and mortality of severe hyponatraemia—a hospital-based study. *Clin Endocrinol (Oxf).* 2006;65(2):246–249.

20. Clayton JA, Le Jeune IR, Hall IP. Severe hyponatraemia in medical in-patients: aetiology, assessment and outcome. *QJM.* 2006;99(8):505–511.

21. Hoorn EJ, Lindemans J, Zietse R. Development of severe hyponatraemia in hospitalized patients: treatment-related risk factors and inadequate management. *Nephrol Dial Transplant.* 2006;21(1):70–76.

22. Waikar SS, Mount DB, Curhan GC. Mortality after hospitalization with mild, moderate, and severe hyponatremia. *Am J Med.* 2009;122(9):857–865.

23. Adrogue HJ, Madias NE. Hyponatremia. *N Engl J Med.* 2000;342(21):1581–1589.

24. Rahman M, Friedman WA. Hyponatremia in neurosurgical patients: clinical guidelines development. *Neurosurgery.* 2009;65(5):925–935.

25. Winzeler B, Lengsfeld S, Nigro N, et al. Predictors of nonresponse to fluid restriction in hyponatremia due to the syndrome of inappropriate antidiuresis. *J Intern Med.* 2016;280(6):609–617.

26. Steer M, Fromm D. Recognition of adrenal insufficiency in the postoperative patient. *Am J Surg.* 1980;139(3):443–446.

27. Jenkins D, Forsham PH, Laidlaw JC, et al. Use of ACTH in the diagnosis of adrenal cortical insufficiency. *Am J Med.* 1955;18(1):3–14.

28. Hagg E, Asplund K, Lithner F. Value of basal plasma cortisol assays in the assessment of pituitary-adrenal insufficiency. *Clin Endocrinol (Oxf).* 1987;22(2):221–226.

29. Marko NF, Gonugunta VA, Hamrahian AH, et al. Use of morning serum cortisol level after transsphenoidal resection of pituitary adenoma to predict the need for long-term glucocorticoid supplementation. *J Neurosurg.* 2009;113(3):540–544.

30. Hamilton DD, Cotton BA. Cosyntropin as a diagnostic agent in the screening of patients for adrenocortical insufficiency. *Clin Pharmacol.* 2010;2:77–82.

31. Garrahy A, Moran C, Thompson CJ. Diagnosis and management of central diabetes insipidus in adults. *Clin Endocrinol (Oxf).* 2019;90(1):23–30.

32. Sterns RH. Evidence for managing hypernatremia. is it just hyponatremia in reverse? *Clin J Am Soc Nephrol.* 2019;14(5):645–647.

33. Chauhan K, Pattharanitima P, Patel N, et al. Rate of correction of hypernatremia and health outcomes in critically ill patients. *Clin J Am Soc Nephrol.* 2019;14(5):656–663.

Questions

A 62-year-old male with a history of lung cancer, emphysema, coronary artery disease, and tobacco abuse is treated in the neurologic intensive care unit after presenting with altered mental status and a severe SAH. Two days after admission, the patient remains disoriented and lethargic.

His heart rate is elevated at 116 bpm, his blood pressure is normal, and he has a temperature of 100.4°F. Labs reveal a serum sodium level of 129 mmol/L, but the remainder of his basic metabolic panel is normal.

1. Which of the following is the best first step in the workup of this patient's hyponatremia?
   a. Echocardiogram
   b. Morning cortisol level
   c. Urine sodium level
   d. Ultrasound of the kidneys

2. All the following are true in this case, except:
   a. Fluid restriction should be avoided when treating this patient's hyponatremia.
   b. Hyponatremia is the most likely cause of this patient's disorientation and lethargy.
   c. Even mild hyponatremia is associated with an increased risk for mortality.
   d. CSW, SIADH, and AI are all potential causes of the hyponatremia.

3. What is the most significant diagnostic difference between CSW and SIADH?
   a. Urine osmolality
   b. Early morning cortisol level
   c. Urine sodium
   d. ECV status

A 55-year-old female undergoes pituitary surgery for resection of a pituitary adenoma. On postop day 2, she mentions that she has been urinating constantly and feeling very thirsty. There is an empty pizza box on her bedside table but no water in the room. Her blood tests reveal a sodium level of 148 mmol/L, increased from 143 mmol/L the previous day.

4. Which of the following is most likely true in this scenario?
   a. The patient has developed some degree of CDI, and the physician should be notified.
   b. The patient has a urinary tract infection.
   c. The hypernatremia is caused by dietary salt intake.
   d. These findings are not clinically significant, and the physician does not need to be notified.

5. What is the best first step in management of this patient?
   a. Start hypotonic IVF
   b. Increase oral water intake
   c. Start desmopressin
   d. MRI brain

Answers

1. c

2. b

3. d

4. a

5. b

CHAPTER 21

Identification and Management of Hypopituitarism

Hadi Abou-Rass, BS, DO   ■   Allison M. Lang, MSN, CRNP, AGACNP-BC

Introduction

The pituitary gland is responsible for the release of several hormones, including adrenocorticotrophic hormone (ACTH), thyroid-stimulating hormone (TSH), and growth hormone (GH). Pituitary disease can lead to deficiency in all hormones (panhypopituitarism) or can selectively target an individual hormone. Adrenal insufficiency (AI) is a disorder of the hypothalamic-pituitary-adrenal (HPA) axis and can be classified as primary, secondary, or tertiary disease. AI can be an acute or chronic disorder. Identifying patients who are at risk for AI in the preoperative period is important for preventing adrenal crisis, a life-threatening condition that occurs when the body does not produce adequate amounts of cortisol. Understanding the basic pathophysiology of AI will help nurses identify the signs, symptoms, and lab findings of AI and anticipate treatment options that may be indicated.[1]

Anatomic Structures and Hormone Production

The adrenal glands are located above each kidney and consist of an outer cortex and an inner medulla. The inner medulla secretes the catecholamines norepinephrine and epinephrine. The outer cortex consists of three layers that each secrete different hormones.[2]
- Adrenal gland outer cortex (Fig. 21.1)
  - Outermost layer: secretes mineralocorticoid (aldosterone)
    - Aldosterone release is controlled by the renin-angiotensin system (RAS) and acts to influence blood pressure through sodium and potassium regulation
  - Middle layer: secretes glucocorticoids (cortisol)
    - Cortisol release is triggered by ACTH, which is released by the anterior pituitary gland
  - Innermost layer: secretes androgens

The pituitary gland is located at the base of the brain beneath the hypothalamus and is connected to the hypothalamus by the pituitary stalk. The pituitary gland is divided into anterior and posterior portions, each of which is responsible for the production and regulation of different hormones (Fig. 21.2, Table 21.1).

Hormone Significance

ACTH secretion from the anterior pituitary is stimulated by corticotropin-releasing hormone (CRH), which is produced by the hypothalamus. Once released into bloodstream circulation, ACTH travels to the adrenal glands and increases their cortisol output. This sequence of hormone secretion and activity occurs in a pulsatile fashion following a circadian rhythm. Consequently,

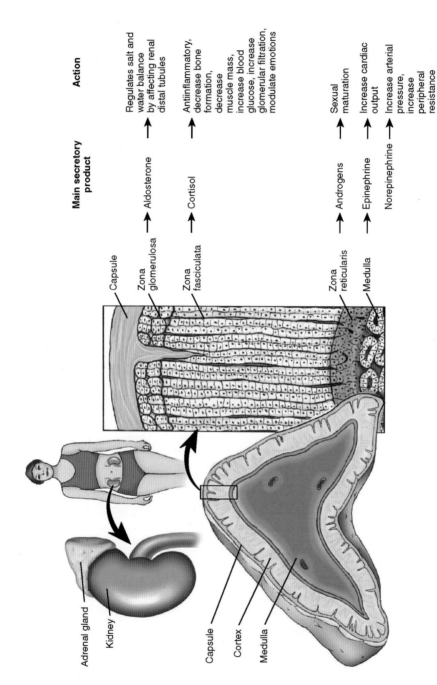

Fig. 21.1 Anatomy of the adrenal gland. (Adapted from Thibodeau GA, Patton KT. *Anatomy and Physiology*, 7th ed. Mosby; 2010.)

TABLE 21.1 ■ **Pituitary Regulated Hormones**

Anterior Pituitary	Luteinizing hormone and follicle-stimulating hormone:	Adrenocorticotrophic hormone:	Thyroid-stimulating hormone:	Growth hormone:	Prolactin:
	• Testosterone, estrogen production • Ovarian follicle production, spermatogenesis	• Controls cortisol release	• Stimulates the production of thyroid hormone	• Responsible for the growth of many tissues within the body, stimulates protein synthesis, regulates energy and metabolism	• Necessary for lactation, suppressed by dopamine
Posterior Pituitary	Oxytocin: • Causes uterine contractions, releases milk when breastfeeding, assists in ejaculation in males	Antidiuretic hormone: • Responsible for water homeostasis			

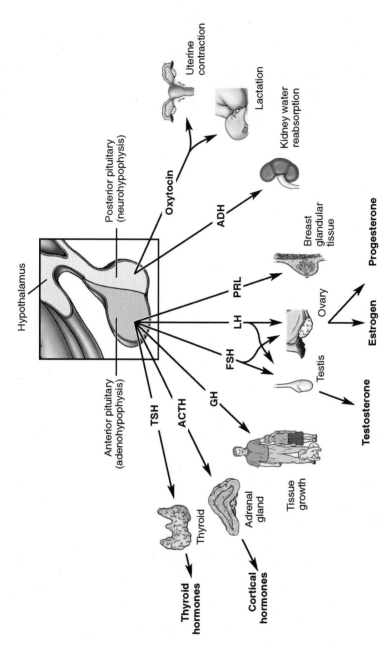

Fig. 21.2 Anatomy of the pituitary gland. *ACTH*, Adrenocorticotrophic hormone; *ADH*, antidiuretic hormone; *FSH*, follicle-stimulating hormone; *GH*, growth hormone; *LH*, luteinizing hormone; *PRL*, prolactin; *TSH*, thyroid-stimulating hormone. (Adapted from Herlihy B, Maebius NK. *The Human Body in Health and Illness*, 3rd ed. Saunders; 2007.)

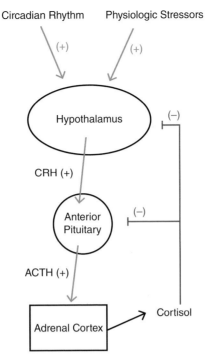

Fig. 21.3 Hypothalamic-pituitary-adrenal axis with feedback inhibition of cortisol on the hypothalamus. *ACTH*, Adrenocorticotrophic hormone; *CRH*, corticotropin-releasing hormone.

cortisol levels are highest in the morning and lowest at night. Interestingly, emotional or physical stress (including fever, hypoglycemia, and hypotension) can also stimulate the hypothalamus to release CRH, which raises cortisol levels even further.[3]

Under healthy conditions, elevated levels of cortisol signal the hypothalamus and anterior pituitary to decrease their release of CRH and ACTH, respectively. This self-regulatory process is called negative feedback (Fig. 21.3). It is important to remember that mineralocorticoid (aldosterone) production is not dependent on the hypothalamus or pituitary, but on RAS, which entails renin secretion by the kidney in response to decreased renal perfusion pressure.[1,3,4]

Luteinizing hormone (LH) and follicle-stimulating hormone (FSH) are released by the anterior pituitary and are integral to testosterone and estrogen production, ovarian follicle stimulation, and spermatogenesis. Cycles of LH and FSH activity are regulated by the pulsatile secretion of gonadotropin-releasing hormone (GnRH) from the hypothalamus. Prolactin production and secretion is suppressed by dopamine secreted from the hypothalamus. Thyrotropin-releasing hormone from the hypothalamus stimulates release of TSH, which stimulates production and release of thyroid hormone from the thyroid gland. GH release is stimulated by GH-releasing hormone and inhibited by somatostatin, both of which are secreted by the hypothalamus. The posterior pituitary secretes oxytocin and antidiuretic hormone (ADH) required for water homeostasis.[1,2]

Adrenal Insufficiency

AI is a disorder of the HPA axis and is classified as either primary, secondary, or tertiary.

PRIMARY ADRENAL INSUFFICIENCY

Primary AI is the dysfunction of all three layers of the adrenal cortex. This results in loss of both mineralocorticoid and glucocorticoid production because the adrenal glands themselves are dysfunctional. Decreased cortisol levels subsequently lead to an increase in ACTH. Because all the layers of the adrenals are affected in primary AI, the patient will show signs and symptoms associated with both glucocorticoid and mineralocorticoid deficiency. ACTH also acts on melanocytes, and excess ACTH leads to overstimulation of melanocytes, which causes hyperpigmentation. This is best seen in skin areas exposed to friction and sunlight such as the creases on the palm of the hand, toes, and axillary folds. These patients may also have vitiligo, especially in patients with an autoimmune cause of primary AI.[3,5]

The most common cause of primary AI in the United States is autoimmune. Many of these patients will also develop another autoimmune endocrine disorder in their lifetime (such as primary hypothyroidism, primary ovarian insufficiency, celiac disease, hypoparathyroidism, or type 1 diabetes mellitus). Other causes include infection (such as tuberculosis, fungal infections, or human immunodeficiency virus), sarcoidosis, lymphoma, certain drugs, bilateral adrenal hemorrhage, and metastatic cancers (less common).[1,6]

Medications that decrease cortisol synthesis (such as mitotane, ketoconazole, suramin, etomidate, and aminoglutethimide) or accelerate the metabolism of cortisol/synthetic steroids (such as phenytoin, rifampin, and barbiturates) can cause AI in at-risk patients. Bilateral adrenal hemorrhage, the bleeding of ruptured vessel into the adrenal glands, is a rare but serious cause of AI. Risk factors for adrenal hemorrhage include protein c deficiency, anticoagulation, disseminated intravascular coagulopathy, and sepsis.[1,5]

SECONDARY ADRENAL INSUFFICIENCY

Secondary AI occurs due to dysfunction of the anterior pituitary gland that influences secretion of ACTH. ACTH deficiency leads to decreased release of corticosteroids (cortisol) from the adrenal glands. Because the adrenal glands are intact, there is still functional release of mineralocorticoids (aldosterone) that are stimulated by the RAS. Thus the patients will primarily show signs/symptoms associated with mainly glucocorticoid deficiency, especially hypoglycemia. They may also present with alabaster-colored pale skin due to deficiency of ACTH and decreased melanocyte activation.[3]

Common causes of secondary AI include panhypopituitarism, which can be from pituitary tumors or craniopharyngiomas, infection, infiltrative diseases, head trauma/traumatic brain injury (TBI), pituitary surgery or radiotherapy, intracranial artery aneurysms, and Sheehan syndrome. Up to 30% of patients with head trauma experience pituitary dysfunction, which can last for several months or years. This type of AI is commonly seen in the neurosurgical population.[1,3]

TERTIARY ADRENAL INSUFFICIENCY

Like secondary AI, tertiary AI is associated with glucocorticoid deficiency but not mineralocorticoid deficiency. It occurs due to decreased CRH secretion from the hypothalamus, which subsequently leads to decreased ACTH and cortisol secretion. This occurs most commonly in patients who are on prolonged glucocorticoid (commonly referred to as steroids) therapy. These patients who have an abrupt discontinuation of prolonged glucocorticoid therapy or experience periods of increased physiologic stress are unable to mount an adequate cortisol response for normal body homeostasis. Patients who are on chronic steroids develop atrophied adrenal glands, so when their steroids are abruptly discontinued for any reason their adrenal glands will be unable to produce enough cortisol. These patients tend to develop adrenal crisis, which is a medical emergency. Therefore patients with chronic steroid use will often receive stress-dose steroids perioperatively to help prevent this from occurring.[1,3,5]

As discussed, patients on chronic daily oral glucocorticoids (steroids such as prednisone) are at largest risk for developing tertiary AI. However, it is important to note that it can also happen to patients on intermittent oral corticosteroids, inhaled steroids, and even patients receiving frequent musculoskeletal steroid injections. Prolonged therapy involving taking >5 mg/day of prednisone (or its equivalent) places patients at increased risk for developing tertiary AI. Patients taking <5 mg/day of prednisone are less likely to develop AI.[1,3]

Clinical Presentation

In the inpatient setting, AI might occur in a patient on long-term corticosteroid therapy who is not receiving equivalent dosing while admitted or in a patient in physiologic stress who is not receiving necessary increased dosing, such as ill patients with sepsis. Common causes of AI to watch for in the neurosurgical setting include pituitary tumors or craniopharyngioma, head trauma/TBI, pituitary surgery or radiotherapy, and intracranial artery aneurysms.[2]

- Glucocorticoid deficiency can manifest as a variety of symptoms[1-3]:
    - Fatigue, lack of energy, weight loss, joint pains, fever
    - Anemia, hypotension (including postural hypotension), increased TSH, and hypercalcemia
    - Hypoglycemia
        - This occurs because glucocorticoids promote gluconeogenesis, the process of glucose generation and release from the liver.
- Mineralocorticoid deficiency can manifest as a variety of symptoms[1-3]:
    - Abdominal pain/nausea/vomiting, dizziness, salt craving
    - Low blood pressure (including postural hypotension)
    - Increased serum creatinine and hyperkalemia
    - Hyponatremia more common in mineralocorticoid deficiency
        - This occurs because aldosterone release (which is deficient in primary AI) is responsible for promoting sodium retention and potassium excretion.
- Androgen deficiency can be present in both primary and secondary AI[1-3]:
    - Symptoms: dry and itchy skin, loss of libido, loss of pubic hair
- Primary AI commonly presents gradually with vague and nonspecific signs and symptoms.
    - It is important to watch for the findings associated with glucocorticoid, mineralocorticoid, and androgen deficiencies noted earlier.
- Secondary and tertiary AI will show findings primarily associated with glucocorticoid deficiency.

In the inpatient setting it is especially important to watch for acute primary AI, also known as adrenal crisis. Adrenal crisis can be the initial presentation of a patient with previously undiagnosed primary AI. Adrenal crisis is considered a medical emergency due to the subsequent risk for hypotension and shock, which is more commonly seen in patients with primary AI.

- Patients in adrenal crisis often present with severe hypotension not responsive to fluids and vasopressors, hypoglycemia, fever, confusion, or coma.
- Onset is often precipitated by an acute illness or a stressful situation, such as major surgery.
- Initiation of thyroid replacement therapy can also trigger an adrenal crisis.
    - Providers will therefore often start corticosteroid replacement before thyroid replacement.[1]

Diagnosis

It is essential to understand that in an unstable patient with suspected adrenal crisis, diagnosis should not delay treatment. In these cases, providers will likely order intravenous (IV) steroids, such as hydrocortisone, and subsequently may order stat cortisol, ACTH, and renin:aldosterone ratio levels to further evaluate. On the other hand, in patients with suspected AI who are hemodynamically stable, a morning cortisol level drawn between 6 and 8 am (recall that endogenous cortisol levels are highest in the morning) can assist with diagnosis. When interpreting the lab value:

- A cortisol level <3 µg/dL rules in AI.
- A cortisol level >15 µg/dL rules out AI.
- Patients with levels between 3 and 15 µg/dL are considered nondiagnostic and should undergo a 250-µg cosyntropin stimulation test.
  - Cosyntropin is a synthetic version of ACTH.
  - Nurses will be expected to draw a subsequent cortisol level 30–60 minutes after administration of cosyntropin.
  - Levels <18 µg/dL indicate AI (a cutoff of 9 µg/dL is often used in the critical setting).

When the cortisol level is reflective of AI, the provider will also order ACTH levels to differentiate the type of AI. ACTH levels >100 pg/mL indicate primary AI. The provider may also order a 48-hour ACTH stimulation test to confirm the results. Furthermore, secondary AI can be differentiated from tertiary AI by use of a CRH test, which is done in the same manner as the cosyntropin stimulation test explained earlier. Administration of the CRH should boost ACTH levels in the blood in tertiary AI but not in secondary AI.[1,2]

Treatment

ACUTE ADRENAL INSUFFICIENCY/CRISIS

In patients with suspected acute AI/adrenal crisis, treatment should not be delayed. Nurses should expect the provider to order baseline cortisol/ACTH/renin levels and start steroids immediately, opting not to wait until the morning to obtain labs. Baseline labs can be obtained as treatment is initiated. The nurse will need to gain IV access urgently as the provider will likely order isotonic fluids, such as normal saline, and IV steroids. Steroid treatment will often entail either a continuous infusion or scheduled IV pushes.

The nurse will need to continue to assess the patient and monitor vitals for improvement. Nursing assessments should include hydration status, intake and output, and mental status. Nurses should urgently report to the provider fevers >101°F, persistent hypotension, weight increase >3 lb/day, abnormal cardiac rhythms, and hypoglycemia. If the patient's course improves and is uncomplicated, expect the provider to order a tapering IV regimen over 1–3 days before transitioning to maintenance oral (PO) dosing.[2,3,7]

CHRONIC ADRENAL INSUFFICIENCY

In treatment of chronic AI, glucocorticoid replacement should simulate natural release of cortisol. This is done in the form of morning and evening doses. The morning dose should be ordered to be taken as close to waking up as possible. The evening dose should be given about 6–8 hours after the morning dose. Providers will monitor the response to therapy based on clinical presentation rather than lab findings. The overall goal is to adequately treat the symptoms of disease with the lowest dose possible to avoid adverse effects of excessive corticosteroid replacement. Patients with primary AI will also be ordered fludrocortisone. The response to this mineralocorticoid replacement includes measuring orthostatic vitals, sodium, potassium, and renin:aldosterone ratio levels.[8]

Patient Education

It is important that patients are instructed on how to manage their chronic AI with respect to stressors. They must be instructed on what constitutes a stressor and how to classify the severity.

Patients may be able to treat their AI with stress dosages at home in minor stress situations (mild fever, minor infections) but in more severe situations should seek medical care for steroid replacement (if the severe stressor has not already prompted them to seek medical care). Nurses play a significant role in providing crisis management education to patients with a history of AI. Nurses must educate patients on wearing medical alert identification, carrying a medical information card, using emergency intramuscular steroid medication, and when to seek medical attention.[7,9]

Hypopituitarism

The pituitary is composed of an anterior and posterior gland. The anterior pituitary gland secretes six hormones: LH, FSH, ACTH, prolactin, TSH, and GH. The posterior pituitary does not produce hormones but instead stores and secretes hormones produced in the hypothalamus, including oxytocin and ADH[10] (see Fig. 21.3).

Hypopituitarism is defined as deficiency in one or more of the pituitary hormones. Decreased function of the pituitary gland can occur due to disease of the pituitary gland itself or disease of the hypothalamus. Hypopituitarism can result from metastatic cancer, lymphoma, infiltrative diseases (e.g., sarcoid), inflammation, surgery, radiation, or medication. In the neurosurgical population, it can result from a pituitary adenoma, meningioma, craniopharyngioma, pituitary infarction or apoplexy, or TBI. Panhypopituitarism is a lack or deficiency of all pituitary hormones. This usually occurs due to large tumors or from pituitary surgery.[2,4,11]

PRESENTATION AND DIAGNOSIS

The presenting symptoms will differ depending on which hormones are affected.[8,12]
- GH
  - Reduced energy, muscle mass, and strength
  - Increased central fat distribution
  - Decreased sweating and impaired thermal regulation
    - Evaluation for GH deficiency includes checking insulin-like growth factor 1 levels, but a normal test does not rule out the disease.
- ACTH
  - Fatigue, weakness, anorexia, weight loss, nausea, vomiting, abdominal pain, hypoglycemia
- FSH/LH
  - Men: erectile dysfunction, soft testes, reduced muscle mass, reduced energy
  - Women: oligomenorrhea or amenorrhea, dyspareunia, breast atrophy
    - Both: loss of libido, hot flashes, infertility
- TSH
  - Fatigue, apathy, cold intolerance, constipation, weight gain, dry skin
    - Evaluation involves checking TSH and free T4 (thyroxine)
- ADH
  - Polyuria, polydipsia, nocturia
  - Loss of ADH leads to diabetes insipidus (DI)
  - Patients who lack an intact thirst mechanism are at risk for hypernatremia
    - Evaluation involves checking serum osmolality and electrolyte levels
- Prolactin
  - Inability to breastfeed

While overall screening for hypopituitarism includes testing FSH, LH, cortisol, TSH, and free T4, clinicians should order the appropriate lab tests depending on the clinical scenario and presenting symptoms. Additional workup may require imaging, including brain computed tomography and magnetic resonance imaging, to look for pituitary tumors. If found, surgery may be required.[4,10,11]

TREATMENT

If hypopituitarism is suspected, treatment will depend on which hormones are affected[4,11]:
- ACTH deficiency
  - Steroids and fluids
- TSH deficiency
  - Daily administration of levothyroxine
  - Monitoring free T4 levels and not TSH
- Gonadotropin deficiency (GnRH, LH, FSH)
  - Treatment decided on an individual basis, in individuals without contraindications
  - Testosterone replacement in men
  - Combined estrogen-progesterone in premenopausal women
  - Replacement necessary in men and women who desire fertility
- GH deficiency
  - Diagnosis and treatment of GH deficiency: complex, should involve an endocrinologist
  - Benefits of treatment: increased exercise capacity, body composition, bone density
  - Hormone replacement contraindicated in the setting of malignancy

Central Diabetes Insipidus

In neurosurgical patients, central DI can result from brain tumors, TBI, and surgical resection of pituitary tumors. DI is due to a deficiency in ADH. This causes the kidneys to be unable to concentrate urine, and the patient will produce copious amounts of diluted urine. This results in an increase in serum sodium, also known as hypernatremia. Conscious patients may compensate with polydipsia, which is the increased consumption of fluids due to increased thirst. Neurosurgery nurses will commonly see DI in patients who recently underwent surgery to resect brain tumors. These at-risk patients should have frequent access to free water and be encouraged to drink to thirst. If the patient is unable to drink or has impaired thirst mechanisms, water can be given enterally through a feeding tube.

In at-risk patients, neuroscience nurses should monitor for changes in neurologic status as well as increased urine output, excess polydipsia, hypotension, and hypernatremia. The provider should be alerted to changes in any of these findings. Treatment for DI includes replacement with desmopressin and fluid administration. When a patient with DI is discharged from the hospital, nurses should provide education on increasing fluid intake and monitoring for any increased thirst and urination. Nurses should ensure patients understand the need for follow-up and are comfortable with new medication/method of administration. Patients should also be encouraged to wear medical alert identification.[2,7,9]

Conclusion

The pituitary gland is a very complex organ that helps regulate important hormones that are involved in many functions within the body. Hormone dysregulation, resulting from pituitary gland dysfunction, can cause deleterious effects and must be recognized and treated quickly. Neurosurgical patients, due to the nature of their disease processes, are especially at increased risk for pituitary gland dysfunction. Neurosurgical nurses play a key role in recognizing dangerous symptoms related to hypopituitarism and should be able to quickly identify these signs and notify the provider to initiate prompt treatment. Nurses are also pivotal in implementing therapeutic interventions to treat the disease process.

References

1. Arlt W. Disorders of the adrenal cortex. In: Loscalzo J, Fauci A, Kasper D, et al., eds. *Harrison's Principles of Internal Medicine*, 21st ed. McGraw Hill; 2022.
2. Burns CA. *MKSAP 17 Endocrinology and Metabolism*. American College of Physicians; 2015.
3. Huecker MR, Bhutta BS, Dominique E. *Adrenal Insufficiency*. StatPearls Publishing; 2023.
4. Jain SH, Katznelson L. Pituitary disease. In: McKean SC, Ross JJ, Dressler DD, et al., eds. *Principles and Practice of Hospital Medicine*, 2nd ed. McGraw Hill; 2017.
5. Passini JC, Liew E, Sheehy AM, et al. Adrenal Insufficiency. In: McKean SC, Ross JJ, Dressler DD, et al., eds. *Principles and Practice of Hospital Medicine*, 2nd ed. McGraw Hill; 2017.
6. Michels AW, Eisenbarth GS. Immunologic endocrine disorders. *J Allergy Clin Immunol.* 2010;125(2):S226–S237. doi:10.1016/j.jaci.2009.09.053.
7. Hinkle JL, Cheever KH. Assessment and management of patients with endocrine disorders. In: Hinkle JL, Cheever KH, eds. *Brunner & Suddarth's Textbook of Medical-Surgical Nursing*, 14th ed. Wolters Kluwer; 2018.
8. Ross JJ, Dressler DD, Scheurer DB, eds. *Principles and Practice of Hospital Medicine*. 2nd ed. McGraw Hill; 2017.
9. Konick-McMahan J. Crisis management: acute adrenal insufficiency. *Nursing Crit Care.* 2006;1(5): 52–57.
10. Melmed S, Jameson J. Hypopituitarism. In: Loscalzo J, Fauci A, Kasper D, et al., eds. *Harrison's Principles of Internal Medicine*, 21st ed. McGraw Hill; 2022.
11. Esposito D, Olsson DS, Ragnarsson O, et al. Non-functioning pituitary adenomas: indications for pituitary surgery and post-surgical management. *Pituitary.* 2019;22:422–434. doi:10.1007/s11102-019-00960-0.
12. Prabhakar VKB, Shalet SM. Aetiology, diagnosis, and management of hypopituitarism in adult life. *Postgrad Med J.* 2006;82(966):259–266. doi:10.1136/pgmj.2005.039768.

Questions

1. Fred, a 56-year-old male with a past medical history (PMH) of rheumatoid arthritis on daily prednisone, is about to undergo spine surgery. You see that he is ordered IV hydrocortisone. The patient questions why he is getting a different steroid than the one he takes at home. What do you tell him?
   a. You are not allowed to eat and drink before surgery and should therefore not get your oral steroid.
   b. You are in a high-stress situation, and your body needs more steroids than what you usually get to prevent crisis.
   c. Hydrocortisone is the only steroid the pharmacy has available in the hospital.
   d. Assume it is a mistake and hold the medication.

2. Mary is a 67-year-old female with a history of chronic obstructive pulmonary disease who was admitted several days ago for postoperative pneumonia as a transfer from an outside hospital. Records are not available from the transferring facility. The provider is concerned about adrenal insufficiency and orders an early morning cortisol level. The patient is currently hemodynamically stable. Which of the following is appropriate?
   a. Draw cortisol level with 1 am labs.
   b. Draw early morning cortisol between 6 and 8 am.
   c. Plan to draw an early morning cortisol level but start ordered steroids first.
   d. Draw cortisol level with 4 am labs.

3. Sarah is a 43-year-old female with recent diagnosis of secondary adrenal insufficiency after pituitary surgery. She has been initiated on IV hydrocortisone with a taper to PO dose. She is ready for discharge and has plans for outpatient follow-up with endocrinology. What education should be provided to the patient prior to discharge?
   a. Explanation of stressors to look out for, including infection, fever, trauma, and surgery, and the need to follow the physician's instructions on increasing corticosteroid dosing with these stressors
   b. Recommendation for wearing a medical alert bracelet
   c. Confirming the physician has provided a prescription for emergency hydrocortisone kit
   d. All the above

4. John is a 42-year-old male who recently underwent pituitary resection for an adenoma. You have noticed some increased thirst but otherwise his vitals and labs, including basic metabolic panel, are normal. What, if anything, should be done next?
   a. Nothing. The patient is stable and sodium is normal.
   b. Give him IV fluids and encourage him to drink more.
   c. Report findings to provider and measure accurate input and output.
   d. Hold IV and PO fluids.

5. Sam is a 32-year-old female with recent diagnosis of panhypopituitarism. What education should be given on discharge?
   a. If you wish to have children, you may follow up with an endocrinologist to see if estrogen + progesterone replacement is appropriate for you.
   b. You should continue taking your levothyroxine.
   c. You should obtain a medical alert bracelet.
   d. All the above

Answers

1. b

2. b

3. d

4. c

5. d

CHAPTER 22

Nursing Management of Anemia

Bharath Ganesh, MD, FACP

Introduction

Anemia is defined as a decrease in circulating red blood cell (RBC) mass.[1] The diagnostic criteria for anemia in adults define thresholds according to hemoglobin (Hgb) and hematocrit (Hct) levels. Although the anemia cutoff for these parameters may vary slightly from one hospital laboratory to another, it is generally defined as a Hgb <12 g/dL or Hct <36% in nonpregnant women or Hgb <13 g/dL or Hct <39% in males.[2] Depending on the acuity and severity, patients with anemia often experience changes in the following:

- Vital signs: tachycardia, hypotension
- Appearance: pallor, decreased capillary refill time
- Presentation: lethargy, fatigue, increased shortness of breath

There is an abundance of scientific literature that states that anemia at the time of hospital admission is associated with increased mortality and morbidity, particularly in the elderly.[3,4] Patients with anemia are also more likely to have a prolonged hospitalization and an increased risk of early readmission after discharge.[5,6] The detrimental effects of anemia are exacerbated in patients during the perioperative period of medical care, and the postoperative neuroscience patient is particularly vulnerable.

Relevance to Nursing

The inpatient neurosurgical nurse plays a critical role in the early recognition of symptoms and complications of acute anemia. Nurses are frequently the first among the interprofessional care team to recognize the early signs of anemia even before laboratory results become available. A preoperative diagnosis of anemia before elective spine surgery is a risk factor for poor outcomes during hospitalization, such as increased duration of hospitalization, incidence of postoperative complications, and 30-day mortality after surgery.[7] An accurate admission medication reconciliation, along with a thorough medical history and coagulopathy screen, is crucial for identifying patients who are at an increased risk for adverse bleeding outcomes. Furthermore, significant anemia requiring transfusion is a well-established risk factor for prolonged hospitalization and early readmission after discharge.[8] In the postop spine patient, effective nursing care in the context of anemia may involve:

- Prompt recognition of early signs and symptoms of blood loss
- Effective communication with medical and surgical teams
- Expeditiously obtaining necessary imaging and labs for diagnosis
- Close monitoring of transfusion-related complications

Laboratory Evaluation[1,9]

A variety of laboratory tests are used to determine the etiology and severity of anemia:

1. Complete blood count (CBC) is the most frequently ordered hematologic test in the hospital and often is monitored daily for some patients. The components of CBC directly related to anemia include:

    a. Hgb: the most important lab value in the CBC for diagnosis of anemia. When reviewing Hgb levels in the context of an anemia workup, the absolute number is usually less important than the rate of decrease. The National Cancer Institute grades the severity of anemia as follows:
        i. Mild: Hgb 10.0 g/dL to the lower limit of normal
        ii. Moderate: Hgb 8.0–9.9 g/dL
        iii. Severe: Hgb 6.5–7.9 g/dL
        iv. Life-threatening: Hgb <6.5 g/dL
    b. Hct: the surrogate measure of RBC mass
        i. Normal range: typically 40–50%
    c. Mean corpuscular volume (MCV): the mean measure of the volume of red cells. An abnormal MCV is useful to determine the pathophysiologic process driving the anemia.
        i. Normal MCV range: 80–100 fL
        ii. Microcytic anemias (MCV <80 fL): seen in iron deficiency and thalassemia
        iii. Macrocytic anemias (MCV >100 fL): point toward B12 and folate deficiencies
        iv. Acute anemias (e.g., from blood loss or hemolysis): typically result in normocytic values
    d. Mean corpuscular hemoglobin: average amount of hemoglobin in an RBC; normal range: 27–33 pg
    e. White blood cell (WBC) and platelet counts: Although the WBC and platelet counts are not direct measures of anemia, low counts in all three cell lines may indicate a disease involving the bone marrow (aplastic anemia, metastatic cancer, myelofibrosis, etc.).
    f. Red cell distribution width (RDW): a measure of variation in red cell size. Elevated RDW signifies a greater variability in RBC size and is commonly seen in iron deficiency anemia.
2. Reticulocyte index (RI): Reticulocytes are immature RBCs released into circulation by the bone marrow in response to anemia. It is not part of a routine CBC but is a useful measure of the bone marrow's response to anemia. The RI is a calculated index that incorporates absolute reticulocyte count and is corrected for the patient's hematocrit level.
    a. RI <2 indicates decreased production of RBCs
        i. Seen in hypoproliferative disorders such as bone marrow failure, chronic iron deficiency, B12 deficiency, etc.
    b. RI >2 indicates an adequate bone marrow response to anemia
        i. Commonly seen in acute bleeding and hemolysis
3. Peripheral smear: The microscopic examination of a manually prepared blood smear can provide useful clues to identify the underlying disease process. RBC morphology is altered in most forms of anemia. Experienced reviewers will review RBC size, shape, presence of inclusions, and any abnormal red cell morphology (schistocytes, sickle cells, target cells, teardrop cells, etc.) to help identify the type of anemia.
4. Bone marrow biopsy: This is an invasive study performed by a consulting hematology fellow or attending physician. It is not typically required solely for the workup for anemia but may be performed if there is a high index of suspicion for bone marrow involvement (i.e., other cytopenias, active cancer, low reticulocyte index, unexplained normocytic anemia).

In the case of acute blood loss anemia, laboratory evaluation will demonstrate a characteristic pattern of abnormalities. Hgb and Hct levels fall proportionately with the rapidity and severity of bleeding. With aggressive fluid resuscitation, Hgb and Hct will decrease further because of hemodilution, and lab results should be interpreted with this phenomenon in mind.

- Peripheral smear is not critical for diagnosis but, when available, will typically show a normocytic anemia (normal MCV on CBC) with no abnormal red cell morphology unless there is a preexisting chronic anemia.
- Reticulocyte index, if obtained, will show an adequate bone marrow response (RI >2), thereby differentiating it from primary bone marrow disorders, such as aplastic anemia, myelodysplasia, and metastatic cancer (Table 22.1, Fig. 22.1).

TABLE 22.1 ■ Overview of Common Anemias

Type of Anemia	Additional Workup	Management
Microcytic anemia (MCV <80 fL)		
Iron deficiency anemia[27] • Reduced red blood cell (RBC) production due to lack of iron in the bone marrow	• Low iron, low ferritin, high total iron-binding capacity (TIBC) • Reticulocyte index (RI) normal or low • Bone marrow (BM) biopsy: hypocellular marrow, low iron staining	• Identify anatomic site of bleed (imaging, endoscopy, etc.) • Oral/intravenous iron supplementation
Thalassemia[48] • May be alpha- or beta-thalassemia • Inherited disorder of hemoglobin (Hgb) synthesis	• Peripheral smear: poikilocytosis, nucleated RBCs • Hgb electrophoresis	• Most mild cases need no treatment • Transfusion to keep Hgb >9–10 g/dL • Iron chelation therapy in severe cases
Sideroblastic anemia[49] • Abnormal iron metabolism characterized by presence of ring sideroblasts • Inherited or acquired • Associated with myelodysplastic syndromes, drugs, alcohol use	• BM biopsy: presence of ring sideroblasts	• Remove offending agent • Pyridoxine supplementation
Normocytic anemia (MCV 80–100 fL)		
Anemia of chronic disease[50] • Associated with inflammatory disease, cancer, chronic infection	• Low serum iron, low TIBC • Ferritin may be normal or elevated	• Treat underlying cause • Treat coexisting iron deficiency, if present • Erythropoiesis-stimulating agents (ESAs) for severe symptomatic anemia
Anemia of chronic kidney disease[51] • Due to low erythropoietin production and/or iron deficiency	• Diminished renal function • Ferritin and transferrin saturation help guide therapy	• ESAs • Treat underlying iron deficiency. Oral iron is not effective
Hemolytic anemias[52] • Wide range of causes • May be due to sickle cell disease, drug-induced, autoimmune, infections, RBC microtrauma, etc.	• Peripheral smear: abnormal RBC forms • RI >2 • Elevated lactate dehydrogenase, indirect bilirubin, low haptoglobin • Other: direct/indirect Coombs tests, Hgb electrophoresis, autoantibody testing	• Treatment according to underlying cause • Stop offending drugs, if any
Aplastic anemia[53] • Bone marrow failure resulting in anemia +/- leukopenia and thrombocytopenia • May be idiopathic, infectious, drug induced, or secondary to cancer	• Bone marrow biopsy is diagnostic: low cellularity often involving all blood lines • Cytogenetic testing	• Stop offending drugs • Hematology consultation • Immunosuppressive medications • Treatment of underlying cancer, if present

Continued

TABLE 22.1 ■ Overview of Common Anemias—cont'd

Type of Anemia	Additional Workup	Management
Macrocytic anemia (MCV >100 fL)		
Vitamin B12 deficiency[54]	• Peripheral smear: macro-cytes, hypersegmented neutrophils	• Oral or intramuscular vitamin B12 replacement
• Associated with low intake (e.g., vegan diet) or low absorption (gastric atrophy, bowel disease, malabsorption)	• Elevated methylmalonic acid (MMA) and homocysteine	• Treat coexisting iron deficiency
• Severe disease: neurologic deficits	• Antibodies to intrinsic factor for pernicious anemia	
Folate deficiency[55]	• Peripheral smear: macrocytes	• Oral folate therapy
• Due to low intake, low intestinal absorption, or increased requirement (e.g., pregnancy)	• Normal MMA and low homocysteine	• Treat coexisting iron deficiency
• Does not cause neurologic disease		

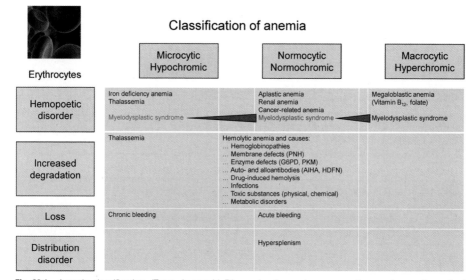

Fig. 22.1 Anemia classification. (From Jansen V. Diagnosis of anemia—a synoptic overview and practical approach. *Transfus Apher Sci.*2019;58[4]:375–385.)

Clinical Features

HISTORY AND SYMPTOMS

A comprehensive history and physical exam can provide important clues regarding the severity and cause of anemia. A major determinant of the signs and symptoms of anemia that a patient may experience is the rate of decrease in Hgb over time. Chronic anemias that develop over several months are frequently asymptomatic despite a severe decrease in Hgb.[1] Common symptoms associated with anemia include[2]:

- Fatigue
- Shortness of breath with exertion

- Chest pain with exertion
- Symptoms of acute blood loss (dizziness, syncope, increased surgical site pain, abdominal pain)
- Jaundice (yellowish discoloration of skin seen in hemolytic anemias)
- Poor exercise tolerance

Additional history that is useful for determining the cause of anemia includes[1]:

- Family history of anemia
- Current use of anticoagulants or antiplatelet drugs (including over-the-counter medications and herbal supplements)
- Other medications
- Menstrual and obstetric history
- Gastrointestinal bleeding (melena, hematochezia, hematemesis)
- History of kidney disease
- History of autoimmune disease
- History of malabsorption syndrome
- Alcohol intake, dietary restrictions (vitamin B12, folate deficiencies)

PHYSICAL EXAMINATION

Physical exam findings vary depending on the abruptness of onset of anemia.

Patients with anemia due to acute ongoing blood loss typically display signs of intravascular volume loss. This can include sinus tachycardia and hypotension and can progress to oliguria, acute kidney injury, and circulatory collapse if not recognized and treated early.[9] In all cases of acute blood loss, nurses should focus their physical exam on finding the anatomic site of the bleed. Bleeding from the operative bed is a common source of blood loss in the postoperative neurosurgical spine patient. Accurate documentation of operative blood loss by the surgical team can predict the severity of postoperative anemia, and surgical drain outputs should be quantified frequently and accurately.

The presence of conjunctival rim pallor is strongly predictive of anemia (likelihood ratio +16.7).[10] Scleral jaundice indicates an underlying hemolytic process caused by the deposition of unconjugated bilirubin (a by-product of hemoglobin degradation) in the scleral connective tissue.

In some patients with significant chronic anemia, auscultation of the heart will reveal a systolic flow murmur typically heard best at the cardiac base (aortic and pulmonic areas).[9] These murmurs are benign and do not indicate valvular damage; they usually resolve with treatment of anemia. Koilonychia (spooning of the nails) of the extremities is suggestive of chronic iron deficiency anemia.[11]

Postoperative Anemia After Spine Surgery

OVERVIEW

Spine surgery is associated with an increased risk of operative blood loss. The extent of blood loss in an individual depends on patient-specific and operative risk factors.[12]

- Patient-specific risk factors include preoperative anemia, female sex, and small body surface area.[13]
- Operative risk factors include multilevel spine procedures, osteotomies, and revision surgeries, as these carry a higher risk for large volume blood loss.[12]

CLINICAL FEATURES OF PERIOPERATIVE BLOOD LOSS

During the perioperative period, hemodynamically significant acute blood loss usually results in overt symptomatology. Vital signs are often abnormal, and routine hematologic lab evaluation reveals a decrease in Hgb compared to preoperative levels. These patients often manifest changes consistent with acute decompensated intravascular volume depletion (hypotension, sinus tachycardia, and end-organ injury). Younger, healthier patients with no underlying cardiac disease tend to be able to compensate for blood loss without significant compromise of their cardiac output within physiologic limits.[9]

It is worth noting that Hgb levels during or immediately after a significant bleeding episode will underestimate the volume of blood loss due to hemoconcentration. Conversely, Hgb levels may precipitously drop following isotonic volume resuscitation due to hemodilution of RBCs.[14] Therefore any estimate of total blood loss should include the patient's overall clinical condition and take into consideration additional objective indicators (such as hemodynamic measures, estimated surgical blood loss, drain output, and urine output) rather than relying on laboratory values alone.

POSTOPERATIVE SPINAL EPIDURAL HEMATOMA

Small, asymptomatic epidural hemorrhage at the operative site is common after spine surgery and is usually self-resolving. It is often only apparent on computed tomography (CT) or magnetic resonance imaging (MRI) in the postoperative period.[15,16] On the other hand, symptomatic postoperative epidural hematoma is a rare but potentially devastating complication, with an incidence of <1% of all spine surgeries.[17] Decompressive procedures of the spine (e.g., laminectomy and laminotomy) expose its neurovascular structures and increase the likelihood of vascular disruption during surgery. This results in continued accumulation of blood within the restricted dural space, eventually causing a mass effect on the spinal cord.[18] Symptomatic epidural hematomas are usually apparent within 24–48 hours after surgery.[19] The nurse caring for a postoperative spine patient should monitor closely for clinical signs of epidural hematoma. The patient may complain of worsening back pain around the surgical site, radicular symptoms (numbness and tingling), and weakness in the extremities. The patient's neurologic exam can progress rapidly to sensory loss, motor deficits, and urinary retention.[18] The primary surgical team should be made aware of any change in neurologic exam immediately.

When deterioration of neurologic exam is dramatic in the immediate postoperative setting, a diagnosis of spinal epidural hematoma is not difficult to determine. In cases where confirmatory imaging is needed, the appropriate study is an urgent MRI of the spine. MRI will reveal a convex fluid collection causing severe thecal sac compression in acutely symptomatic cases.[20] The treatment for epidural hematoma is emergent evacuation of the hematoma, ideally within 6–12 hours of the onset of symptoms.[21]

RETROPERITONEAL HEMATOMA

A retroperitoneal hematoma can develop in a subset of patients who have undergone lumbar spine procedures and should be included in the differential diagnosis when acute blood loss anemia occurs. The retroperitoneum is the space in the abdominal cavity that is located behind the peritoneal lining and anterior to the vertebrae. This space houses important organs and structures, such as the kidneys, aorta, and inferior vena cava. Bleeding from the lumbar spine operative bed can seep into the retroperitoneal space and form a large hematoma before surrounding tissues are able to tamponade the hemorrhage.[22] Besides the usual clinical signs of acute blood loss, patients may also have bruising of the skin around the abdomen and flank. Additionally, the hemorrhage can track down the fascia of the psoas muscle to its insertion in the hip. When this occurs, patients will complain of unilateral hip pain and have a palpable mass.[23]

If retroperitoneal hemorrhage is suspected, evaluation and management should be expedient to prevent mortality and end-organ damage due to tissue hypoperfusion. Diagnosis is made by obtaining a CT scan of the abdomen and pelvis. CT with intravenous (IV) contrast is preferred as it can accurately delineate the size and extent of the hematoma. It also has the added advantage of being able to locate an actively bleeding vessel, which may be amenable to intervention such as embolization.[24] In patients with a contrast allergy or kidney disease that prevents use of IV contrast, a noncontrast study usually is a sufficient diagnostic study.

Treatment

GENERAL PRINCIPLES

A 2018 study demonstrated that more than one-third of patients who did not have anemia on admission developed it at some point during their hospitalization.[6] With this in mind, nurses should discuss with providers the necessity of routine blood draws to decrease the occurrence of hospital-acquired anemia. The primary goals when treating acute anemia in the hospital are to stabilize the patient and to determine the cause. Treatment should be tailored toward the cause of anemia. Frequently, in the case of chronic mild-moderate anemia that is present on admission and is stable throughout hospitalization, detailed workup is often deferred to the outpatient setting. In these cases the importance of outpatient follow-up with the patient's primary care physician must be emphasized.

APPROACH TO A PATIENT WITH IRON DEFICIENCY

Iron metabolism is a carefully regulated physiologic process. In a nondeficient individual, only ~10% of all ingested elemental iron is absorbed by the gastrointestinal tract, most of it occurring in the duodenum.[25] In a state of iron deficiency, the absorbed fraction of ingested iron is increased through feedback mechanisms involving the inhibition of the hormone hepcidin.[26] When iron deficiency is suspected as a cause of anemia, a blood iron panel is ordered to confirm the diagnosis. The panel includes:

- Serum iron
- Serum ferritin
- Total iron binding capacity
- Transferrin saturation

Ferritin is a protein that is bound to elemental iron within cells and is the storage form of iron. Serum ferritin most accurately correlates with total body iron stores. Serum ferritin (<12 µg/mL) is diagnostic of iron deficiency anemia.[27] Serum ferritin levels tend to be overestimated in acute or chronic inflammatory states, such as infections and autoimmune conditions, and therefore must be interpreted with caution in states of acute illness.[28]

ORAL IRON SUPPLEMENTATION

In a stable asymptomatic patient with confirmed iron deficiency anemia, oral iron supplementation is the preferred route of treatment. Ultimately the goal of iron supplementation is not only the resolution of anemia but also replacement of the body's iron stores. Oral iron supplementation is available in several formulations ranging from simple iron salts to more complex compounds that provide sustained absorption from the intestine. The most common formulation is ferrous sulfate due to its wide availability and low cost, and absorption is best when taken on an empty stomach. Common side effects of oral iron therapy are predominantly gastrointestinal in nature. Patients may report bloating, epigastric pain, abdominal cramps, nausea, vomiting, constipation, and dark stools. Nurses should monitor for these side effects and discuss dosage changes with the provider. These side effects are usually dose dependent and can be ameliorated by titrating the frequency of dosing to the patient's tolerated level.[29] Oral vitamin C, when taken together with iron, is known to enhance the iron absorption in the duodenum.[30] A general rule of thumb is to continue iron supplementation for 3–6 months after anemia has resolved.[27]

Historically it was common to prescribe 200 mg of elemental iron daily in 2–3 divided doses.[27] However, in recent years there has been an increasing quantity of evidence that up to 50–65 mg of elemental iron once daily, or even alternate-day dosing, may be as effective (if not more) at repleting iron stores.[31] It is believed that regimens that are more spaced out over time may reduce the stimulation of hepcidin (the hormone that inhibits iron absorption from the gut).[32]

INTRAVENOUS IRON SUPPLEMENTATION

In a minority of patients, oral iron supplementation may not be a feasible option. Patients may be unable to tolerate oral iron due to prohibitive side effects. Others may have a poor response to oral iron, be unable to absorb iron due to prior gastrointestinal surgery or malabsorptive states (e.g., celiac disease), be unable to adhere to therapy, or may require a more acute form of iron replacement. In these patients, IV iron therapy is a suitable alternative to oral formulations.

Iron sucrose is perhaps the most widely used IV iron preparation in the United States, followed by iron gluconate. The advantage of iron sucrose lies mainly in the lower incidence of anaphylactic reactions.[33] A large (>400 mg) single-dose administration of iron sucrose is associated with a higher incidence of adverse effects (fatigue, myalgia, rash) that may persist for a few days after the dose.[1] These reactions are typically self-limiting, and supportive care with nonsteroidal antiinflammatory drugs is sufficient. Iron dextran is an older IV iron formulation that is not commonly used today due to its relatively higher incidence of anaphylaxis. Ferrous carboxymaltose is a newer, more expensive iron formulation that is more common in the outpatient infusion center setting. With this formulation, hypotension during infusion may occur.[1]

A long-standing controversy in the field of IV iron replacement is the potential to cause or exacerbate preexisting infection. Iron is a growth factor used by several bacteria for normal metabolic processes. There is no evidence that IV iron therapy is associated with 30-day postoperative infections or mortality in patients after major surgery.[32] However, in patients who have active infection—particularly with bacteremia—IV iron therapy is often deferred until the infection is treated appropriately.

Blood Transfusions

Packed RBC (PRBC) transfusion is the mainstay of treatment for acute, severe, and symptomatic anemia. Blood transfusions can be lifesaving in patients who are experiencing acute and severe hemorrhage (trauma, acute gastrointestinal bleeding, intraabdominal bleeding). PRBC transfusions are also commonly used in patients who have severe anemia but are otherwise hemodynamically stable. Acutely ill patients with massive ongoing hemorrhage or persistent hypotension should be monitored closely in the intensive care unit with hemodynamic support. These patients will often require multiple units of PRBCs; depending on their comorbidities (e.g., thrombocytopenia or coagulopathy), they may also need platelet transfusions and fresh frozen plasma.

The threshold for PRBC transfusion is usually a Hgb <7 g/dL.[34] Nevertheless, providers should base the decision to transfuse on the overall clinical status of the patient, not by Hgb level alone. Patients with significant preexisting cardiovascular disease, particularly those with ongoing myocardial ischemia, typically have a slightly more liberalized transfusion threshold of Hgb <8 g/dL.[35] This strategy helps prevent worsening of oxygen delivery to the cardiac muscle already at risk for ischemia.

- Any benefit of blood transfusion in a patient with significant cardiac disease must always be weighed against the potential risks of fluid overload.

COMMON COMPLICATIONS OF BLOOD TRANSFUSIONS

Blood transfusions, like any other therapeutic intervention, carry a risk for serious adverse events. The benefits of blood transfusion must be weighed against any potential risk to the patient on a case-by-case basis. There is a risk of transmitting viral infections via transfusion, but these complications are exceedingly rare due to stringent screening of donor blood units for common infectious agents. The rates of transmission are ~1 in 350,000 for hepatitis B, 1 in 1.8 million for hepatitis C, and 1 in 2.3 million for human immunodeficiency virus.[36] Regardless, nurses should be prepared to provide reassurance to patients and monitor for the most common acute transfusion complications.

Acute Hemolytic Reactions[36,37]

- Incidence: 1–5 in 50,000 transfusions
- Immune-mediated destruction of RBCs by antibodies in donor blood in response to a corresponding antigen on recipient RBCs
- ABO blood group incompatibility is the most severe form.
- Clinical features are dramatic and apparent within 24 hours of transfusion.
  - Signs and symptoms: fever, hypotension, hemoglobinuria, acute kidney injury, disseminated intravascular coagulation
- Prevention: routine ABO blood group typing, usage of bar coding to accurately verify recipient information before transfusion, close hemodynamic monitoring
- Treatment is mainly supportive (IV hydration, diuretics, bicarbonate infusion). Blood transfusion must be stopped immediately when acute reaction is suspected, and the hospital blood bank should be notified.

Acute Allergic Reactions[36,38]

- Incidence: 1–3% of transfusions
- Caused by the presence of antibodies in recipient plasma to an antigen in the donor unit
- Signs are apparent within first 15–20 minutes of starting blood transfusion.
- Diagnosed clinically
  - Clinical features: urticarial rash, generalized pruritus, angioedema, laryngeal edema, circulatory collapse/anaphylactic shock
- Treatment: If observed, nurses should immediately stop transfusion and notify the provider.
  - Intramuscular (IM) epinephrine, IV steroids, and antihistamines may be ordered.
- Endotracheal intubation is indicated if the patient is unable to maintain an airway.
- Prevention: Nurses should obtain a thorough allergy history. In patients with a known history of allergic transfusion reactions, washed RBC units may be prepared by the blood bank.

Febrile Nonhemolytic Transfusion Reactions[36,39]

- Defined as an increase in body temperature by 1.8°F above 98.6°F within 24 hours after blood transfusion
- More commonly seen after platelet transfusions; its incidence after PRBC transfusions has decreased significantly since the adoption of leukoreduced blood units
- Diagnosis of exclusion; other, more serious causes of fever after transfusion should be ruled out first
- Treatment: supportive, and fever is typically self-resolving

Transfusion-Associated Circulatory Overload[36,40]

- A syndrome of hypervolemia mostly seen in patients who have preexisting volume overload from cardiac, renal, or liver disease
- Clinical features: dyspnea, tachypnea, hypoxemia, cough, elevated jugular venous pressures (JVP)
- Chest x-ray will reveal bilateral pulmonary infiltrates characteristic of pulmonary edema; N-terminal probrain natriuretic peptide (NT-pro BNP) level can be elevated.
- Prevention: slower infusion rate
- Treatment: IV diuretics, avoid additional transfusion if possible until volume status is optimized

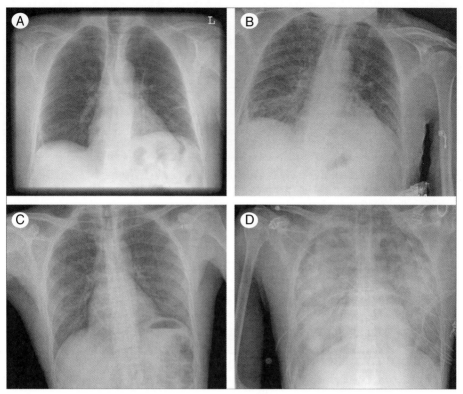

Fig. 22.2 Chest x-ray in transfusion-related acute lung injury (TRALI) comparing pretransfusion x-rays (A, C) and posttransfusion x-rays (B, D) in two patients with TRALI. (From Vlaar VPJ, Juffermans NP. Transfusion-related acute lung injury: a clinical review. *Lancet*. 2013;382[9896]:984–994.)

Transfusion-Associated Acute Lung Injury (TRALI)[36,41]

- Acute respiratory distress syndrome (ARDS) with onset <6 hours since blood transfusion with no preexisting cardiac or lung disease
- Risk factors: critical illness, multiparous female blood donor
- Caused by immune-mediated destruction and capillary leak in the lungs
- Clinical features: fever and hypotension
- Chest x-ray: bilateral pulmonary infiltrates characteristic of ARDS (noncardiogenic pulmonary edema)
- NT-pro BNP is typically normal, JVP is not elevated.
- Treatment: supportive care (oxygen therapy, invasive ventilation if indicated); diuretics can be tried but may not be effective in pure TRALI (Fig. 22.2)

Conclusion

Anemia is extremely common in the hospital, affecting up to half of all inpatient admissions.[42,43] Moderate-severe anemia from any cause leads to significant mortality, morbidity, and increased length of hospital stay.[44] In the perioperative setting, early recognition of anemia is crucial to prevent serious adverse outcomes. During the postoperative period, nurses are key in recognizing signs of symptomatic anemia in patients, assessing for possible causes, carrying out the workup required, and monitoring for blood transfusion complications.

Interestingly, large academic medicals centers will often take a proactive approach by referring at-risk preoperative patients to anemia clinics. Here the cause of anemia will be identified and treatment initiated, thereby optimizing any preoperative risk for bleeding after surgery. Results from quality improvement studies across the country suggest that a preoperative anemia clinic model may help anticipate and reduce the incidence of some of the worst adverse outcomes from anemia.[44-46] Furthermore, another subject of research focus is the increasing emphasis on single-unit PRBC transfusions in patients with stable severe anemia. This approach, as opposed to multiple-unit transfusions (>1 unit ordered at a time), encourages a more judicious and conservative approach to blood unit utilization.[47]

References

1. Crees Z, Fritz C, Heudebert A, et al., eds. *The Washington Manual of Medical Therapeutics*, 36th ed. Wolters Kluwer; 2020.
2. Bhat P, Dretler A, Gdowski M, et al. *The Washington Manual of Medical Therapeutics*, 35th ed. Wolters Kluwer; 2016.
3. Culleton BF, Manns BJ, Zhang J, et al. Impact of anemia on hospitalization and mortality in older adults. *Blood*. 2006;107(10):3841–3846. doi:10.1182/blood-2005-10-4308.
4. Fowler AJ, Ahmad T, Phull MK, et al. Meta-analysis of the association between preoperative anaemia and mortality after surgery. *Br J Surg*. 2015;102(11):1314–1324. doi:10.1002/bjs.9861.
5. Randi ML, Bertozzi I, Santarossa C, et al. Prevalence and causes of anemia in hospitalized patients: impact on diseases outcome. *J Clin Med*. 2020;9(4):e950. doi:10.3390/jcm9040950.
6. Krishnasivam D, Trentino KM, Burrows S, et al. Anemia in hospitalized patients: an overlooked risk in medical care. *Transfusion*. 2018;58(11):2522–2528. doi:10.1111/trf.14877.
7. Seicean A, Seicean S, Alan N, et al. Preoperative anemia and perioperative outcomes in patients who undergo elective spine surgery. *Spine (Phila Pa 1976)*. 2013;38(15):1331–1341. doi:10.1097/BRS.0b013e3182912c6b.
8. Khanna R, Harris DA, McDevitt JL, et al. Impact of anemia and transfusion on readmission and length of stay after spinal surgery: a single-center study of 1187 operations. *Clin Spine Surg*. 2017;30(10):e1338–e1342. doi:10.1097/BSD.0000000000000349.
9. Kasper DL, Fauci AS, Hauser SL et al., eds. *Harrison's Principles of Internal Medicine*, 19th ed. McGraw Hill; 2015.
10. Stern SDC, Cifu AS, Altkorn D. *Symptom to Diagnosis: An Evidence-Based Guide*, 4th ed. McGraw-Hill; 2020.
11. Ghaffari S, Pourafkari L. Koilonychia in iron-deficiency anemia. *N Engl J Med*. 2018;379(9):e13. doi:10.1056/NEJMicm1802104.
12. Qureshi R, Puvanesarajah V, Jain A, et al. Perioperative management of blood loss in spine surgery. *Clin Spine Surg*. 2017;30(9):383–388. doi:10.1097/BSD.0000000000000532.
13. Hayn D, Kreiner K, Kastner P, et al. Data driven methods for predicting blood transfusion needs in elective surgery. *Stud Health Technol Inform*. 2016;223:9–16.
14. Kumar V, Abbas AK, Aster JC, et al., eds. *Robbins & Cotran Pathologic Basis of Disease*, 10th ed. Elsevier; 2021.
15. Ikuta K, Tono O, Tanaka T, et al. Evaluation of postoperative spinal epidural hematoma after microendoscopic posterior decompression for lumbar spinal stenosis: a clinical and magnetic resonance imaging study. *J Neurosurg Spine*. 2006;5(5):404–409. doi:10.3171/spi.2006.5.5.404.
16. Kotilainen E, Alanen A, Erkintalo M, et al. Postoperative hematomas after successful lumbar microdiscectomy or percutaneous nucleotomy: a magnetic resonance imaging study. *Surg Neurol*. 1994;41(2):98–105. doi:10.1016/0090-3019(94)90105-8.
17. Kao FC, Tsai TT, Chen LH, et al. Symptomatic epidural hematoma after lumbar decompression surgery. *Eur Spine J*. 2015;24(2):348–357. doi:10.1007/s00586-014-3297-8.
18. Djurasovic M, Campion C, Dimar JR, et al. Postoperative epidural hematoma. *Orthop Clin North Am*. 2022;53(1):113–121. doi:10.1016/j.ocl.2021.08.006.
19. Schroeder GD, Kurd MF, Kepler CK, et al. Postoperative epidural hematomas in the lumbar spine. *J Spinal Disord Tech*. 2015;28(9):313–318. doi:10.1097/BSD.0000000000000329.
20. Braun P, Kazmi K, Nogués-Meléndez P, et al. MRI findings in spinal subdural and epidural hematomas. *Eur J Radiol*. 2007;64(1):119–125. doi:10.1016/j.ejrad.2007.02.014.
21. Mukerji N, Todd N. Spinal epidural haematoma: factors influencing outcome. *Br J Neurosurg*. 2013;27(6):712–717. doi:10.3109/02688697.2013.793289.

22. Peiró-García A, Domínguez-Esteban I, Alía-Benítez J. Retroperitoneal hematoma after using the extreme lateral interbody fusion (XLIF) approach: presentation of a case and a review of the literature. *Rev Esp Cir Ortop Traumatol.* 2016;60(5):330–334. doi:10.1016/j.recot.2014.12.006.

23. Mondie C, Maguire NJ, Rentea RM. *Retroperitoneal Hematoma.* StatPearls Publishing; 2022.

24. Sunga KL, Bellolio MF, Gilmore RM, et al. Spontaneous retroperitoneal hematoma: etiology, characteristics, management, and outcome. *J Emerg Med.* 2012;43(2):e157–e161. doi:10.1016/j.jemermed.2011.06.006.

25. Andrews NC. Disorders of iron metabolism. *N Engl J Med.* 1999;341(26):1986–1995. doi:10.1056/NEJM199912233412607.

26. Camaschella C, Nai A, Silvestri L. Iron metabolism and iron disorders revisited in the hepcidin era. *Haematologica.* 2020;105(2):260–272. doi:10.3324/haematol.2019.232124.

27. Camaschella C. Iron deficiency: new insights into diagnosis and treatment. *Hematol Am Soc Hematol Educ Program.* 2015;2015:8–13. doi:10.1182/asheducation-2015.1.8.

28. Kernan KF, Carcillo JA. Hyperferritinemia and inflammation. *Int Immunol.* 2017;29(9):401–409. doi:10.1093/intimm/dxx031.

29. Tolkien Z, Stecher L, Mander AP, et al. Ferrous sulfate supplementation causes significant gastrointestinal side-effects in adults: a systematic review and meta-analysis. *PLoS One.* 2015;10(2):e0117383. doi:10.1371/journal.pone.0117383.

30. Lynch SR, Cook JD. Interaction of vitamin C and iron. *Ann N Y Acad Sci.* 1980;355:32–44. doi:10.1111/j.1749-6632.1980.tb21325.x.

31. Rimon E, Kagansky N, Kagansky M, et al. Are we giving too much iron? Low-dose iron therapy is effective in octogenarians. *Am J Med.* 2005;118(10):1142–1147. doi:10.1016/j.amjmed.2005.01.065.

32. Muñoz M, Gómez-Ramírez S, Besser M, et al. Current misconceptions in diagnosis and management of iron deficiency. *Blood Transfus.* 2017;15(5):422–437. doi:10.2450/2017.0113-17.

33. Macdougall IC, Comin-Colet J, Breymann C, et al. Iron sucrose: a wealth of experience in treating iron deficiency. *Adv Ther.* 2020;37(5):1960–2002. doi:10.1007/s12325-020-01323-z.

34. Carson JL, Stanworth SJ, Dennis JA, et al. Transfusion thresholds for guiding red blood cell transfusion. *Cochrane Database Syst Rev.* 2021;12(12):CD002042. doi:10.1002/14651858.CD002042.pub5.

35. Docherty AB, O'Donnell R, Brunskill S, et al. Effect of restrictive versus liberal transfusion strategies on outcomes in patients with cardiovascular disease in a non-cardiac surgery setting: systematic review and meta-analysis. *BMJ.* 2016;352:i1351. doi:10.1136/bmj.i1351.

36. Sharma S, Sharma P, Tyler LN. Transfusion of blood and blood products: indications and complications. *Am Fam Physician.* 2011;83(6):719–724.

37. Panch SR, Montemayor-Garcia C, Klein HG. Hemolytic transfusion reactions. *N Engl J Med.* 2019;381(2):150–162. doi:10.1056/NEJMra1802338.

38. Hirayama F. Current understanding of allergic transfusion reactions: incidence, pathogenesis, laboratory tests, prevention and treatment. *Br J Haematol.* 2013;160(4):434–444. doi:10.1111/bjh.12150.

39. Wang H, Ren D, Sun H, et al. Research progress on febrile non-hemolytic transfusion reaction: a narrative review. *Ann Transl Med.* 2022;10(24):1401. doi:10.21037/atm-22-4932.

40. Semple JW, Rebetz J, Kapur R. Transfusion-associated circulatory overload and transfusion-related acute lung injury. *Blood.* 2019;133(17):1840–1853. doi:10.1182/blood-2018-10-860809.

41. Roubinian N. TACO and TRALI: biology, risk factors, and prevention strategies. *Hematol Am Soc Hematol Educ Program.* 2018;2018(1):585–594. doi:10.1182/asheducation-2018.1.585.

42. Nathavitharana RL, Murray JA, D'Sousa N, et al. Anaemia is highly prevalent among unselected internal medicine inpatients and is associated with increased mortality, earlier readmission and more prolonged hospital stay: an observational retrospective cohort study. *Intern Med J.* 2012;42(6):683–691. doi:10.1111/j.1445-5994.2011.02566.x.

43. Zaninetti C, Klersy C, Scavariello C, et al. Prevalence of anemia in hospitalized internal medicine patients: correlations with comorbidities and length of hospital stay. *Eur J Intern Med.* 2018;51:11–17. doi:10.1016/j.ejim.2017.11.001.

44. Lin Y. Preoperative anemia-screening clinics. *Hematol Am Soc Hematol Educ Program.* 2019;2019(1):570–576. doi:10.1182/hematology.2019000061.

45. Theusinger OM, Spahn DR. Perioperative blood conservation strategies for major spine surgery. *Best Pract Res Clin Anaesthesiol.* 2016;30(1):41–52. doi:10.1016/j.bpa.2015.11.007.

46. Kotzé A, Carter LA, Scally AJ. Effect of a patient blood management programme on preoperative anaemia, transfusion rate, and outcome after primary hip or knee arthroplasty: a quality improvement cycle. *Br J Anaesth.* 2012;108(6):943–952. doi:10.1093/bja/aes135.

47. Warner MA, Schaefer KK, Madde N, et al. Improvements in red blood cell transfusion utilization following implementation of a single-unit default for electronic ordering. *Transfusion.* 2019;59(7):2218–2222. doi:10.1111/trf.15316.
48. Muncie HL, Campbell J. Alpha and beta thalassemia. *Am Fam Physician.* 2009;80(4):339–344.
49. Abu-Zeinah G, DeSancho MT. Understanding sideroblastic anemia: an overview of genetics, epidemiology, pathophysiology and current therapeutic options. *J Blood Med.* 2020;11:305–318. doi:10.2147/JBM. S232644.
50. Madu AJ, Ughasoro MD. Anaemia of chronic disease: an in-depth review. *Med Princ Pract.* 2017;26(1):1–9. doi:10.1159/000452104.
51. Mikhail A, Brown C, Williams JA, et al. Renal association clinical practice guideline on anaemia of chronic kidney disease. *BMC Nephrol.* 2017;18(1):345. doi:10.1186/s12882-017-0688-1.
52. Dhaliwal G, Cornett PA, Tierney LM. Hemolytic anemia. *Am Fam Physician.* 2004;69(11):2599–2606.
53. Brodsky RA, Jones RJ. Aplastic anaemia. *Lancet.* 2005;365(9471):1647–1656. doi:10.1016/S0140-6736(05)66515-4.
54. Langan RC, Goodbred AJ. Vitamin B12 deficiency: recognition and management. *Am Fam Physician.* 2017;96(6):384–389.
55. Green R, Datta Mitra A. Megaloblastic anemias: nutritional and other causes. *Med Clin North Am.* 2017;101(2):297–317. doi:10.1016/j.mcna.2016.09.013.

Questions

Ms. B is a 68-year-old female with a past medical history of class 3 obesity, obstructive sleep apnea not on CPAP, hypertension, and hyperlipidemia. She is now on postoperative day 4 after L2–L3 decompression and fusion. Estimated operative blood loss was 850 cc. She is doing well postoperatively. Her preoperative Hgb level was 12.4, and her Hgb level postoperatively has been drifting down slowly each day, now reaching 7.2 g/dL. She is otherwise hemodynamically stable except for mild orthostasis when working with physical therapy today (blood pressure [BP] dropped to 90/55 mm Hg). Her supine BP is 124/70 mm Hg. She notes mild abdominal pain associated with left-sided groin pain. On physical exam you notice mild bruising in her left groin and mild tenderness to deep palpation over the abdomen diffusely. The attending hospitalist decides to transfuse 1 unit of PRBC to treat acute blood loss anemia. Ten minutes after starting the transfusion, she complains of difficulty breathing and generalized itching. On physical exam, you notice a diffuse urticarial rash. Pulmonary auscultation is notable for inspiratory and expiratory stridor. The patient's BP drops to 85/50 mm Hg.

1. What is the most likely diagnosis for anemia in this patient?
   a. Hemolytic anemia
   b. Aplastic anemia from bone marrow failure
   c. Acute retroperitoneal hemorrhage
   d. Sickle cell anemia

2. You notify the provider of the change in the patient's clinical status. What is the next best step in management?
   a. CT abdomen and pelvis with or without contrast
   b. MRI abdomen and pelvis with contrast
   c. Check vitamin B12 and folate levels
   d. Check lactate dehydrogenase (LDH), haptoglobin levels

3. What is your choice of treatment in this patient with acute, symptomatic, and severe anemia?
   a. IV fluid boluses and maintenance fluids
   b. Single-unit PRBC transfusion
   c. Oral iron supplementation
   d. IV iron supplementation

4. Shortly after starting the blood transfusion, you notice that the patient develops acute dyspnea, urticarial rash, and hypotension. What is the next best step in treatment?
   a. Do not stop the transfusion. Administer IM epinephrine, IV methylprednisolone, and IV Benadryl from the code cart.
   b. Stop the transfusion. Notify the provider and blood bank immediately and anticipate orders for IM epinephrine, IV steroids, and IV antihistamines.
   c. Stop the transfusion and hang an IV fluid bolus. Anticipate orders for obtaining blood cultures, checking lactate, and starting broad-spectrum antibiotics.
   d. Provide symptomatic and emotional support to the patient. Continue the transfusion and continue to monitor vital signs as per protocol.

5. The patient is stabilized and is ready for discharge. Hgb is stable ~9–10 g/dL. Iron panel is suggestive of iron deficiency. You see orders for oral iron supplementation three times a day for 3 months to replete iron stores. What should you do next?
   a. Fill the order from pharmacy at the currently prescribed dose.
   b. Ask the physician why the patient is not getting an additional unit of blood before discharge.
   c. Ask the physician to order repeat imaging to ensure the hematoma is stable in size.
   d. Ask the physician why the patient is not prescribed oral iron once a day or every other day.

Answers

1. c

2. a

3. b

4. b

5. d

CHAPTER 23

Nursing Management of Thrombocytopenia

Eric Gladstone, DO

Introduction

Platelets, or thrombocytes, are small cell fragments in the blood that are central to the process of hemostasis (i.e., clot formation). When activated by blood vessel injury, platelets will aggregate and form a platelet plug to control bleeding. The normal range for platelet count is 150,000–450,000/µL of blood. Thrombocytopenia is defined as a platelet count <150,000/µL. Having a low platelet count predisposes patients to bleeding at any site in the body. It is useful to categorize the severity of thrombocytopenia for the purpose of assessing bleeding risk.[1]

- Mild thrombocytopenia (>70,000/µL) is generally asymptomatic and often incidentally discovered.
- Severe thrombocytopenia (<20,000/µL) imparts a significantly higher risk of excessive bleeding.[2]

Because bleeding complications in neurosurgical patients can be particularly devastating, thrombocytopenia must never be overlooked. Bleeding within the brain or spinal cord can damage essential life-sustaining structures. Generally, neurosurgical procedures warrant a platelet count of at least 100,000/µL to ensure adequate hemostasis in the operating room (OR).[3]

Initial Evaluation

The first step in the workup of thrombocytopenia is to establish the diagnosis by excluding pseudothrombocytopenia. Pseudothrombocytopenia is of no clinical significance. It is caused by in vitro platelet clumping, usually due to ethylenediaminetetraacetic acid (EDTA) in collection tubes. Pseudothrombocytopenia is confirmed when the platelet count normalizes after collection in a tube with heparin or citrate, without EDTA. This test will likely be ordered for any patient with an unexpectedly low platelet count without a prior history of thrombocytopenia, and nurses can assist with ensuring that the correct test tube is provided for the lab draw.

Thrombocytopenia may be driven by decreased platelet production, increased platelet destruction, or platelet sequestration. Normally, approximately one-third of circulating platelets are contained within the spleen.[4] In platelet sequestration, this fraction is increased. This generally occurs as a consequence of cirrhosis of the liver, which leads to the pooling of platelets within the spleen. Abnormal platelet production or destruction can be triggered by numerous processes (Fig. 23.1).

Providers will utilize the patient's history, physical exam, and lab results to pinpoint the underlying cause(s) of thrombocytopenia. Initial testing frequently includes a complete blood count with differential, blood smear, complete metabolic profile, coagulation profile, serum B12 and folate levels, as well as screening for human immunodeficiency virus and hepatitis C virus. An abdominal ultrasound may be ordered to check for splenomegaly or cirrhosis. Additional testing may be performed after consultation with hematology. As a patient is undergoing workup, nursing staff can help educate patients and their families regarding the basic rationale behind the testing that is ordered.

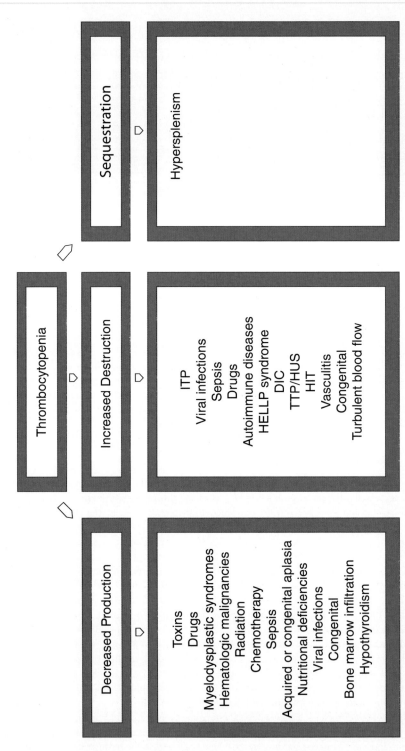

Fig. 23.1 Common etiologies of thrombocytopenia. *DIC,* Disseminated intravascular coagulation; *HELLP,* hemolysis, elevated liver enzymes, and low platelet count; *HIT,* heparin-induced thrombocytopenia; *ITP,* immune thrombocytopenia; *TTP/HUS,* thrombotic thrombocytopenia purpura/hemolytic uremic syndrome.

Treatment Strategy

When the underlying cause of a patient's thrombocytopenia is established, an individualized treatment strategy can be formulated. A patient-specific approach to management is imperative to achieve and maintain platelet counts in the targeted range. Recall that thrombocytopenia can be caused by decreased platelet production, increased platelet destruction, or platelet sequestration. Unsurprisingly, treatment of thrombocytopenia is not a one-size-fits-all paradigm.

DECREASED PLATELET PRODUCTION

Patients who are suffering from decreased platelet production tend to respond more favorably to platelet transfusion. Nevertheless, it is prudent to also identify and treat the cause of decreased platelet production, as platelets have a relatively short life span of 7–10 days in circulation.[5] Treating the underlying cause of decreased platelet production may be relatively straightforward in some cases. For example, it may only be a matter of supplementing a deficient nutrient or discontinuing a medication that can suppress the bone marrow. Many medications that are regularly prescribed to neurosurgical patients, including various antibiotics and anticonvulsants, can inhibit platelet production. All providers should review the patient's list of medications and potentially discontinue or replace any offending agents to aid in the restoration of platelet production.

PLATELET SEQUESTRATION

Treating thrombocytopenia due to sequestration poses a unique challenge. Typically, this pertains to patients who have cirrhosis and who respond only transiently to platelet transfusion. Transfused platelets will be rapidly sequestered in the spleen. In patients with platelet counts <100,000/μL who need invasive neurosurgical procedures, a common strategy is to transfuse platelets slowly intraoperatively. In this case platelets may be ordered on call for the OR and not given preoperatively by the floor nurse. Postoperatively, the platelet goal may need to be liberalized as the immediate risk of bleeding decreases. This strategy, which requires close collaboration with the neurosurgical team, seeks to avoid repeated and excessive transfusion of platelets that are providing only a short-lived benefit. In rare cases, thrombopoietin receptor agonists will be given to stimulate platelet production, and splenic embolization or splenectomy may also be considered.[6,7]

INCREASED PLATELET DESTRUCTION

Treating thrombocytopenia due to increased platelet destruction can be equally challenging. In this case, thrombocytopenia can be refractory to platelet transfusion and may be driven by an acute, life-threatening process, such as disseminated intravascular coagulation (DIC). Treatments to suppress platelet destruction are tailored to the underlying cause of the destruction. For example, platelet destruction that is driven by sepsis is treated very differently than platelet destruction caused by immune thrombocytopenic purpura (ITP). ITP is a disease in which the immune system attacks and destroys platelets. Platelet transfusion alone for ITP typically does not achieve a sustained response; immunosuppressants are often used.[8] In contrast, immunosuppressants would do more harm than good in a patient with thrombocytopenia that is caused by sepsis. In this case, providers must treat the underlying infection.

In certain cases of thrombocytopenia, transfusing platelets actually is contraindicated. For instance, platelets are not given for heparin-induced thrombocytopenia (HIT), thrombotic thrombocytopenic purpura (TTP), or DIC without major bleeding. These patients are prone to developing thromboses, and platelet transfusion will only increase this risk.[9] Heparin must be discontinued immediately in cases of suspected HIT, and plasma exchange is the mainstay of treatment for TTP.

Platelet Transfusion

When platelet transfusion is indicated, the number of units ordered is determined by each patient's particular conditions and circumstances. Considerations include the severity and chronicity of thrombocytopenia and the patient's weight and volume status. Platelet transfusion responsiveness should also be taken into account. Compared to other blood products, platelets are associated with an increased risk of bacterial contamination because they must be stored at room temperature.[10] When refrigerated, platelets rapidly lose their function. Transfusion reactions can also occur, including hemolytic reactions, febrile nonhemolytic reactions, allergic reactions, transfusion-related acute lung injury, and transfusion-associated circulatory overload.[11]

Symptoms of a transfusion reaction may include subjective fevers or chills, itching, difficulty breathing, abdominal discomfort, nausea, diarrhea, and flank pain. Concerning signs include hypothermia, fever, tachycardia, hypotension, hypoxia, lip or tongue swelling, facial flushing, wheezing, and hematuria. Any sign of a transfusion reaction should be reported immediately to both the provider and blood bank for guidance. It is the responsibility of the nurse to monitor the patient's vital signs and lung sounds during and immediately after platelet transfusion. Nurses should notify providers if they identify abnormal lung sounds or peripheral edema. Providers may prescribe a diuretic in these situations to combat fluid overload.

Nursing Considerations

The neurosurgical nurse should vigilantly monitor patients with thrombocytopenia for bleeding complications. Tachycardia and hypotension warrant prompt evaluation, as they can be signs of blood loss, and patients should be frequently examined for bruising and petechiae. Nonspecific signs and symptoms such as fatigue, dizziness, skin pallor, or lethargy should not be overlooked, as they may be an indicator of anemia. These patients should have an active type and screen on file to prevent delays in blood product transfusion. Postoperatively, frequent wound checks should be performed. Swelling near the surgical site may suggest the presence of a hematoma. Drain outputs should be monitored and recorded. The surgeon should be alerted of any overtly sanguineous drainage, which is deep red in color and indicates fresh bleeding. Frequent neurologic exams should be performed to ensure that any new neuro deficits do not go unnoticed. Changes in exam findings, especially in the postoperative period, can indicate acute bleeding, which should be further evaluated with blood work and imaging.

Thrombocytopenia can predispose a patient to bleeding anywhere in the body. The neurosurgical nurse should monitor for epistaxis, hemoptysis, melena, hematochezia, hematuria, and menorrhagia. Nurses should assess mucous membranes and the skin around intravenous catheters for bleeding or trauma. Good oral care keeps mucous membranes moist and will prevent bleeding. Nurses should limit the use of dental floss and only use a soft-bristle toothbrush. Additionally, nurses should exercise increased caution with rectal tubes and suctioning equipment. Firm pressure should be applied following any venipuncture, and intramuscular injections should be avoided. If injections are necessary, nurses should use a small-gauge needle. Patients should be taught to avoid blowing their nose forcefully, and electric shavers or clippers are preferred over razors.[12] Behaviors that can cause bleeding, such as straining with bowel movements, vomiting, and coughing, should be controlled. When appropriate, patients should be counseled on avoiding activities that can cause injury. Fall prevention is especially crucial. Nurses should implement fall precaution protocols, such as the use of bed/chair alarms and nonslip slippers. Nurses can suggest a consult with physical therapy to determine any special equipment a patient needs to prevent injury.

Many neurosurgical patients receive glucocorticoids, such as dexamethasone, to control edema. High doses of steroids can predispose a patient to gastrointestinal (GI) bleeding.[13] If not already

---

BOX 23.1 ■ Thrombocytopenia Care Plan

- Establish and treat underlying cause of thrombocytopenia
- Monitor for bleeding and thrombosis
- Frequent neurologic exams
- Fall prevention
- Good oral hygiene
- Symptom control—straining with bowel movements, coughing, retching
- Patient education
- Maintain active type and screen
- Monitor for and report platelet transfusion reactions
- Use only small-gauge needles
- Avoid intramuscular injections

---

ordered, GI prophylaxis with an H2-blocker (e.g., famotidine) or proton pump inhibitor (e.g., pantoprazole) may be indicated and should be discussed with the provider. Patients with recent exposure to anticoagulants or antiplatelet agents may be at higher risk of bleeding. In the setting of moderate or severe thrombocytopenia, pharmacologic prophylaxis against deep vein thrombosis (DVT) is often held at the provider's discretion, as its use can provoke unwanted bleeding. In cases of HIT, heparin should be listed as an allergy in the patient's medical record. Patients with HIT, DIC, and TTP should be observed closely for signs and symptoms of DVT, such as swelling, pain, or redness in an extremity (Box 23.1).

Conclusion

Thrombocytopenia, a platelet count <150,000/μL, may be a result of different processes in the body. Having a low platelet count predisposes patients to bleeding at any site in the body and can lead to disastrous complications in neurosurgical patients. A thorough understanding of thrombocytopenia and bleeding risks is necessary to help manage the care of these patients, both inpatient and outpatient. Nurses should be comfortable with the testing and workup for thrombocytopenia, know the warning signs to monitor for (both preop and postop) that hint at uncontrolled bleeding, and be comfortable administering platelet transfusions and monitoring for transfusion reactions. Lastly, nurses should be able to provide adequate discharge instructions to these patients to ensure a safe transition out of the hospital setting.

References

1. Williamson DR, Albert M, Heels-Ansdell D, et al. Thrombocytopenia in critically ill patients receiving thromboprophylaxis: frequency, risk factors, and outcomes. *Chest*. 2013;144(4):1207–1215. doi:10.1378/chest.13-0121.
2. Gauer RL, Braun MM. Thrombocytopenia. *Am Fam Physician*. 2012;85(6):612–622.
3. Li D, Glor T, Jones GA. Thrombocytopenia and neurosurgery: a literature review. *World Neurosurg*. 2017;106:277–280. doi:10.1016/j.wneu.2017.06.097.
4. Wadenvik H, Kutti J. The spleen and pooling of blood cells. *Eur J Haematol*. 1988;41(1):1–5. doi:10.1111/j.1600-0609.1988.tb00861.x.
5. Cho J. A paradigm shift in platelet transfusion therapy. *Blood*. 2015;125(23):3523–3525. doi:10.1182/blood-2015-04-640649.
6. Nilles KM, Caldwell SH, Flamm SL. Thrombocytopenia and procedural prophylaxis in the era of thrombopoietin receptor agonists. *Hepatol Commun*. 2019;3(11):1423–1434. doi:10.1002/hep4.1423.
7. Wang YB, Zhang JY, Zhang F, et al. Partial splenic artery embolization to treat hypersplenism secondary to hepatic cirrhosis: a meta-analysis. *Am Surg*. 2017;83(3):274–283.

8. Neunert C, Terrell DR, Arnold DM, et al. American Society of Hematology 2019 guidelines for immune thrombocytopenia. *Blood Adv.* 2019;3(23):3829–3866. doi:10.1182/bloodadvances.2019000966.

9. Goel R, Ness PN, Takemoto CM, et al. Platelet transfusions in platelet consumptive disorders are associated with arterial thrombosis and in-hospital mortality. *Blood.* 2015;125(9):1470–1476. doi:10.1182/blood-2014-10-605493.

10. Levy JH, Neal MD, Herman JH. Bacterial contamination of platelets for transfusion: strategies for prevention. *Crit Care.* 2018;22(1):271. doi:10.1186/s13054-018-2212-9.

11. Kaufman RM, Djulbegovic B, Gernsheimer T, et al. Platelet transfusion: a clinical practice guideline from the AABB. *Ann Intern Med.* 2015;162(3):205–213. doi:10.7326/M14-1589.

12. Radovich P. The multiple causes and myriad presentations of thrombocytopenia. *Am Nurse.* 2011. https://www.myamericannurse.com/the-multiple-causes-and-myriad-presentations-of-thrombocytopenia. Accessed June 6, 2023.

13. Narum S, Westergren T, Klemp M. Corticosteroids and risk of gastrointestinal bleeding: a systematic review and meta-analysis. *BMJ Open.* 2014;4(5):e004587. doi:10.1136/bmjopen-2013-004587.

Questions

Michael is a 64-year-old male with a history of alcohol abuse, who is admitted after a fall while intoxicated. He was found to have traumatic fractures of his L3 and L4 vertebrae with retropulsion causing severe spinal canal stenosis. Neurosurgery plans to perform a lumbar decompression and fusion. His preoperative labs are largely unremarkable aside from a low platelet count of 40,000/μL. He says that he has not seen a primary care provider in two decades.

1. The patient's provider explains to him that his platelet count is likely low because of his alcohol abuse, but some additional blood work is warranted to confirm this before he goes to the OR. Later, when phlebotomy comes to draw his blood, he has forgotten this conversation and becomes very irritated, saying that he is tired and already had blood work. How can the nurse best respond in this scenario?
   a. Explain the need to rule out pseudothrombocytopenia.
   b. Ask the provider to order antianxiety medications for the patient.
   c. Empathize with the patient, but remind him that because of his low platelet count, additional blood work was ordered to ensure the procedure is performed safely.
   d. Both a and c

2. The patient consents to receive 2 units of platelets to be transfused just before he goes to the OR. While the platelets are running, he develops a fever of 102°F. What is the most appropriate course of action?
   a. Notify the provider and blood bank, and stop the transfusion.
   b. The fever is likely due to the speed of infusion, and it should be slowed down.
   c. Reassure him that there is nothing to worry about because, unlike red blood cell transfusions, platelet transfusions cannot cause serious reactions.
   d. Run the 2 units of platelets in at the same time at a quicker rate to end the transfusion as soon as possible.

3. The patient's procedure is completed without complications. Postoperatively, labs are ordered to check his platelet count. The patient asks why this is necessary if he did not experience any serious bleeding intraoperatively. What is an appropriate response?
   a. "We need to check your labs to determine when it is safe to start DVT prophylaxis."
   b. "If your platelet count is <200,000/μL, you will need another platelet transfusion."
   c. "It is important that we continue to monitor your platelet count until we know that it is stable because you are still at risk of bleeding."
   d. Both b and c

4. The patient's postprocedural platelet count is 55,000/µL. His neurologic assessment is unchanged, but you notice significant bruising and swelling to one side of his flank, which is new. Why is it important to immediately notify the provider?
   a. There is no need to tell the provider at this point because the patient's neurologic assessment is unchanged.
   b. The patient may have a hematoma.
   c. There is no need to tell the provider at this point because the patient's platelet count is >50,000/µL.
   d. Both a and c

5. The patient has stabilized and is ready to go home. In addition to alcohol cessation resources and fall precaution education, what additional education should you provide to the patient?
   a. Avoid straight razors and hard-bristled toothbrushes.
   b. Monitor for bruising and bleeding, and check wound frequently for drainage.
   c. Avoid aggressive nose blowing and straining when having bowel movements.
   d. All of the above

Answers

1. d

2. a

3. c

4. b

5. d

Nursing Management of Dysautonomia: Autonomic Dysreflexia and Paroxysmal Sympathetic Hypersensitivity

Crystal Pak, BSN, MSN, CRNP

Introduction

Dysautonomia is a disorder of the autonomic nervous system, which is composed of the sympathetic, parasympathetic, and enteric nervous systems. The sympathetic nervous system is most commonly associated with the fight-or-flight response. Its functions include increasing the heart rate, causing vasoconstriction and bronchodilation, and decreasing gut motility.[1,2] Generally speaking, the parasympathetic nervous system works to generate the opposite physiologic outcomes. Typically these two systems work to balance each other and achieve homeostasis within the body. Dysautonomia entails either the failure or overactivity of the sympathetic or parasympathetic nervous system.

Dysautonomia can be divided into two categories: primary and secondary. Primary dysautonomia occurs due to a degenerative or genetic disease that affects the nervous system. Examples of primary dysautonomia include pure autonomic failure, familial dysautonomia, and multiple system atrophy.[3] Secondary dysautonomia is the result of other injuries or conditions, such as spinal cord injury (SCI), traumatic brain injury (TBI), diabetes, or other central nervous system diseases.[2,3] Although there are various types of dysautonomia, neurosurgery patients most often experience either autonomic dysreflexia or paroxysmal sympathetic hyperactivity.

Autonomic Dysreflexia

BACKGROUND

Autonomic dysreflexia is a potentially life-threatening condition that can develop in patients with SCI and is usually associated with injuries at or above the T6 level of the spine. Patients with higher levels of injury and more severe injuries have an increased risk of developing this disorder.[4,5] The hallmark sign of autonomic dysreflexia is an exaggerated elevation of blood pressure usually triggered by a noxious stimulus below the level of injury, which activates the sympathetic response, causing vasoconstriction.[4-7] If not treated quickly and correctly, severe cases can lead to hypertensive encephalopathy, stroke, and cardiac arrest.[4,6,8]

CAUSES

One of the most common triggers for autonomic dysreflexia is bladder distention, which is often due to blocked or kinked indwelling urinary catheters. This is easily reversible and can be fixed with either flushing or repositioning the catheter. Other common causes include fecal impaction, rectal distention, and skin breakdown or pressure injuries below the level of injury.[9]

CLINICAL SIGNS

The most recognizable sign of autonomic dysreflexia is a rise in systolic blood pressure (at least 20–40 mm Hg above baseline) paired with bradycardia, though tachycardia has also been reported.[4,6,8,9] Patients may develop symptoms of severe headache, nasal congestion, blurred vision, and increased anxiety, along with signs of diaphoresis, skin flushing, cool skin, and constricted pupils.[4–6]

MANAGEMENT

Nonpharmacologic

In the event of autonomic dysreflexia, patients should be moved quickly into an upright seated position in an attempt to stimulate an orthostatic drop in blood pressure. Patients should be thoroughly assessed for bladder distention, bowel distention, sores, lacerations, or even tight clothing.

- Patients without indwelling urinary catheters, who are unable to empty their bladder independently, should either have one inserted, or undergo straight catheterization. Insertion, however, may be difficult due to increased tone in the urethral sphincter, so nurses should have a curved-tip catheter available if needed.
- Patients with indwelling urinary catheters already in place should have them flushed with warm fluid to remove any potential blockage, then repositioned to remove any kinks.[9]
- Patients should be asked about their last bowel movement and assessed for abdominal distention. If necessary, bowel interventions, such as suppositories or small-volume enemas, should be administered.

When removing noxious stimuli, blood pressures should be monitored to see whether patients effectively respond to treatment. If the stimuli cannot be identified and blood pressures continue to be elevated (systolic pressures >150 mm Hg), providers should be contacted because pharmacologic management should be considered.[4,7,9]

Pharmacologic

Nitrates are the drug of choice when treating autonomic dysreflexia. They promote the release of nitric oxide, which relaxes smooth muscles, causing vasodilation and ultimately a reduction in blood pressure. Application of 2% nitroglycerin paste (1–2 inches thick) above the level of injury is a commonly ordered intervention. This is often the method of choice to rapidly reduce blood pressure (due to its easy application by caregivers) and easy removal when resolution of the hypertensive crisis has been achieved.[4,6,7] Sublingual and chewable nitrates are also available. In the hospital setting, sodium nitroprusside may be administered intravenously for severe cases.[6] A contraindication for nitrates is the use of phosphodiesterase type 5 inhibitors (e.g., sildenafil, tadalafil) within 24–48 hours of the onset of autonomic dysreflexia, due to the possibility of severe hypotension.[4,7,9]

- Nifedipine, a calcium channel blocker, is another commonly used medication to treat hypertensive crisis in autonomic dysreflexia.
  - Providers may order 10-mg tablets that can be administered every 20–30 minutes for a maximum dosage of 40 mg/24 hours.[4,6]
- Sublingual administration of captopril or clonidine is another treatment available especially if there is a contraindication to nitrates.
  - Captopril is often ordered in 25-mg dosages every hour as needed for a maximum 50 mg/24 hours.
  - Initially, 0.2 mg of sublingual clonidine should be given followed by 0.1 mg every hour as needed for a maximum 0.8 mg/24 hours.[4]

If transdermal and oral medications do not effectively treat hypertension, providers may consider 20 mg intravenous (IV) hydralazine (administered slowly) or a bolus of 20 mg diazoxide.[4,7] Regardless, rebound hypotension is a common side effect that may occur up to 5 hours after receiving nitrates or nifedipine, so nurses should continue frequent blood pressure monitoring even after the episode has resolved.

COMPLICATIONS

If left untreated, complications of autonomic dysreflexia are similar to those of hypertensive crisis. The most serious complication is hemorrhagic stroke, which can cause severe neurologic damage and death. Other complications include myocardial infarction, renal failure, seizure, or pulmonary edema.[4]

PREVENTION

Because bowel and bladder distention are common precipitating factors of autonomic dysreflexia, it is important for patients to maintain regular bowel and bladder management protocols. Patients may be asked to perform self-catheterization intermittently five to six times a day and adhere to a daily bowel regimen.[4] Use of lidocaine gel to numb the area of insertion prior to indwelling urinary catheter changes or straight catheterizations has been shown to reduce the occurrence of autonomic dysreflexia.[4] Nurses should educate patients on the use of pressure-relieving cushions and mattresses and encourage routine skin checks to reduce the risk of any skin breakdown. Additionally, prazosin, an adrenergic receptor antagonist (taken twice a day), has been shown to reduce the severity of autonomic dysreflexia and its symptoms when taken prophylactically.[6]

Paroxysmal Sympathetic Hypersensitivity

BACKGROUND

Paroxysmal sympathetic hypersensitivity (PSH), also known as storming or dysautonomic crisis, is caused by a dysfunction of the sympathetic nervous system. The pathophysiology of PSH is not well understood, but studies have shown that it results from disconnection or disruption in the cortical and subcortical regions of the brain secondary to brain injury.[10,11] Since different parts of the brain can be involved, presentation and severity among patients can differ greatly. Episodes can last from minutes to hours, occur intermittently or continuously, and may persist in patients for weeks, months, or even years.[12]

CAUSES

Most patients who develop PSH have suffered from a TBI, anoxic brain injury, or stroke. Tumors, hydrocephalus, and infection are less common conditions that may result in PSH.[11,13] Patients with PSH typically overreact to nonnoxious stimuli, such as bathing, repositioning, passive motion, and noise. Extraneous stimuli can precipitate episodes of PSH by leading to an uncontrolled sympathetic nervous response.[14]

CLINICAL SIGNS

PSH is a complex disorder that varies clinically in every patient. The most common symptoms associated with PSH include tachycardia, tachypnea, hypertension, hyperthermia, hyperhidrosis, and posturing.[10,13] However, when patients are first admitted to a hospital after a brain injury, they are often medically sedated. This will lead to the masking of symptoms, making diagnosis difficult, as patients will rarely exhibit all of the most common symptoms. Instead, patients will more commonly have some combination of symptoms, with tachycardia being present in most cases.[10]

Ultimately, PSH is a diagnosis of exclusion. Since symptoms of PSH can present similarly to other neurologic sequelae, diagnosis can be difficult. Sepsis, infection, seizure, and withdrawal should all be ruled out and, if necessary, treated before diagnosing PSH. Due to varying opinions on definitions and criteria of PSH, a clinical scoring system was developed to help provide consistency among clinicians for diagnosis.[15] It features two parts: clinical feature scale (CFS) and a diagnosis likelihood tool (DLT).

The CFS is based on six criteria, each of which are scored from 0 to 3[15]:

- Heart rate: <100 = 0, 100–119 = 1, 120–139 = 2, >140 = 3
- Respiratory rate: <18 = 0, 18–23 = 1, 24–29 = 2, >30 = 3
- Systolic blood pressure: <140 = 0, 140–159 = 1, 160–179 = 2, >180 = 3
- Temperature: <37C = 0, 37–37.9C = 1, 38–38.9C = 2, >39C = 3
- Sweating: absent = 0, mild = 1, moderate = 2, severe = 3
- Posturing: absent = 0, mild = 1, moderate = 2, severe = 3

The DLT is calculated by giving 1 point for each of the following clinical features present[15]:

- Paroxysmal episodes
- Clinical features present for ≥3 days consecutively
- Clinical features present for ≥2 weeks after initial brain injury
- ≥2 episodes a day
- Overreactive sympathetic response to normally nonpainful stimuli
- Clinical features still present even with treatments of alternative diagnoses
- Pharmacologic intervention to reduce sympathetic features
- No parasympathetic features during episode
- No other presumed causes
- Brain injury directly prior
- Clinical features happen simultaneously

Adding both the scores of the CFS and DLT, clinicians are able to determine the likelihood of PSH in a patient. If the combined score is <8, PSH is unlikely; 8–16 is possible PSH; if ≥17, PSH is probable.[15]

MANAGEMENT

Ultimately because the etiology of PSH is not completely understood, treatment is focused on the management of symptoms through nonpharmacologic and pharmacologic methods. There is no preferred method of treatment, and each intervention should be adjusted to the patient's symptoms, experiences of side effects, and tolerance.

Nonpharmacologic

The first step in nonpharmacologic management involves controlling environmental factors. Nurses should aim to provide a calm environment and prevent overstimulation. The room should be maintained at a comfortable temperature,[10] and patients should be assessed for any untreated pain. It is also important to optimize nutrition and manage any fluid and electrolyte imbalances that may result from increased caloric needs, higher metabolic rates, and hyperhidrosis.[13] Patients may benefit from supplemental oxygen, even with adequate oxygenation levels on pulse oximetry, as PSH can result from cerebral hypoxia.[10] Overall, interventions should be customized to each patient but are all aimed to help lessen the occurrence and duration of PSH.

Pharmacologic

There are three focus points in pharmacologic management: treat symptoms, prevent symptoms, and treat refractory symptoms.[10,12]

- Nonselective beta receptor blockers are effective in treating hypertension and tachycardia present in PSH. Propranolol is the preferred beta blocker not only for its potent cardiovascular effect but also for its ability to reduce the hyperthermic response secondary to brain injury.[10,12,14] It also has the advantage of lipophilicity, which allows it to cross the blood-brain barrier.[11]
- Alpha-2 receptor agonists are second-line drugs used to treat hypertension and tachycardia.
    - Clonidine is the preferred drug in this class. Transdermal clonidine patches have been shown to be effective in controlling PSH; oral doses have been shown to cause hypotension and bradycardia.[11,12]
    - Dexmedetomidine is a viable option when continuous IV infusion is possible, especially in an intensive care unit (ICU) setting.[12] Nurses should continue to monitor heart rate and blood pressure while on the infusion.
- Opioid receptor agonists, particularly morphine, are first-line drugs in the treatment of PSH. The analgesic effect is helpful, but the cholinergic effects (causing bradycardia) and release of histamine (leading to vasodilation) make these drugs quite effective in treating PSH. IV administration of morphine is suggested at the start of therapy, with the plan to switch to an oral dose of morphine or oxycodone for maintenance.[10,12,14] Dosing should be adjusted for individual patients.
- Dopamine receptor agonists, specifically bromocriptine, can be used in conjunction with other medications, as it has not been shown to be effective as a monotherapy. Though the exact mechanism is unknown, bromocriptine has been shown to be effective in reducing temperature and sweating in patients with PSH.[11–13]
- Gamma-aminobutyric acid (GABA) receptor agonists are another line of treatment used in conjunction with other medications to treat PSH.
    - Baclofen is a $GABA_B$ receptor agonist that is used to treat spasticity and reduce the frequency of spasms that are often associated with PSH. For a more long-term solution in patients with persistent spasticity, baclofen can be administered via intrathecal infusion.[10,12]
    - Gabapentin, a GABA analog, can treat pain from neuropathies, reduce spasticity, and provide a sedative effect.[12,14]
    - Benzodiazepines, a type of $GABA_A$ receptor agonists, can be used to manage hypertension, tachycardia, and agitation. Most commonly, clonazepam, diazepam, and lorazepam are used. The use of short-acting benzodiazepines is preferable in immediate treatment of PSH.[10,12,14]
        - Abrupt discontinuation of benzodiazepine, when used long term, can cause withdrawal and lead to seizures and worsening symptoms of PSH. Therefore patients should be tapered appropriately.
- Ryanodine receptor antagonists, specifically dantrolene, disrupt the release of calcium, resulting in weaker contractions of the muscle. Therefore dantrolene is used to treat posturing and spasticity that persists when other drugs have failed, and it can be safely combined with benzodiazepines and opiates for treatment.[11,12,14]
    - Providers should frequently monitor liver function tests as there is a risk of hepatotoxicity.[10,12,14]

COMPLICATIONS

Unrecognized and/or refractory PSH may increase length of stay and prevent patient progression to rehabilitation centers. Prolonged admissions are often associated with increased risk of infection, deconditioning, and skin breakdown. Furthermore, if symptoms remain uncontrolled, PSH can lead to secondary brain injury, cardiac damage, or even death.[14]

Conclusion

Though there are various types of dysautonomia, the most common in the neurosurgical population are autonomic dysreflexia and paroxysmal sympathetic hyperactivity. Autonomic dysreflexia is commonly seen in patients with SCI at the level of T6 or above; PSH is seen in patients suffering from TBI, anoxic brain injury, or stroke. Both conditions affect the sympathetic nervous system and are associated with tachycardia, hypertension, and diaphoresis. Pharmacologic treatment is targeted toward managing the symptoms and abnormal vitals experienced, and patient response to treatment should be monitored closely. Nonpharmacologic treatment is centered on the removal of stimuli and creating a calm, pain-free environment. Overall, being able to recognize the signs and symptoms of dysautonomia and being knowledgeable in monitoring for triggers will improve quality of care and patient outcomes.

References

1. Lonsdale D. Dysautonomia, a heuristic approach to a revised model for etiology of disease. *Evid Based Complement Alternat Med.* 2009;6(1):3–10. doi:10.1093/ecam/nem064.
2. Novak P. Autonomic disorders. *Am J Med.* 2019;132(4):420–436. doi:10.1016/j.amjmed.2018.09.027.
3. Reichgott MJ. Clinical evidence of dysautonomia. In: Walker HK, Hall WD, Hurst JW, eds. *Clinical Methods: The History, Physical, and Laboratory Examinations,* 3rd ed. Butterworths; 1990.
4. Allen KJ, Leslie SW. *Autonomic Dysreflexia.* StatPearls Publishing; 2018.
5. Solinsky R, Svircev JN, James JJ, et al. A retrospective review of safety using a nursing driven protocol for autonomic dysreflexia in patients with spinal cord injuries. *J Spinal Cord Med.* 2016;39(6):713–719. doi:10.1080/10790268.2015.1118186.
6. Eldahan KC, Rabchevsky AG. Autonomic dysreflexia after spinal cord injury: systemic pathophysiology and methods of management. *Auton Neurosci.* 2018;209:59–70. doi:10.1016/j.autneu.2017.05.002.
7. Morgan S. Recognition and management of autonomic dysreflexia in patients with a spinal cord injury. *Emerg Nurse.* 2020;28(1):22–27. doi:10.7748/en.2019.e1978.
8. Wan D, Krassioukov AV. Life-threatening outcomes associated with autonomic dysreflexia: a clinical review. *J Spinal Cord Med.* 2014;37(1):2–10. doi:10.1179/2045772313Y.0000000098.
9. Bycroft J, Shergill IS, Chung EA, et al. Autonomic dysreflexia: a medical emergency. *Postgrad Med J.* 2005;81(954):232–235. doi:10.1136/pgmj.2004.024463.
10. Zheng RZ, Lei ZQ, Yang RZ, et al. Identification and management of paroxysmal sympathetic hyperactivity after traumatic brain injury. *Front Neurol.* 2020;11:81. doi:10.3389/fneur.2020.00081.
11. Meyfroidt G, Baguley IJ, Menon DK. Paroxysmal sympathetic hyperactivity: the storm after acute brain injury. *Lancet Neurol.* 2017;16(9):721–729. doi:10.1016/S1474-4422(17)30259-4.
12. Samuel S, Allison TA, Lee K, et al. Pharmacologic management of paroxysmal sympathetic hyperactivity after brain injury. *J Neurosci Nurs.* 2016;48(2):82–89. doi:10.1097/JNN.0000000000000207.
13. Perkes I, Baguley IJ, Nott MT, et al. A review of paroxysmal sympathetic hyperactivity after acquired brain injury. *Ann Neurol.* 2010;68(2):126–135. doi:10.1002/ana.22066.
14. Choi HA, Jeon SB, Samuel S, et al. Paroxysmal sympathetic hyperactivity after acute brain injury. *Curr Neurol Neurosci Rep.* 2013;13(8):370. doi:10.1007/s11910-013-0370-3.
15. Baguley IJ, Perkes IE, Fernandez-Ortega JF, et al. Paroxysmal sympathetic hyperactivity after acquired brain injury: consensus on conceptual definition, nomenclature, and diagnostic criteria. *J Neurotrauma.* 2014;31(17):1515–1520. doi:10.1089/neu.2013.3301.

Questions

You are starting your shift and receive sign-out on your assignment. You are getting a neurosurgical patient coming out of the neuro ICU.

1. Which of these patients is at risk for autonomic dysreflexia?
    a. A 45-year-old male who came in with an ischemic stroke
    b. A 73-year-old female with a brain mass

   c. A 69-year-old male with a spinal cord injury above T6

   d. A 32-year-old male who had a subarachnoid hemorrhage

2. A 55-year-old male with a prior traumatic spinal cord injury with resultant quadriplegia is exhibiting signs and symptoms of autonomic dysreflexia, including hypertension. What are the appropriate environmental factors for the nurse to address? Select all that apply.

   a. Raise the head of the bed.

   b. Lay the patient flat.

   c. Check for kinks in the indwelling urinary catheter.

   d. Assess for abdominal distension.

3. Which is the drug of choice in treating autonomic dysreflexia?

   a. Nitrates

   b. Beta blockers

   c. Morphine

   d. Benzodiazepines

4. Which best describes PSH?

   a. A potentially life-threatening condition that can present in patients with a spinal cord injury at the spine level of T6 or above

   b. A condition where the sympathetic nervous system is activated causing frequent panic attacks

   c. A dysfunction of the sympathetic nervous system, usually a diagnosis of exclusion

   d. A condition in which the patient experiences sudden onset of hypotension, hypothermia, and posturing caused by a brain bleed

5. Which medication is preferred for PSH due to its effective treatment for hypertension and tachycardia?

   a. Bromocriptine

   b. Baclofen

   c. Propranolol

   d. Clonidine

Answers

1. c

2. a, c, d

3. a

4. c

5. c

CHAPTER 25

Medical Management of Constipation

Lauren Malinowski-Falk, MSN, BA, CRNP, AGACNP-BC

Introduction

Constipation is characterized by abnormal bowel function. The Rome III criteria diagnoses a person as constipated when experiencing at least two of the following symptoms during ≥25% of defecations[1]:

- Straining
- Lumpy or hard stools
- Sensation of incomplete evacuation
- Sensation of anorectal obstruction or blockage
- Relying on manual maneuvers to promote defecation
- Having less than three unassisted bowel movements per week

Constipation can cause psychosocial distress and negatively impact a patient's quality of life.[2] Constipation is uncomfortable for the patient and can cause a burden on health care resource utilization.[3] Untreated constipation can lead to fecal impaction, incontinence, or colon perforation.[4] A thorough understanding of the causes and treatment of constipation can help decrease its negative impact. Nurses are in the best position to screen for constipation by accurately documenting the date of the patient's last bowel movement, provide education to patients on how to prevent constipation from occurring, and advocate for treatment of constipation on the patient's behalf.

Symptoms

Patients who are constipated often produce stools that are lumpy, hard, or sausage shaped (Fig. 25.1). Patients may complain of abdominal pain, distention, rectal discomfort, feelings of incomplete emptying, or incontinence.[5,6] Patients may also have urinary incontinence or retention, as large amounts of retained stool in the colon can put pressure on the bladder, preventing it from contracting and relaxing as normal.[5] On abdominal exam, patients will exhibit distention and pain with palpation and may have a palpable colonic mass.[5]

Workup

While most cases of constipation are benign and treatable, providers should complete a thorough history and physical exam to ensure that a serious, life-threatening disease is not the underlying cause of the constipation. A physical examination should focus on the abdomen and rectal area.[1] Red flag symptoms from the history and physical exam include[1]:

- Rectal bleeding
- Blood in stool
- Recent unintentional weight loss
- Anemia

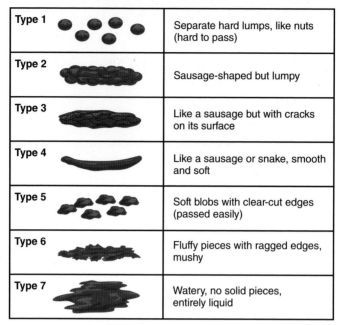

Type 1		Separate hard lumps, like nuts (hard to pass)
Type 2		Sausage-shaped but lumpy
Type 3		Like a sausage but with cracks on its surface
Type 4		Like a sausage or snake, smooth and soft
Type 5		Soft blobs with clear-cut edges (passed easily)
Type 6		Fluffy pieces with ragged edges, mushy
Type 7		Watery, no solid pieces, entirely liquid

Fig. 25.1 Characteristics of stool production correlate with degree of constipation. (From Harding MM, Kwong J, Hagler D, et al. *Lewis's Medical-Surgical Nursing: Assessment and Management of Clinical Problems*, 12th ed. Elsevier; 2022.)

TABLE 25.1 ■ Risk Factors for the Development of Constipation

Extrinsic Factors	Intrinsic Factors
Poor general health	Females
Impaired mobility	Nonwhites
Psychosocial issues	Those age >65 years
Metabolic or neurologic disorders	Those with lower socioeconomic status
Inadequate toilet facilities	
Ignoring the urge to defecate	
Drugs	
• Most common: opioids, antidepressants, anticholinergics, calcium channel blockers, nonsteroidal antiinflammatories, and calcium supplements	

- Family history of colorectal cancer
- Recent unexplained changes in stool habits

Once life-threatening causes have been ruled out, providers should try to uncover any behaviors or medications that are contributing to constipation.[1] The etiology of constipation is often multifactorial and can be caused by a combination of extrinsic and intrinsic factors (Table 25.1)[1,5,7].

Opioid-Induced Constipation

Opioids activate the mu receptors in the small intestine and colon.[8] This activation decreases bowel tone, decreases bowel contractility, increases colonic fluid absorption, increases anal sphincter tone, and reduces rectal sensation.[9] The combination of these leads to the development of harder stools that are difficult to pass, straining, decreased stool frequency, and incomplete evacuation.[3,8] The Rome IV criteria characterizes a patient as experiencing opioid-induced constipation (OIC) when new or worsening symptoms of constipation occur when initiating, changing, or up-titrating opioid therapy.[9] This can include changes in stool consistency, stool frequency, and difficulty passing stool.[10]

The development of OIC does not correlate directly with the dose or route of opioids. In fact, OIC can occur in patients who are prescribed opioids chronically, or in patients who are started on opioids after a surgical procedure for short-term use, such as after a neurosurgical procedure.[3] The risk of developing OIC is increased in postoperative surgical patients, as these patients also have increased pain, decreased mobility, and decreased oral intake, which all contribute to worsening constipation.[3] OIC can also occur in patients who use and abuse opioids that are obtained illegally and at dosages that tend to be higher than dosages typically prescribed by medical providers.

Nonmedical Management of Constipation

Constipation is associated with dietary fiber deficiency.[2] In general, fiber is used to soften the stool, increase stool bulk/volume, and accelerate stool transit time.[5] Patients should be encouraged to increase their intake of dietary fiber or supplement their intake with commercially available soluble fiber. Common sources of dietary fiber include whole wheat bread, unrefined cereals, fruits with high sugar content, vegetables, and wheat bran, and commercially available fiber includes over-the-counter supplements, such as psyllium husk.[2,5] However, patients need to be educated to increase their fluid intake as well, to allow fiber to work the most efficiently and avoid worsening their constipation.[4,11]

Overall, increasing fiber and hydration works to increase bowel frequency, fecal bulk/volume, and fecal softness, but adverse effects of excess fiber intake can result in abdominal pain, bloating, and flatulence.[1,4,8,9] Increasing physical activity has also been shown to decrease colonic transit time and reduce symptoms of constipation.[11] This is one important reason why postoperative patients should be encouraged to mobilize as soon as possible.[8] Furthermore, patients should set aside a regular time for defecation daily and be encouraged to defecate immediately when the urge is felt. At that time, the gastrocolic reflex, which controls the peristalsis of the intestinal tract, is activated and colonic motor activity is at its highest.[11]

Medical Management of Constipation

Numerous medications are available for the treatment and prevention of constipation. These are categorized according to their mechanism of action, and used in combination to maximize their intended effect (Fig. 25.2). These medications, overall, are considered safe and are easily accessible over the counter, but they can cause increased abdominal pain, nausea, and diarrhea when used.[9,11] As a result, prescribing should be individualized to the patient's comorbidities, and take possible side effects into account.

OSMOTIC LAXATIVES

These agents act by drawing water into the gastrointestinal tract to promote intestinal motility.[9,12]
- Common types
  - Polyethylene glycol (PEG): a metabolically inert substance that, when ingested, promotes water retention in the intestine
    - Moviprep, which is PEG combined with ascorbic acid, is commonly prescribed before colonoscopy procedures to thoroughly clean out the bowels.[12,13] Moviprep contains electrolytes to replete those that are excreted in the large amount of stool that results.

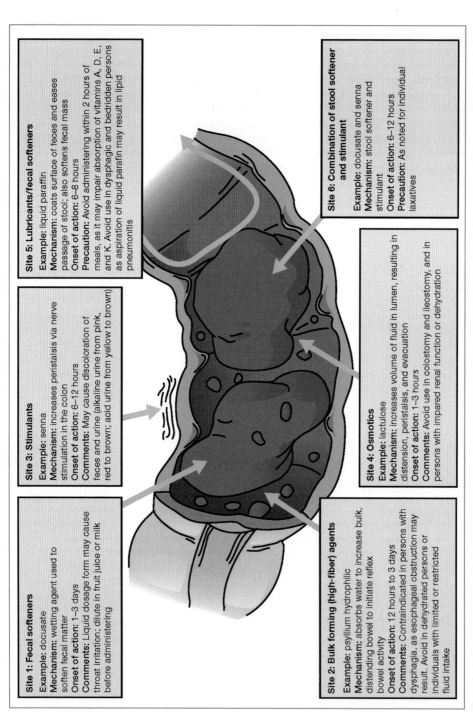

Site 1: Fecal softeners
Example: docusate
Mechanism: wetting agent used to soften fecal matter
Onset of action: 1–3 days
Comments: Liquid dosage form may cause throat irritation; dilute in fruit juice or milk before administering

Site 2: Bulk forming (high-fiber) agents
Example: psyllium hydrophilic
Mechanism: absorbs water to increase bulk, distending bowel to initiate reflex bowel activity
Onset of action: 12 hours to 3 days
Comments: Contraindicated in persons with dysphagia, as esophageal obstruction may result. Avoid in dehydrated persons or individuals with limited or restricted fluid intake

Site 3: Stimulants
Example: senna
Mechanism: increases peristalsis via nerve stimulation in the colon
Onset of action: 6–12 hours
Comments: May cause discoloration of feces and urine (alkaline urine from pink, red to brown; acid urine from yellow to brown)

Site 4: Osmotics
Example: lactulose
Mechanism: increases volume of fluid in lumen, resulting in distension, peristalsis, and evacuation
Onset of action: 1–3 hours
Comments: Avoid use in colostomy and ileostomy, and in persons with impared renal function or dehydration

Site 5: Lubricants/fecal softeners
Example: liquid paraffin
Mechanism: coats surface of feces and eases passage of stool; also softens fecal mass
Onset of action: 6–8 hours
Precaution: Avoid administering within 2 hours of meals, as it may impair absorption of vitamins A, D, E, and K. Avoid use in dysphagic and bedridden persons as aspiration of liquid paraffin may result in lipid pneumonitis

Site 6: Combination of stool softener and stimulant
Example: docusate and senna
Mechanism: stool softener and stimulant
Onset of action: 6–12 hours
Precaution: As noted for individual laxatives

Fig. 25.2   Different types of agents to combat constipation and where they work in the intestinal lumen. (Adapted from Salerno E. *Pharmacology for Health Professionals*, 1st ed. Mosby; 1999.)

- Lactulose: poorly absorbed synthetic sugar that alters the intestinal microbiome and is broken down in the bowel to increase stool frequency and promote intestinal motility[2,8]
  - Also used in patients with hepatic encephalopathy to reduce the amount of ammonia in the blood
  - PEG has been shown to have same efficiency as lactulose.[10]
- Side effects: bloating, flatulence, abdominal cramping, distension

STIMULANT LAXATIVES

These agents are used to activate and encourage intestinal motility.[8] They work by increasing the transport of electrolytes into the colonic lumen, which encourages water to enter the intestinal lumen.[2] Ultimately, this causes irritation of the nerve endings of the colon, which increases intestinal motility, stimulates gut peristalsis, and reduces colonic water absorption.[4,9–11]

- Common types
  - Bisacodyl: induces almost immediate, powerful, propulsive motor activity to cause bowel movements[2]
  - Senna: allows water to enter the stool mass, which softens the stool, and increases the weight of the stool to increase stool frequency[2]
- Side effects: abdominal cramping, abdominal pain, electrolyte abnormalities[6]

STOOL SOFTENERS

These allow water and lipids to penetrate the stool to hydrate and change the consistency of stool.[10] They are less effective than laxatives in promoting bowel movements.[4] More frequently, they are used in conjunction with other therapies when patients report persistently hard stools.[11]

- Common types
  - Docusate sodium: stimulates fluid secretion by the small and large intestine to soften stool
    - Recent studies have demonstrated that docusate sodium is ineffective and adds increased costs and risks to hospitalized patients.[14]
  - Mineral oil: an indigestible lipid that is used to provide lubrication and emulsification of the fecal mass and lubricate the gut lining to enhance the progression of stool[2,10]
- Should be given cautiously in patients with impaired swallowing, as aspiration can lead to lipoid pneumonia[6]

ENEMAS

These act by causing rectal distention and irritation of the intestine.[2]

- Can include commercially made enemas (sodium phosphate, fleet, lactulose) as well as saline, tap water, soap suds enema, or milk-of-molasses enema
  - Care should be taken when inserting the enema to prevent trauma to the anorectal mucosa.[2]
  - Enemas can cause electrolytes abnormalities and should be used cautiously in patient with ascites, congestive heart failure, and kidney disease.[5]

SUPPOSITORY

These work by stimulating an osmotic effect in the rectum. They lubricate the rectum and stimulate the colonic reflex to promote defecation.[8]

METHYLNALTREXONE

This subcutaneous injection/oral medication is approved for opioid-induced constipation. It is a peripheral mu-opioid receptor antagonist, which acts to displace opioids from the mu receptors in the gut. Displacing the opioids allows the gut to function normally again and results in a bowel movement. By favoring the receptors in the intestine, this medication has not been shown to precipitate opioid withdrawal.[2]

DIGITAL DISIMPACTION

This procedure involves inserting a lubricated finger into the rectum and using digital manipulation to break up and remove the stool in pieces until the rectum is empty.[15] This procedure is often followed up with enema or suppository administration to ensure clear bowels.

- Digital manipulation is contraindicated in patients with inflamed bowels, those who are immunocompromised, patients who have undergone recent rectal surgery or trauma, or those who recently received radiation to the pelvic area.[5]
- Frequent digital stimulation can cause injury to the anal canal, hemorrhoids, and infection,[15] so repeated manipulation should be avoided.

Conclusion

Constipation can be an acute or chronic problem. It is psychologically distressing to the patient and can cause increased abdominal bloating and discomfort. The mainstay of management is prevention.[3] Nurses are in the best position to provide education to patients about increasing fiber intake and hydration, promote increased physical activity, and encourage patients to take prescribed laxatives. A multifactorial approach, including a combination of nonmedical and medical techniques, is often most effective to combat symptoms of constipation successfully.

Please note, while this chapter discusses the most common types of agents used in the hospital setting to treat constipation, there are additional medications being trialed in the outpatient setting, as well as different surgical options available. These outpatient/alternative therapies are used to combat constipation refractory to the most common medications described.

References

1. Paquette IM, Varma M, Ternent C, et al. The American Society of Colon and Rectal Surgeons' clinical practice guideline for the evaluation and management of constipation. *Dis Colon Rectum.* 2016;59(6):479–492.
2. Portalatin M, Winstead N. Medical management of constipation. *Clin Colon Rectal Surg.* 2012;25(1):12–19.
3. Saha S, Nathani P, Gupta A. Preventing opioid-induced constipation: a teachable moment. *JAMA Int Med.* 2020;180(10):1371–1372.
4. Pont LG, Fisher M, Williams K. Appropriate use of laxatives in the older person. *Drugs Aging.* 2019;36:999–1005.
5. Mitchell A. Administering an enema: indications, types, equipment and procedure. *Brit J Nurs.* 2019;28(3):154–156.
6. Costilla VC, Foxx-Orenstein AE. Constipation: understanding mechanisms and management. *Clin Geriatr Med.* 2014;30(1):107–115.
7. Kamm MA. Constipation and its management. *BMJ.* 2003;327(7413):459–460.
8. Diebakate-Scordamaglia L, Voican CS, Perlemuter G. Iatrogenic constipation in gastrointestinal surgery. *J Visc Surg.* 2022;159(1S):S51–S57.
9. Rao VL, Micic D, Davis AM. Medical management of opioid-induced constipation. *JAMA.* 2019;322(22):2241–2242.
10. Crockett SD, Greer KB, Heidelbaugh JJ, et al. American Gastroenterological Association Institute guideline on the medical management of opioid-induced constipation. *Gastroenterology.* 2019;156(1):218–226.

11. Corsetti M, Brown S, Chiarioni G, et al. Chronic constipation in adults: contemporary perspectives and clinical challenges. 2: Conservative, behavioural, medical and surgical treatment. *J Neurogastroenterol Motil.* 2021;33(7):e14070.
12. Kang SJ, Cho YS, Lee TH, et al. Medical management of constipation in elderly patients: systematic review. *J Neurogastroenterol Motil.* 2021;27(4):495.
13. Haas S, Andersen LM, Sommer T. Randomized controlled trial comparing Moviprep and Phosphoral as bowel cleansing agents in patients undergoing colonoscopy. *Tech Coloproctol.* 2014;18:929–935.
14. Shair KA, Espinosa SM, Kwon JY, et al. A quality improvement approach to decrease the utilization of docusate in hospitalized patients. *Quality Manage Healthcare.* 2023;10-97. doi:10.1097/QMH.0000000000000406.
15. Bolen PD. How digital disimpaction is used to relieve constipation. Verywell Health. January 11, 2022. https://www.verywellhealth.com/digital-evacuation-1945037. Accessed March 14, 2023.

Questions

Madeline is a 67-year-old female with a past medical history of chronic pain after sustaining a back injury in a car accident 25 years ago. She is paralyzed from the waist down. After the recent passing of her husband, she has become more sedentary and relies on food delivery services for meals. She regularly takes 20 mg of oxycodone every 4 hours at home for pain. She is presenting today for revision spinal surgery.

1. What factors place her at an increased risk for constipation?
   a. Female gender and age >65
   b. Sedentary lifestyle and poor diet
   c. Regular opioid use
   d. All the above

2. As her nurse, what should you do initially?
   a. Ask her about her bowel habits and document the date of her last bowel movement.
   b. Request a decreased dose of her pain medicine immediately.
   c. Request the provider to order daily laxatives while she continues to take her oxycodone.
   d. Both a and c

3. Postoperatively, the patient is placed on a hydromorphone patient-controlled analgesia (PCA) pump. She is adherent with taking oral laxatives but still has not had a bowel movement since admission. She is hesitant to take anything by the rectal route. What education can you provide to the patient?
   a. Enemas and suppositories exert their effect on the mu-opioid receptor in the gut.
   b. Enemas and suppositories work by increasing fecal bulk.
   c. Enemas and suppositories work to irritate and draw water into the colon to stimulate bowel movements.
   d. Enemas and suppositories are not effective in patients who are paralyzed, so they can be avoided in this case.

4. Despite taking the scheduled laxatives and enema, the patient's last bowel movement was over a week ago, and she is starting to feel uncomfortable. What medication can you request to combat opioid-induced constipation?
   a. Continue the current medications as prescribed; eventually she will have a bowel movement.
   b. Methylnaltrexone
   c. IV fluids to increase hydration
   d. Request that the gastrointestinal consult service evaluate the patient.

5. The patient is weaned off the hydromorphone PCA pump and back to her home oxycodone dose. When she is being discharged, which instruction should you *not* provide?
   a. Increase your mobility at home.
   b. Increase your fiber and fluid intake.
   c. Once you have a bowel movement, you can stop your bowel regimen.
   d. Continue to take your stool softeners while you are on oxycodone.

Answers

1. d

2. d

3. c

4. b

5. c

CHAPTER 26

Nursing Management of the Patient With Postoperative Ileus

Rebecca Belfonti, MSN, CRNP, AGACNP-BC, PCCN ■ Shannon Feldman, MSN, CRNP, AGACNP-BC

Introduction

Postoperative ileus (POI) is a syndrome of impaired gastrointestinal (GI) transit that frequently occurs after surgery. It is unfortunately a common but clinically challenging problem that leads to patient discomfort, prolonged hospitalization, increased health care costs, and significant morbidity.[1] Although the exact definition of POI is controversial, it commonly refers to a form of constipation in which patients are unable to pass stool and become intolerant of oral intake. This occurs due to nonmechanical factors that disrupt the normal coordinated peristalsis of the GI tract following surgery. Many factors contribute to the development of POI, such as dehydration, fluid overload, use of narcotics, and decreased mobility.[2] The incidence of POI is difficult to find in the literature because it is believed that many cases go undocumented. In one study, which involved a large multihospital database of patients who underwent a colectomy, POI increased the length of the hospital stay 4.9 days and increased costs by ~$8000.[3] Although the incidence of POI is highest for intraabdominal surgery cases, it can also develop after neurosurgery. A study published in 2022 determined that POI is a common complication after spinal surgery, with an incidence range of 10–30%.[4] It is imperative that bedside nurses be able to recognize the signs and symptoms of POI and initiate timely intervention if ileus is suspected.

Pathophysiology

POI is a problematic and frequent complication of surgery. Ultimately, surgical manipulation, the use of anesthetic agents, and the use of postoperative opioids have a compounding effect on the motility of the entire GI tract. Although the exact pathogenesis of POI remains unclear, it is understood that the formation of POI involves various inhibitory neural reflexes and inflammatory mediators. There are three main reflexes involved with POI:

- Ultrashort reflexes confined to the gut wall
- Short reflexes encompassing prevertebral ganglia
- Long reflexes involving the spinal cord

Inhibitory transmitters, such as nitric oxide and vasoactive peptide, are also known to play a role in the slowing of gastric motility and lead to POI.[1,5]

Although POI is thought to be predominantly due to neural dysfunction, inflammatory factors also play a large role. Increased inflammation in the walls of the intestine can be multifactorial, often caused by intestinal manipulation or trauma at the surgical site. Fluid overload following elective surgery is associated with an increased time until the first passage of flatus and stool, prolonged gastric emptying time, and increased time to tolerance of solid foods.[1,5] Furthermore, opioids, which are commonly used for pain relief in the postoperative setting, act as

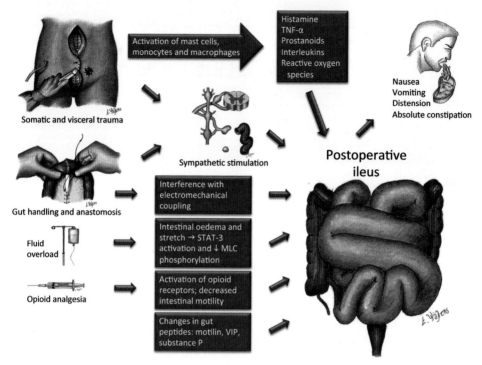

Fig. 26.1 Pathophysiology of postoperative ileus development. *MLC*, Myosin light chain; *TNF*-α, tumor necrosis factor-alpha; *VIP*, vasoactive intestinal peptide. (From Bragg D, El-Sharkawy AM, Psaltis E, et al. Postoperative ileus: recent developments in pathophysiology and management. *Clin Nutr*. 2015;34[3]:367–376.)

potent modulators of the central and peripheral neural system and can affect gastric emptying and smooth muscle contraction in the GI tract (Fig. 26.1).[1,5]

Risk Factors

There are multiple risk factors for POI that are important to identify in the neurosurgical patient. Risk factors include but are not limited to prolonged abdominal surgery, lower GI surgery, open surgery, intraabdominal inflammation (peritonitis/sepsis), intra- and postoperative bleeding requiring transfusion, factors that increase bowel wall edema (such as hypoalbuminemia and aggressive administration of intravenous fluids), perioperative opioid use, and obesity.[2] A systematic review indicated that POI occurrence after lumbar surgery has a statistically significant association with increased patient age, prolonged surgical time, significant blood loss, and longer length of hospital stay. It was also discovered that patients who were male, underwent an anterior surgical approach, or underwent a spinal fusion had increased occurrences of POI.[4]

Presentation/Clinical Features

Failure of peristalsis results in the accumulation of GI contents within the lumen of the gut. Patients will experience abdominal pain, abdominal distension, anorexia, nausea or vomiting, and fail to pass stool or flatus. Physical examination typically reveals abdominal distention and tympany, a reduction of bowel sounds, and often some degree of mild diffuse tenderness.[2]

TABLE 26.1 ■ Labs Ordered When Postoperative Ileus Is Suspected, With Rationale

Labs	Normal Values	Rationale
Hemoglobin	Female: 12.1–15.1 Male: 13.8–17.2	Looks for anemia, rules out bleeding
White blood cell (WBC)	4.0–11.0	Looks for infection • Elevated WBC could mean infection or intestinal ischemia
Potassium	3.5–5 mmol/L	Low potassium can worsen ileus • Should be repleted as needed
Magnesium	1.3–2.1 mEq/L	Low magnesium can affect gut motility • Should be repleted as needed
Creatinine	0.70–1.40 mg/dL	Uremia from acute kidney injury can lead to ileus
Liver function tests	ALP: 25–120 IU/L ALT: <30 IU/L AST: 7–35 IU/L	Postoperative gallbladder dysfunction or pancreatitis can lead to ileus

ALP, Alkaline phosphatase; *ALT,* alanine transaminase; *AST,* aspartate transaminase.

A thorough assessment of the neurosurgical patient is vital to recognize an ileus. Left untreated, an ileus can cause bowel necrosis. The patient's abdomen can provide critical information when assessing for POI. When assessing, nurses should always follow the sequence:

- Inspection: visualization of the abdomen
- Auscultation: listening to the abdomen with a stethoscope
- Percussion: tapping of the abdomen
- Palpation: exerting pressure on the abdomen

Changing the order of these assessment techniques could alter the frequency and characteristics of bowel sounds and make findings less accurate. In the setting of an ileus, the abdomen is usually distended and tympanic with hypoactive bowel sounds, and patients will complain of diffuse, persistent tenderness on physical exam.[2]

Diagnosis

Although POI is usually diagnosed clinically, imaging and laboratory evaluation are used to exclude other diagnoses, such as bowel obstruction or bowel perforation. If an ileus is suspected, it is important to relay this to the patient's provider. A plain film x-ray is the first-line image study in the diagnosis of ileus. On x-ray, dilated loops of small bowel and colon indicate a possible ileus. If inconclusive, a computed tomography scan may give the clinician a better view of the bowels.[2] Lab work, including blood count and a metabolic panel, should be ordered when ileus is suspected to help identify any potentially reversible causes (Table 26.1).

Complications

Complications of POI can be very serious and cause a multitude of adverse effects for patients. Because POI involves decreased gastric mobility, it is often associated with nausea and vomiting, which are both risk factors for pulmonary aspiration. POI can also cause dehydration and electrolyte imbalances.[6] The development of POI following surgery has been found to cause a significant burden on the health care system. Patients who develop POI can increase the median cost of an inpatient stay by ~71%.[7] This cost can be attributed to the increased need for further nursing care, lab work, imaging, and overall prolonged length of stay (LOS) until the resolution of symptoms.

Increased costs are also associated with the possibility of further procedures, such as central line placement for total parenteral nutrition (TPN) and/or nasogastric tube (NGT) placement for gastric decompression. In patients who underwent anterior approach for lumbar interbody fusion, studies demonstrated that the diagnosis of POI was associated with an additional LOS of almost 2.8 days and an additional cost of >$2000.[8] With prolonged hospitalizations, patients are also predisposed to hospital-acquired infections that can further complicate their stay.

Management/Treatment

When treating a patient with POI, it is first important to correct any reversible causes, such as any electrolyte imbalances. Otherwise, supportive care is the mainstay of treatment for patients with POI. For pain management, opioids should be used sparingly, and pain control should involve the utilization of multimodal analgesia, including nonopioid medications, such as nonsteroidal anti-inflammatory drugs and acetaminophen. Any medications that can cause constipation should be withheld if possible, such as narcotics, anticholinergics, and iron supplementation. Early ambulation is also important to stimulate GI motility.

Bowel rest can help a patient with POI. Patients may be on no oral intake or placed on a diet of only sips of clear fluids, if tolerated. If the patient is having moderate to severe continuous vomiting and/or significant abdominal distention, a NGT can be placed for gastric decompression. Patients may also require parenteral nutrition until they can be transitioned to oral feedings. TPN is recommended if the patient is unable to tolerate adequate oral intake after 7 days.[2] If patients are awake and alert, they can be encouraged to chew gum. Chewing gum has the potential to help with ileus resolution, as it stimulates the cephalocaudal reflex, which promotes peristalsis and inhibits inflammation.[2]

Patients should be closely monitored with serial abdominal examinations for improvement or worsening of their condition. Additional imaging studies are warranted if conservative measures do not improve the patient's condition in 48–72 hours. While the patient is on bowel rest, it is imperative to stop all bowel medications to prevent further dilation, obstruction, and possible bowel perforation until GI motility returns and there is resolution of symptoms.

Nursing Considerations

When caring for neurosurgical patients, it is crucial for nurses to perform a thorough history and physical assessment to determine if their patients are at risk of developing a POI. For example, a history of postoperative nausea or vomiting or a history of gastroparesis can contribute to elevated risk of POI. Nurses should also be mindful that patients who undergo anterior approach spine surgeries with bowel manipulation have a higher chance of developing POI.

Nurses should assess if a patient is experiencing abdominal pain, nausea, or vomiting. Additionally, it is important to know if the patient has passed flatus, is complaining of belching following surgery, or is experiencing abdominal distention, bloating, or discomfort. Abdominal assessment following the order of inspection, auscultation, percussion, and palpation is helpful in recognizing a potential ileus forming. Taking note of a patient's appetite and ability to take in adequate PO fluid is helpful in assessing the patient's level of hydration. Overall, any findings that would raise concern for an ileus (i.e., abdominal pain, distention, hypoactive or absent bowel sounds, nausea, vomiting) should be brought to the provider's attention immediately.

Conclusion

POI is a syndrome of impaired GI transit that frequently occurs after surgery. Surgery and anesthesia slow the motility of the entire GI tract, which can lead to nausea and vomiting and the inability to tolerate oral intake. Prolonged abdominal surgeries put patients at risk for developing an ileus, but other types of surgeries are known to cause POI as well. Multiple nonmechanical factors such as dehydration, fluid overload, use of narcotics, and decreased mobility also predispose patients to the development of POI. It is imperative for nurses to be able to promptly recognize early signs of POI through physical assessment and history of present illness to prevent further complications for the patient. Once an ileus occurs, it can lead to further hospital complications, prolonged LOS, the need for additional imaging and testing, and increased patient costs.

References

1. Vather R, O'Grady G, Bissett IP, et al. Postoperative ileus: mechanisms and future directions for research. *Clin Exp Pharmacol Physiol.* 2014;41(5):358–370. doi:10.1111/1440-1681.12220.
2. Beach EC, De Jesus O. *Ileus.* StatPearls Publishing; 2023.
3. Barletta JF, Senagore AJ. Reducing the burden of postoperative ileus: evaluating and implementing an evidence-based strategy. *World J Surg.* 2014;38(8):1966–1977. doi:10.1007/s00268-014-2506-2.
4. Reed LA, Mihas AK, Fortin TA, et al. Risk factors for postoperative ileus after thoracolumbar and lumbar spinal fusion surgery: systematic review and meta-analysis. *World Neurosurg.* 2022;168:e381–e392. doi:10.1016/j.wneu.2022.10.025.
5. Ay AA, Kutun S, Ulucanlar H, et al. Risk factors for postoperative ileus. *J Korean Surg Soc.* 2011;81(4):242–249. doi:10.4174/jkss.2011.81.4.242.
6. Venara A, Neunlist M, Slim K, et al. Postoperative ileus: pathophysiology, incidence, and prevention. *J Visc Surg.* 2016;153(6):439–446. doi:10.1016/j.jviscsurg.2016.08.010.
7. Mao H, Milne TGE, O'Grady G, et al. Prolonged postoperative ileus significantly increases the cost of inpatient stay for patients undergoing elective colorectal surgery: results of a multivariate analysis of prospective data at a single institution. *Dis Colon Rectum.* 2019;62(5):631–637. doi:10.1097/DCR.0000000000001301.
8. Horowitz JA, Jain A, Puvanesarajah V, et al. Risk factors, additional length of stay, and cost associated with postoperative ileus following anterior lumbar interbody fusion in elderly patients. *World Neurosurg.* 2018;115:e185–e189. doi:10.1016/j.wneu.2018.04.006.

Questions

John Smith is a 72-year-old male with a past medical history significant for severe lumbar spinal stenosis, who underwent anterior L2–S1 interbody fusion 2 days ago. Postoperatively, he had high drain output, his hemoglobin dropped, and he required two units of packed red blood cells. He has not yet worked with physical therapy following his surgery due to low blood pressure. Today his vitals have stabilized, and the plan is for him to mobilize. He has been receiving continuous IV fluids in addition to his clear liquid diet because of his lack of appetite.

1. Given the clinical information, what risk factors would predispose this patient to developing a postoperative ileus?
   a. Anterior approach for spine surgery
   b. Age
   c. Prolonged immobilization
   d. Both a and c

2. You are just beginning your shift with this patient. What is the first thing you should do as his nurse when you meet him?
   a. Set him up with breakfast and encourage him to eat so he will have energy to work with physical therapy.
   b. Bring in his morning meds and assess him after you have seen your entire assignment.
   c. Perform your head-to-toe assessment to get a baseline abdominal exam and note if the patient is experiencing abdominal pain, distention, nausea, or vomiting.
   d. Have NGT at bedside in preparation for stomach decompression.

3. When performing your abdominal assessment, which order do you perform each assessment technique?
  a. Inspection, percussion, palpation, auscultation
  b. The order does not matter if you perform all assessment techniques during your assessment
  c. Auscultation, inspection, palpation, percussion
  d. Inspection, auscultation, percussion, palpation

4. About 3 hours into your shift, John is now complaining of abdominal distention and has had two large episodes of projectile vomiting. Upon assessment, his abdomen is distended and bowel sounds absent, which is a change from this morning's assessment. What is the first action you would take for this patient?
  a. Insert NGT because he looks uncomfortable.
  b. Give nausea medication and continue to monitor.
  c. Notify the doctor of new assessment findings to see if abdominal x-ray is warranted.
  d. Call a rapid response.

5. John's symptoms continue to worsen, and he cannot tolerate anything by mouth. The doctor states to preemptively treat him as if this is an ileus. Select the appropriate intervention(s) for management of ileus. (Select all that apply.)
  a. Use narcotics sparingly.
  b. Hold all bowel medications.
  c. Lie the patient flat.
  d. Bowel rest, only allowing ice chips and small sips of clear fluids.

Answers

1. d

2. c

3. d

4. c

5. a, b, d

CHAPTER 27

Nursing Management of Nutrition in Neurosurgical Patients

Alexandra Pisani, BSN, RN, SCRN ▪ Madeline Schuler, BSN, RN, SCRN

Introduction

Nutritional assessment of neurologic patients begins at the time of hospital admission and is a shared responsibility among all members of the interprofessional care team. Patients admitted to the neurologic ward may have had a stroke, brain tumor, cerebral vascular malformation, meningitis or encephalitis, traumatic brain injury, or one of many other diagnoses that create a barrier to healthy nutrition. Developing a comprehensive plan of care, which includes optimization of nutrition, is essential to each patient's well-being and successful recovery. Nurses play a central role in nutritional optimization and must be prepared to perform daily assessments, utilize effective screening tools, identify risk factors for malnutrition, monitor for clinical changes that may change their patient's risk for developing malnutrition, and advocate for their patient to the interprofessional care team.

Enteral Nutrition: Normal Physiology and Common Complications

Caring for patients at risk for malnutrition requires a fundamental understanding of normal gastrointestinal anatomy and physiology. Processing food by mouth or *per orum* (PO) involves oral mastication (chewing), swallowing through oropharyngeal structures, descent via the esophagus and past the lower esophageal sphincter, and collection in the stomach. Peristalsis is the sequential muscular contractions that move food through the digestive system—down the esophagus and into the stomach, through the small intestine, large intestine, and into the rectal vault. Residual material is then excreted as a bowel movement. At first glance, digestion may seem straightforward, but each bite of food initiates a complex process, and nurses must be prepared to identify dysfunction at every level before it causes significant problems for the patient.

The process of mastication, swallowing, and digestion involves cranial nerves V (trigeminal), VII (facial), IX (glossopharyngeal), X (vagus), and XI (spinal accessory).[1] Neurologic patients frequently suffer cranial nerve injuries that compromise their ability to nourish themselves safely and effectively. This includes nerve injuries that cause dysphagia, which can lead to malnutrition and aspiration. Patients with dysphagia due to neurologic injury will often need modified consistency diets to prevent aspiration, and some require a temporary or permanent feeding tube to ensure adequate nutritional intake.[2]

In addition to dysphagia caused by their neurologic injury, hospitalized neurologic patients are at risk for malnutrition due to multifactorial impairment of peristalsis. Medications (e.g., opioids and iron supplements), dehydration, decreased ambulation, and stress can decrease the muscular contractions of the bowel and result in constipation. Untreated constipation can lead to decreased appetite, nausea, vomiting, and bowel impaction, which may require manual, pharmaceutical, or even surgical intervention to correct. Proactive care and communication are essential for preventing constipation and its complications. Nurses should diligently document the patient's date of last bowel movement (LBM) and fluid intake/output volumes and perform abdominal examinations regularly. Patients should be encouraged to mobilize and ambulate and to adhere to a prescribed bowel regimen. Any clinical changes or concerning findings should be communicated to the physician and shared with the interprofessional team.

Bedside nurses are uniquely positioned to make nuanced assessments, provide holistic care, and advocate for their patients' needs. In many ways, nurses are the first-line defense against malnutrition and its devastating consequences. Overall nursing assessments should include considerations such as:

- What is the patient's cognitive status, and can the patient safely eat independently?
- Are there any risk factors for difficulty with swallowing, such as medical devices, body positioning, or neurologic injury?
- How is the patient's dentition? Does the patient normally use dentures or require a modified consistency diet?
- When was the patient's LBM, and does the patient show any signs of constipation, ileus, or inability to tolerate PO nutrition?

Screening Tools: Nutrition and Dysphagia

MALNUTRITION SCREENING TOOL

Many hospitals require that a nutrition assessment be performed at the time of admission, and standardized nutritional screening tools are highly effective for identifying malnutrition. Nevertheless, every screening tool has limitations in practice. In some cases patients with malnutrition or risk factors for malnutrition will test normal according to the screening tool. Nurses should use clinical judgment in combination with the screening protocol result to recommend ordering consultations to nutrition to the interprofessional team so that timely care and interventions can be pursued for patients at high risk for malnutrition.

There are numerous accredited resources available to aid in the assessment of patient nutritional status. Many experts in the field agree that, among the currently available screening tools, the Malnutrition Screening Tool (MST) is the strongest predictor of malnutrition. The MST consists of two questions regarding weight loss and appetite. A score ≥2 indicates risk for malnutrition.[3] When screening, nurses must ensure that the patient has adequate cognitive function to answer the questions appropriately (Fig. 27.1).

The European Society for Clinical Nutrition and Malnutrition defines "at risk" for malnutrition as a positive finding on at least one nutritional screening tool (such as the MST), coupled with one of the following factors:

1. Body mass index (BMI) <18.5 kg/m²
2. Combination of weight loss and reduction in BMI[4]

It is important to note that nutritional status cannot always be visually assessed. No patient should be exempt from nutritional screening based solely on their appearance or BMI. Malnourished patients are not always thin and do not always have a low BMI; they can have a normal BMI or even be overweight. While physical examination can reveal important features suggestive of malnourishment (e.g., thin, gaunt, bloating, pallor, muscle wasting, edema), their absence does not exclude the possibility of malnutrition. In cases of malnutrition or uncertain nutritional status, consulting a dietician is an excellent resource for improving patient care.

YALE SWALLOW PROTOCOL

The Yale Swallow Protocol (YSP) was developed to screen for dysphagia and proactively identify patients at risk for aspiration events. Though not technically part of the nutrition evaluation, early

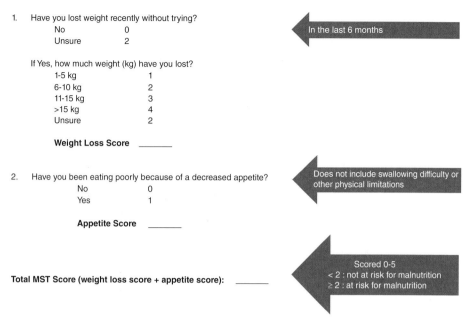

1. Have you lost weight recently without trying?
   No   0
   Unsure   2

   In the last 6 months

   If Yes, how much weight (kg) have you lost?
   1-5 kg   1
   6-10 kg   2
   11-15 kg   3
   >15 kg   4
   Unsure   2

   Weight Loss Score _____

2. Have you been eating poorly because of a decreased appetite?
   No   0
   Yes   1

   Does not include swallowing difficulty or other physical limitations

   Appetite Score _____

Total MST Score (weight loss score + appetite score): _____

Scored 0-5
< 2 : not at risk for malnutrition
≥ 2 : at risk for malnutrition

Fig. 27.1 Malnutrition Screening Tool. (From Ferguson M, Capra S, Bauer J, et al. Development of a valid and reliable malnutrition screeening tool for adult acute hospital patients. *Nutrition*. 1999;15[6]:458–464.)

Yale Swallow Screen

Exclusion Criteria
- Unable to remain alert
- Baseline modified diet
- Tube feeding in place
- HOB restricted <30 degrees
- Tracheostomy
- NPO ordered

Cognitive Screen
- What is your name?
- Where are you?
- What year is it?

Oral Mechanism Exam
- Lingual range of motion-stick tongue out, move it side to side
- Facial symmetry- smile
- Labial closure- puff cheeks with air

3 oz Water Swallow Assessment
Able to:
- Sit upright
- Drink 3 oz of water without stopping
Coughing indicates a fail

Fig. 27.2 Yale Swallow Protocol. (From Leder S, Suiter D. *The Yale Swallow Protocol: An Evidence-Based Approach to Decision Making.* Springer International Publishing. Cham; 2014.)

recognition of dysphagia and aspiration risk factors through the YSP allows nurses to advocate for a nutrition regimen that will be safe and effective. When utilized correctly, the YSP has a sensitivity of 95% and is an important tool for the nursing assessment of neurologic patients.[5] Patients without exclusions to undergoing the YSP (e.g., inability to remain alert, tracheostomy, or head of bed restriction <30 degrees) are evaluated in three consecutive phases:

- Begins with a cognitive screen
- Proceeds to an oral mechanism exam
- Ends with a 3-ounce water swallow assessment (Fig. 27.2)

If patients fail any step in the assessment, they have failed the entire YSP and should not proceed any further in the evaluation. Upon failure of the YSP, patients should be given nothing by mouth (NPO). They should be evaluated by the speech-language pathology (SLP) team, who may perform a fiberoptic endoscopic evaluation of swallowing (FEES) before making recommendations regarding PO intake and a modified consistency diet.[5] If a patient's neurologic function changes at any point during the hospitalization, the YSP should be repeated, and results should be documented and clearly communicated to the interprofessional team.

There are many reasons why neurologic patients may be unable to swallow safely, including cognitive impairment, decreased mobility, severe deconditioning, and neurologic deficits (e.g., facial hemiplegia due to stroke). Aspiration can cause pulmonary edema, respiratory failure, pneumonitis, pneumonia, and sepsis, ultimately leading to an increased risk of death in severe cases.

Modified Consistency Diets

Patients who fail the YSP, FEES, or who otherwise are at risk for aspiration may require a modified consistency oral diet. The International Dysphagia Diet Standardization Initiative includes a scale that systematically grades PO dietary textures by a score of 0–7.[6] These textures range from thin liquids (score of 0) to regular food (score of 7), but it is important to remember that the numerical score does not indicate a level of difficulty. In fact, thin liquids (water or broth) are often the most challenging for patients with swallowing disorders, whereas moderately thickened liquids (think the consistency of honey) may be more safely tolerated.[6] The scale is ordered by grouping of textures and types of PO intake (e.g., solids vs liquids and everything in between). A patient may perform best at different levels of food consistency and fluid consistency (Fig. 27.3).

Regardless of the recommended PO dietary consistency, nurses must be alert to risks or signs of aspiration, such as coughing, choking, pocketing of food, and drooling. Best practices to implement while eating and drinking are to ensure that the patient is fully alert, sitting in upright posture, and waiting enough time in between bites/sips. Nurses can encourage swallowing twice to ensure complete clearance, limit distractions, and offer reminders and cues throughout the swallowing process.[2] Nurses should check that oral suctioning equipment is available and ready for use at bedside in the event of choking. If the nurse notes any evidence of aspiration or other concerns, the nurse should hold off on further PO intake, notify the physician team, and consider reconsulting the SLP team for repeated evaluation.

Tube Feeding

Tube feeding is indicated for patients who are unable to safely meet their nutrition and hydration requirements by PO intake, even with a modified-consistency diet. This commonly occurs in patients with critical illness, severe dysphagia, recurrent aspiration, cognitive impairment,

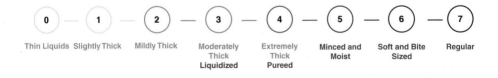

Fig. 27.3 International Dysphagia Diet Initiative liquid-to-food progression. (From International Dysphagia Diet Initiative (IDDSI) framework 2019. https://iddsi.org/IDDSI/media/images/Complete_IDDSI_Framework_Final_31July2019.pdf.)

immobility, physical and functional limitations, neurologic deficits, and persistent inadequate intake, even when safely performed. Patients who can tolerate enteral nutrition but are unable to eat or drink adequately by mouth may need a temporary feeding tube. Nasogastric and orogastric tubes are inserted through the nose or mouth, respectively, passed down through the esophagus, and used to deliver nutrition directly into the stomach. These feeding tubes are placed at bedside, but before using the tube, providers must verify that the tip has advanced beyond the lower esophageal sphincter and is appropriately positioned within the stomach. This is typically done by checking an upright abdominal radiograph to visualize the tip of the tube.

Permanent or semipermanent enteral access is achieved by percutaneous endoscopic gastrostomy or jejunostomy (PEG/PEJ) tubes, which are inserted directly through the abdominal wall and into the stomach or jejunum, respectively. The external portion of these tubes has a soft rubber bumper at the end nearest to the abdominal wall and a nozzle at the open end where feeding formula is attached for infusion. The purpose of the rubber bumper is to prevent migration of the tube, and longer tubes should also be secured with an external fixation device separate from the bumper. Bumpers should be rotated daily to prevent skin breakdown and callusing, promote healing of internal tissues, and decrease the risk of dislodgment. The bumper's location should be carefully marked, monitored, and documented to ensure consistency.

- In the first 24 hours after PEG/PEJ tube placement, nurses should clean the area with gauze and sterile water, later transitioning to gentle soap and water. To protect skin integrity, a thin dressing, such as a layer of split gauze, should be placed between the bumper and the skin. This dressing should be changed if it becomes wet from drainage or cleaning.

When cleared by the procedural team for initiation of tube feeds, "start low and go slow" is the best rule of thumb to follow. The rate of tube feeding often starts around 15 mL/hour and increases by 10 mL/hour every 4 hours until the goal rate is reached (e.g., 45 mL/hour). During this time of progressive increase, nurses should monitor closely for signs of tube feeding intolerance, such as nausea, vomiting, abdominal pain or distention, and high gastric residual volumes. Nurses may need to slow the tube feeding rate or stop the infusion altogether, depending on how their patient appears to be tolerating the process. If any concerns do arise, nurses should notify the physician team immediately. It is important that the tube feed titration schedule is communicated clearly to each oncoming shift, including any problems that may have occurred during the previous shift.

While feeding formula or medications are being administered, nurses should flush 15–30 mL water through the PEG/PEJ tube every 4–6 hours. Flushing should also be performed whenever the tube feeds are stopped and after every medication administration. This protocol aims to minimize the risk of clogging in the tube. To prevent aspiration of refluxed gastric contents, the head of the bed should be raised to 30–45 degrees, kept in reverse Trendelenburg or in semi-Fowler while administering nutrition or medications, and maintained in that position for 1 hour after completion.[7] Nurses should monitor PEG/PEJ sites for drainage, skin discoloration, increased abdominal tenderness, and changes in bowel sounds that could indicate a problem with the tubing's function or position.

There are many varieties of tube feed formulas, and each has different compositions and indications for use depending on the patient's nutritional requirements and medical comorbidities. Fig. 27.4 summarizes the main categories of feeding formula and their common indications.[8]

Parenteral Nutrition

Although enteral feeding is preferred to maintain overall gut function, patients who cannot tolerate enteral nutrition—whether due to acute or chronic pathologies—may be candidates for parenteral nutrition. In practice, parenteral nutrition is treated more like a medication than a meal. It must be ordered by the physician or advanced practice provider, prepared by the pharmacist, monitored for complications, and administered at a specific rate for a predetermined duration of time. Peripheral parenteral nutrition is a temporary nutritional supplement that can be administered

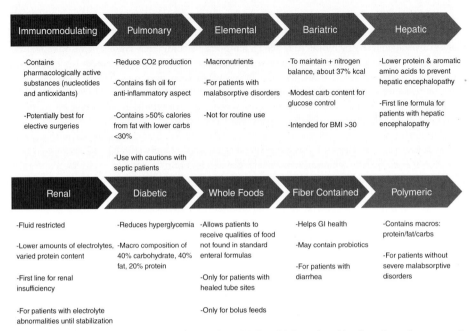

Fig. 27.4 Types of enteral feeds. (From Brown B, Roehl K, Betz M. Enteral nutrition formula sections: current evidence and implications for practice. *Nutr Clin Pract.* 2015:30[1]72–85.)

through a peripheral line; total parenteral nutrition (TPN) provides a full range of macronutrients for a longer term, but it must be administered through a central line.

■ There is no mortality difference between enteral and parenteral nutrition regimens, but prolonged and exclusive use of parenteral nutrition is associated with an increased risk of infections, increased length of stay in the intensive care unit, loss of intestinal integrity and microbiome diversity, and compromised gut-mediated immunity.[9]

Like patients with tube feeding devices, parenterally nourished patients must have their site of infusion monitored for signs of complications or dysfunction. Because the method of administration is an intravenous catheter, it is important to monitor for complications (e.g., redness, streaking, inflammation of the skin and insertion site). Daily external tubing changes, dressing changes, routine site assessments, and periodic blood tests are all part of a safety-centered protocol for patients receiving parenteral nutrition.

Conclusion

Studies consistently demonstrate that nutritional status and individualized nutritional care plans have significant implications for a patient's overall health and well-being.[10] Unfortunately, neurologic patients may be unable to advocate for their own nutritional well-being due to medical comorbidities such as stroke, cognitive impairment, and acute illness. Nurses play an important role in caring for these patients not only through their clinical knowledge, technical skills, and bedside expertise but also through their advocacy and representation to the interprofessional team. Timely nutritional assessments, early identification of high-risk patients, and proactive interventions are essential to correcting and preventing malnutrition, reducing hospitalization length of stay, and improving overall patient outcomes.[11]

A nutrition screen should be performed for every patient at the time of hospital admission. Current best practice according to the Academy of Nutrition and Dietetics is to use the MST for nutritional assessment of adult patients,[12] along with the YSP to monitor for dysphagia. Overall, screening on admission allows nurses to collect valuable information that guides decisions regarding nutrition optimization, food and fluid consistency, and whether consultation with a dietician or the SLP team is indicated.

Nutrition encompasses a vast body of knowledge, and implementing best practice guidelines can feel overwhelming in a fast-paced inpatient environment. Nurses must advocate for their patients and keep nutrition at the forefront of communication with the interprofessional team. Attentive assessments, detailed documentation, clear communication, and early interventions can go a long way in promoting nutritional gains and improving outcomes for hospitalized patients.

References

1. Malone JC, Arya NR. *Anatomy, Head and Neck, Swallowing*. StatPearls Publishing; 2021.
2. Donahue PA. When it's hard to swallow: feeding techniques for dysphagia management. *J Gerontol Nurs*. 1990;16(4):6–9. doi:10.3928/0098-9134-19900401-05.
3. Ferguson M, Capra S, Bauer J, et al. Development of a valid and reliable malnutrition screening tool for adult acute hospital patients. *Nutrition*. 1999;15(6):458–464. doi:10.1016/s0899-9007(99)00084-2.
4. Cederholm T, Barazzoni R, Austin P, et al. ESPEN guidelines on definitions and terminology of clinical nutrition. *Clin Nutr*. 2017;36(1):49–64. doi:10.1016/j.clnu.2016.09.004.
5. Leder S, Suiter D. *The Yale Swallow Protocol: An Evidence- Based Approach to Decision Making*. Springer International Publishing; 2014.
6. The International Dysphagia Diet Initiative (IDDSI) framework 2016. https://iddsi.org/IDDSI/media/images/FrameworkDocuments/IDDSIFramework-EvidenceStatement.pdf. Accessed June 14, 2023.
7. Roveron G, Antonini M, Barbierato M, et al. Clinical practice guidelines for the nursing management of percutaneous endoscopic gastrostomy and jejunostomy (PEG/PEJ) in adult patients: an executive summary. *J Wound Ostomy Continence Nurs*. 2018;45(4):326–334. doi:10.1097/WON.0000000000000442.
8. Brown B, Roehl K, Betz M. Enteral nutrition formula selection: current evidence and implications for practice. *Nutr Clin Pract*. 2015;30(1):72–85. doi:10.1177/0884533614561791.
9. Elke G, van Zanten AR, Lemieux M, et al. Enteral versus parenteral nutrition in critically ill patients: an updated systematic review and meta-analysis of randomized controlled trials. *Crit Care*. 2016;20(1):117. doi:10.1186/s13054-016-1298-1.
10. Xu X, Parker D, Ferguson C, et al. Where is the nurse in nutritional care? *Contemp Nurse*. 2017;53(3):267–270. doi:10.1080/10376178.2017.1370782.
11. Allard JP, Keller H, Jeejeebhoy KN, et al. Malnutrition at hospital admission-contributors and effect on length of stay: a prospective cohort study from the Canadian Malnutrition Task Force. *JPEN J*. 2016;40(4):487–497.
12. Skipper A, Coltman A, Tomesko J, et al. Position of the Academy of Nutrition and Dietetics: malnutrition (undernutrition) screening tools for all adults. *J Acad Nutr Diet*. 2020;120(4):709–713. doi:10.1016/j.jand.2019.09.011.

Questions

1. What is the gold standard for verifying nasogastric tube placement?
   a. Measuring gastric residuals
   b. Checking the tip location on abdominal x-ray
   c. Measuring its position externally
   d. All of the above

2. How can nurses support patient tolerance of new enteral tube feeding?
   a. Trialing different feeds
   b. Increasing the infusion rate slowly
   c. Frequent water flushes
   d. Assessing patient's appetite

3. Which is *not* a benefit of enteral nutrition compared to parenteral nutrition?
   a. Decreases risk of mortality
   b. Preserves intestinal tract integrity
   c. Lower risk of infectious complications
   d. Promotes gut-mediated immunity

4. You are orienting a new nurse, Tracy, to the unit. After receiving report from the previous shift, Tracy asks how the patient could be receiving TPN when he does not have a PEG tube listed in his electronic medical record (EMR) documentation. You remind Tracy that TPN is administered
   a. orally.
   b. through a nasogastric tube.
   c. through an intravenous device.
   d. through a PEG tube, and show her how to add the device into the EMR.

5. You walk into your patient's room and see that the nasogastric tube is sitting at 40 cm. During report you were told it was inserted to 23 cm. What should you do?
   a. Place a STAT consult for SLP to evaluate the patient.
   b. Decrease the rate of tube feed infusion and auscultate the patient's abdomen.
   c. Stop the tube feed infusion, wait 2 hours, and resume tube feed infusion at 15 mL/hour.
   d. Stop the tube feed infusion and alert the team of a possibly dislodged nasogastric tube.

Answers

1. b

2. b

3. a

4. c

5. d

CHAPTER 28

Wound Care in the Surgical Setting

Jinah Yoo, MSN, AGPCNP-BC, CWOCN ■ René Daniel, MD, PhD, FACP, FHM

Introduction

Surgical wounds are the most common type of wound seen in the acute care setting.[1] While the management of these wounds often includes an interdisciplinary team of health care professionals, nurses have historically been tasked to make critical decisions related to interventions and direct care of these wounds.[2] Nurses play a critical role in identifying and preventing intra- and postoperative complications, such as surgical site infections (SSIs) and pressure injuries, as they care for patients 24 hours a day in the acute care setting. Nurses should be familiar with methods of prevention and common medications used for wound treatment and feel comfortable providing education to patients and families to continue wound management in the outpatient setting.

Principles of Wound Healing

There are three main classifications in wound healing: primary, secondary, and tertiary healing.

■ Primary wound healing involves wound closure by bringing the wound edges together and keeping them approximated by using sutures, staples, or a skin adhesive. The wound heals under the closed incision by filling with granular tissue. Primary healing is considered the least complex process to wound healing and leaves the least amount of scarring.[3]

■ In secondary wound healing, the wound bed must fill in with granular tissue because there is too much tissue damage and tissue loss to close and heal via primary intention. Secondary wound healing takes longer to heal, increases the risk of wound infection, and requires a longer healing time compared to primary wound healing.[4] Secondary healing usually results in scarring because more granulation tissue is needed for wound healing.

■ Tertiary wound healing occurs when wound closure is intentionally delayed. There are times when a wound may need to be kept open for a prolonged period. This is typically used for wounds with infection, severe crush injuries, when the wound is still present for a long time after an initial injury/surgery, or when wound observation is needed, such as after a wound debridement.[3]

Stages of Wound Healing

Wound healing is the body's automatic response to tissue injury. In surgical wounds, the injury is often purposeful and created with surgical instruments. Acute wounds typically go through four physiologic stages of healing within ~4–12 weeks.

■ First is the hemostasis phase, occurring immediately after injury. In the hemostasis phase, the body works to stop bleeding by vasoconstricting the area of injury, while platelets, collagen, and other factors begin clotting the area to stop the bleeding. Vasoconstriction is quickly followed by vasodilation, allowing critical cells, such as white blood cells, to travel to the site of injury.[5] This cascade of cells begins the second phase of wound healing, the inflammatory phase.

- In the inflammatory phase, the body's focus is to prevent further tissue damage, clean up any debris, and prepare the wound bed for regeneration and healing. White blood cells, such as neutrophils and macrophages, travel to the site of injury to remove debris and destroy harmful microorganisms. Other immune response mediators, such as serotonin and histamine, increase cellular permeability. Fibroblasts synthesize collagen and promote angiogenesis, the formation of new blood vessels.[6]
  - The inflammatory phase is associated with erythema and edema to the site and pain and warmth to touch. It is important to note that these signs can sometimes be mistaken for signs of wound infection.
- The third phase of wound healing is the proliferative phase. In this stage new blood vessels form, enabling oxygenation and healthy granulation tissue formation, and reepithelialization begins.[6]
- The fourth phase of wound healing is the remodeling (maturation) phase. During this phase new epithelium begins to increase in tensile strength. This phase can last weeks to years.
  - The tensile strength of new epithelium will never be as strong as the original preinjury tissue. It can be up to 80% of its original strength. Because of this, areas of new epithelium, even at its most mature, will still be vulnerable to reinjury.[6]

Surgical Site Complications

SURGICAL SITE INFECTIONS

SSIs are common surgical wound complications worldwide. The Centers for Disease Control and Prevention defines an SSI as an infection occurring within 30 days of surgery without an implant or within 90 days with implant involvement. In the United States, SSIs occur in ~2–5% of all surgical procedures and are the leading cause of readmission to the hospital after surgery.[7] Approximately 3% of patients with SSIs will die.[8] SSIs also have significant fiscal implications. Treating patients with SSIs costs billions of dollars annually, while readmissions and extended hospital stays create a financial burden.[9] Although certain factors can increase the risk of SSI, it is generally considered a preventable complication in most cases. Patient risk factors for developing SSI include tobacco use, malnutrition, existing medical comorbidities, and older age. Emergent surgical procedures may also increase the risk of SSI.[8]

Nurses play a critical role in the prevention, identification, and management of surgical site infections. In the preoperative setting, nurses can educate patients on preoperative SSI prevention interventions, such as chlorhexidine gluconate bathing preoperatively and avoiding the use of razors to remove hair at the surgical site.[10] Nurses should also assist with the administration of any prophylactic antibiotic before surgery. Accurate application of antiseptic products, the use of adhesive drapes to create a physical barrier to isolate the surgical site, and the use of topical dressings can all help to prevent SSIs.[9]

Early diagnosis of an SSI is often key in reducing the severity and negative outcomes. Because nurses provide 24-hour care to patients in the hospital setting, any change in a patient's baseline wound is often first identified by nursing. Clinical assessment is more reliable than laboratory tests in determining the presence of SSIs, as laboratory tests, such as a wound culture, only test for superficial microorganisms on the wound surface.[2] Nurses need to know the clinical signs and symptoms of wound infection and educate their patients on what to look for upon discharge to indicate impending infection. Common signs and symptoms of wound infection include swelling, redness, and increase in pain at the wound site. Other signs of infection include the presence of increased purulent and/or malodorous drainage.

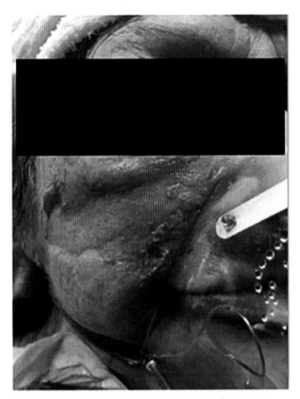

Fig. 28.1 Epidermal stripping from medical adhesive–related skin injury caused by improper endotracheal tube attachment adhesive removal. (Courtesy Jinah Yoo.)

WOUND DEHISCENCE

Surgical wound dehiscence occurs when a closed surgical incision reopens partially or completely. Causes of wound dehiscence include infection, increased wound pressure and excess tension, poor perfusion to the wound site, prior radiation to the site, malnutrition, smoking, steroid use, and obesity.[11] Preceding surgery, patients may benefit from addressing nutritional needs and smoking cessation to help decrease the risk of postoperative wound dehiscence.

MEDICAL ADHESIVE–RELATED SKIN INJURY

Medical adhesive is used to approximate wound edges or to affix an external device (e.g., tape, dressing, catheter, electrode, pouch, patch) to the skin. Although medical adhesives are used frequently in health care settings, adhesive-related skin injury is poorly reported among health care professionals.[12] A medical adhesive–related skin injury (MARSI) occurs when erythema and/or other manifestation of cutaneous abnormalities, such as a vesicle, bulla, erosion, or tear, persists for ≥30 minutes after adhesive removal (Fig. 28.1).[13]

MARSI occurs when the attachment to the adhesive is stronger than the skin's structural integrity, causing a separation between the epidermal layers or the dermal layer of skin. Skin damage can appear as partial or full thickness tissue loss and may result in scarring. MARSI may increase pain, risk of infection, and length of stay. MARSI can also occur to the periwound with frequent dressing changes and improper removal of adhesives. MARSI may present as a mechanical injury, such as a skin tear, dermatitis, or other forms of irritation/injury (e.g., folliculitis, macerated skin).[12]

Commonly used devices causing MARSI in the surgical setting include medical adhesive tapes (often used to close the eyes or affix endotracheal tubes in place during surgery) and wound dressings with an adhesive border. The effectiveness of adhesive tapes containing acrylate increases the longer it is applied to the skin. Therefore the risk of MARSI increases as the duration of surgery increases.[12]

Intrinsic risk factors for MARSI include dehydration, malnutrition, certain medical conditions (e.g., diabetes), immunosuppression, and edema. MARSI also occurs more commonly in the very young (neonate) or the elderly. Extrinsic risk factors include dry skin, radiated skin, skin with prolonged exposure to moisture, and certain medications, such as chemotherapeutic drugs, anticoagulants, and the long-term use of corticosteroids.[12]

Education of health care professionals on the prevention of MARSI is crucial. The use of skin barrier products, use of adhesive removers, proper prepping of skin, and proper removal of adhesives can help prevent these injuries. Patient education includes encouraging the use of moisturizer if the skin is dry before surgery, teaching the patient how to improve nutrition preoperatively, and emphasizing the importance of hydration.[12] A preoperative skin assessment should be performed immediately prior to surgery to set a baseline and help differentiate any new skin changes after surgery. Postoperatively, a daily head-to-toe skin assessment should be performed, with close attention paid to areas where adhesives were placed during surgery. Any areas of new erythema, blistering, skin color changes, or skin tears should be noted.[14]

Topical Wound Management

In their qualitative study on nurses' and surgeons' experiences with open surgical wounds, McCaughan et al. found that nurses were often tasked with making decisions regarding topical management in the postoperative setting and that physicians often rely on nursing insight.[15] Their study shed light on the importance for nurses having a basic understanding of the topical products commonly used for wound management. Factors to consider when choosing a topical wound dressing include the level of tissue injury, wound depth, amount of exudate, presence of necrotic or nonviable tissue, presence of tunneling or undermining, and how often a dressing can be changed. Decisions in topical management may change depending on the progression of the wound.

COMMON TYPES OF WOUND DRESSINGS

- Contact layers: Often impregnated with petrolatum or made entirely of silicone, contact layer dressings are typically nonadherent and placed directly onto the wound bed to protect the wound and/or maintain a moist wound environment. Because of their porous nature, wound exudate can pass through the contact layer, so a secondary dressing is needed to absorb exudate. This dressing is most appropriate for clean superficial wounds with minimal to moderate drainage.[5]
- Hydrogels: These contain hydrophilic polymers designed to add moisture to wounds and allow for the autolytic debridement of necrotic tissue. It is best to use hydrogels on wounds with a small amount of drainage or wound beds that need moisture. Hydrogels come in a variety of mediums, including gel, impregnated gauze, and sheets, and have the added benefit of conforming to any wound shape.[16]
- Hydrocolloid dressings: Hydrocolloids most often come in sheet form but also exist as powder and paste. Hydrocolloid dressings generally contain a matrix of gelatin, pectin, and sodium carboxymethylcellulose. They work to create a moist wound environment and an optimal temperature for wound healing because they absorb exudate, lower wound pH, and

decrease bacterial load.[5] This type of dressing is occlusive or semiocclusive, and the outer layer is impermeable to water.[16] Hydrocolloids should not be used for moderate to heavily exudating wounds because they cannot absorb a large amount of exudate.[5]

- Alginates: Alginate dressings are used primarily for highly exudative wounds and to fill in dead space. They are made of extracts of algae, which contain ingredients that provide an absorptive ability and tensile strength. Alginates create a moist wound environment by absorbing exudate and turning it into a gel-like consistency. This prevents wounds from becoming too dry. Alginate dressings can absorb ~20–30 times their weight in exudate. Depending on the amount of drainage, most alginates can be left in a wound for days. A secondary dressing is needed over the alginate.[5]

- Hydrofibers: Like alginates, hydrofibers are highly absorptive. The main ingredient is sodium carboxymethylcellulose, which forms a gel as it absorbs exudate. A secondary dressing is required. Hydrofibers often come in sheet or ribbon/rope form for packing tunnels and undermining.[5]
  - Both alginates and hydrofiber dressings are good products to use for packing a wound because the gel will not cause tissue trauma upon removal.

- Foams: Foam dressings come in a variety of sizes, shapes, and layers. Foam dressings are primarily made of polyurethane and can absorb a small to moderate amount of exudate. In recent years, foam dressings have been used as a method to prevent pressure injuries by padding bony prominences during long surgical procedures.[5]

- Silver-impregnated dressings: All the topical dressings mentioned also come in a silver-impregnated form. Silver is an antimicrobial used on locally infected wounds to prevent systemic spread. Silver is bactericidal and effective against both gram-negative and -positive bacteria, especially common nosocomial pathogens, such as *Pseudomonas aeruginosa*, methicillin-resistant *Staphylococcus aureus*, and vancomycin-resistant enterococci. The silver is released slowly over time, enough to be an effective antimicrobial while preventing healthy tissue damage. However, silver must be used cautiously in the pediatric population, in which the systemic absorption of topical products is greater.[5]

- Collagenase: Collagenase is an enzymatic debriding agent derived from clostridium bacteria. It is the only enzymatic debriding agent available currently in the United States. Collagenase is a good choice for wounds with necrotic tissue because the enzyme breaks down and digests it. It is not compatible with iodine products and with some silver products, depending on the amount of silver. It is important to apply collagenase to the entire surface of the wound, even if there is clean tissue, as it will not harm healthy tissue and may even help keep clean tissue clean. Collagenase is by prescription only in the United States.[16]

- Medical grade honey: Honey has antimicrobial properties due to its very high sugar content and low amount of water. It also has an acidic pH, which inhibits bacterial growth and contributes to angiogenesis, the formation of new blood vessels. The high sugar content also creates an osmotic effect, pulling fluid from the wound. This creates a moist wound environment, while promoting autolytic debridement, and helps reduce pain during dressing changes because there is less adherence to the wound surface. Medical grade honey comes in paste, gel, alginate-impregnated sheet, and hydrocolloid sheet formulations and should not be used on any patient with a honey allergy.[17]

- Negative pressure wound therapy (NPWT): This type of therapy promotes wound healing by facilitating granulation tissue formation, increasing blood flow to the site of injury, managing exudate and inflammation, and is good for infection prevention.[5] The NPWT system involves placing an open-foam reticulated sponge directly on the wound bed, covered with a semiocclusive transparent dressing to get a vacuum seal, followed by the application of continuous or intermittent negative pressure directly to the wound bed.[18] Indications for traditional NPWT include acute and chronic wounds, dehisced surgical wounds, and split thickness skin graft recipient sites. NPWT is particularly useful in wounds with significant depth because it aids in granulation tissue formation. Contraindications for NPWT include wounds with necrotic tissue, underlying malignancy, untreated osteomyelitis, and uncontrolled bleeding.[18] Although not an absolute contraindication, particular attention must be paid if a wound has exposed structures, such as fascia, blood vessels, tendons, or organs.[18] It is within the scope of nursing practice to apply NPWT dressings; however, specific training and education on correct application techniques are critical because improper use and application may lead to complications.

- Traditional NPWT has also been adapted to include fluid instillation. A solution such as saline or antimicrobial solution is directly instilled into the wound bed in conjunction with negative pressure. NPWT with fluid instillation facilitates wound irrigation and removal of infectious and nonviable material, such as slough. NPWT with instillation may be a good option for patients who ideally need surgical wound debridement but are not candidates for surgery.[19]

- In recent years NPWT has been utilized on closed surgical incisions to reduce edema, promote perfusion, and prevent surgical site infections and dehiscence in high-risk patients.[18] High-risk patients include those with diabetes, obesity (body mass index [BMI] >30 kg/m^2), hypoalbuminemia (serum albumin level <3 g/dL), chronic renal insufficiency, chronic obstructive pulmonary disease, current tobacco use, corticosteroid use, and recent or current chemotherapy.[20] In these cases NPWT is often applied to high tension incisions, areas of repeated incisions, edema, incision to presurgical radiation areas, or area of poor perfusion.[20]

- Wet-to-dry gauze/packing: Historically considered a mechanical means of debridement, saline-moistened gauze is now considered a suboptimal means of debridement because studies have shown it to be painful and to damage healthy tissue in the process. The idea that a moistened gauze dressing helps to keep a wound moist and promote autolytic debridement is also not based on current evidence. Furthermore, some studies have shown that this type of dressing increases the risk of infection.[21]

Pressure Injury

DEFINITION

The National Pressure Injury Advisory Panel defines a pressure injury as damage to the skin or soft tissue either over a bony prominence or related to a device.[22] Prolonged pressure results in poor vascular and lymphatic perfusion, causing tissue ischemia and eventual tissue death. Therefore pressure injuries are considered ischemic in etiology. They develop from the bottom up, with deeper structures, such as muscle, being more vulnerable to ischemia rather than superficial layers, such as the epidermis and dermis. Other factors affecting the development of pressure injuries include nutrition status, the presence of comorbidities, and the general condition of the skin and soft tissue.[23] Patient-specific risk factors include poor nutrition ahead of surgery, age >60 years, increased BMI, active smoking, and comorbidities such as hypertension and diabetes. Patients who are critically ill have added risk factors, such as the need for ventilator support, vasopressors, and general poor perfusion.[24]

CLASSIFICATION OF PRESSURE INJURIES

Pressure injuries are categorized based on the amount of tissue damage involved.[22]

- Stage 1: intact skin with nonblanchable erythema. It is important to note that erythema may appear differently in darkly pigmented skin. There may also be changes to the skin's temperature and sensation. The skin may also feel firmer or softer than adjacent skin (Fig. 28.2).

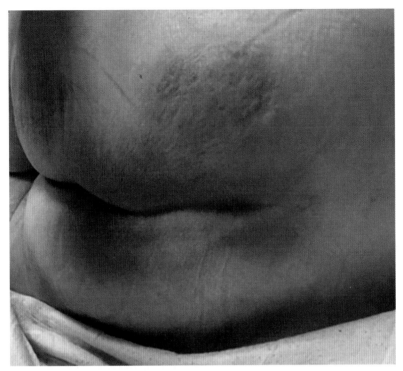

Fig. 28.2   Stage 1 pressure injury: intact skin with nonblanchable erythema. (Courtesy Jinah Yoo.)

- Stage 2: partial-thickness tissue loss involving the dermis. It may present as a superficial open wound with a pink nongranular wound bed. A stage 2 pressure injury can also present as an intact or open serum-filled blister (Fig. 28.3). Because they are caused by pressure, these wounds should not be documented as superficial cutaneous injuries, such as skin tears, abrasions, or moisture-associated skin damage. Stage 2 pressure injuries generally do not have depth because the tissue damage does not go past the dermal layer.
- Stage 3: full-thickness tissue loss, with the presence of granular tissue or adipose tissue. There may be some nonviable tissue present such as slough and/or eschar; however, the nonviable tissue does not cover the wound bed (Fig. 28.4). There may also be undermining and/or tunneling present. The depth of the wound depends on the anatomic location.
- Stage 4: full-thickness tissue loss with exposed structures, such as fascia, muscle, tendon, or bone. There may be nonviable tissue and undermining/tunneling present. The depth of the wound depends on the anatomic location (Fig. 28.5).
- Unstageable: full-thickness tissue loss with the extent of tissue loss undetermined, as the wound bed is covered by eschar or slough (Fig. 28.6). Unstageable pressure injuries may also appear as dry stable eschar. When the nonviable tissue is removed and the tissue underneath is exposed, the wound can be staged.
- Deep tissue: an area of nonblanchable maroon or purple discoloration. It can also present as a blood-filled blister. These wounds indicate there is extensive tissue injury below the epidermal layer that is not yet visible. The wound may improve without the skin opening to a full-thickness wound, or the injury may worsen and evolve into a full-thickness pressure injury.

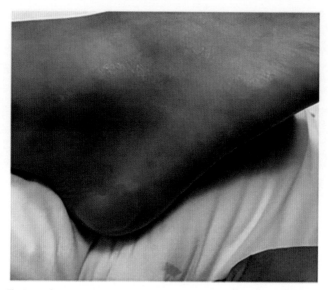

Fig. 28.3   Stage 2 pressure injury: serum-filled blister. (Courtesy Jinah Yoo.)

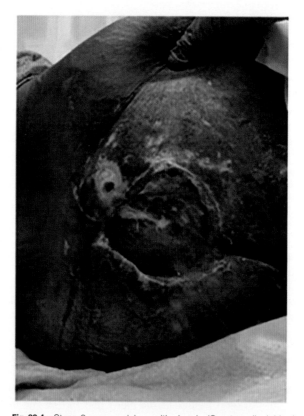

Fig. 28.4   Stage 3 pressure injury, with slough. (Courtesy Jinah Yoo.)

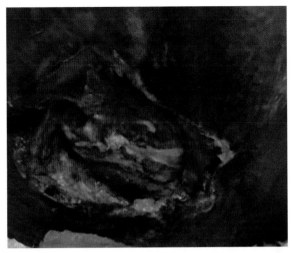

Fig. 28.5   Stage 4 pressure injury, bone exposed. (Courtesy Jinah Yoo.)

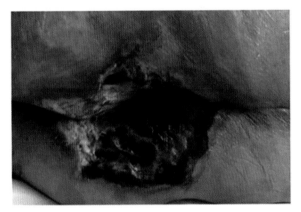

Fig. 28.6   Unstageable pressure injury. (Courtesy Jinah Yoo.)

- Mucosal membrane: injury to mucous membranes due to pressure. Examples of mucous membranes include lips, inside of the mouth, inside the nostrils, the vaginal canal, the urethra, and the gastrointestinal mucosa. Mucosal membrane pressure injuries are often caused by medical devices, although medical device–related pressure injuries can occur anywhere. Mucosal membrane pressure injuries are not staged because mucosal tissue is different from other areas of the body.
- Medical device related: Although this is not a classification of pressure injury, it is important to note whether the pressure injury was caused by a medical device (Fig. 28.7).

Pressure Injuries in the Perioperative Setting

A perioperative pressure injury occurs during a surgical procedure and is detected within 72 hours of the procedure.[25] However, some studies have shown the injury may not be visible until ≥5 days after a procedure.[25] Perioperative pressure injuries can result in significant repercussions to the patient and hospitals. The incidence of perioperative pressure injuries ranges from 3.5–45% of

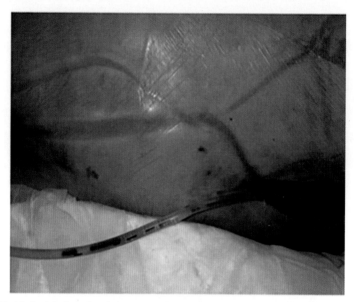

Fig. 28.7 Medical device–related stage 1 pressure injury from device tubing. (Courtesy Jinah Yoo.)

patients. Additionally, perioperative pressure injuries increase the cost of hospitalization by an estimated 44%, adding $1.3 billion in health care costs annually in the United States.[25]

Due to the nature of immobility during a surgical procedure, all perioperative patients should be considered at risk for developing a pressure injury especially with longer procedures.[25] Risk increases in the operating room, with procedures >4 hours, general anesthesia, surgical blood loss, patient position during the procedure, and moisture. Prevention of perioperative pressure injuries should include a risk assessment and thorough skin assessment prior to surgery, protection of bony prominences and at-risk areas of the skin during the surgery, and assessment and communication postoperatively. A root cause analysis program should also be established so potential issues and areas that need improvement can be discussed and institutional changes to policy and procedure can be made.

NURSING INTERVENTIONS DURING THE PREOPERATIVE/ INTRAOPERATIVE PERIOD[25]

- Before the surgery date, discuss with the patient the importance of optimizing nutrition, smoking cessation (if applicable), adequate hydration, and management of chronic conditions such as diabetes and hypertension (if applicable).
- Perform a head-to-toe skin assessment, noting areas of existing skin injury or areas that may be prone to pressure during the surgery.
- Discuss with the surgical team the expected positioning and relay this to the patient.
- If applicable, apply padding to bony prominences to minimize pressure and shearing, such as a five-layer silicone foam dressing. If possible, offload any potential areas of pressure such as heels.
- Communicate any at-risk findings with the team.

NURSING INTERVENTIONS DURING THE POSTOPERATIVE PERIOD[24]

- Perform a head-to-toe skin assessment, paying particular attention to areas that sustained prolonged pressure during surgery.

- Offload areas of prolonged pressure during surgery as well as bony prominences.
- Communicate and document any areas of injury or potential injury.
- Initiate pressure injury prevention interventions.
  - Does the patient need a pressure redistributive support surface for a bed and/or a chair?
  - Are nutrition/hydration needs addressed?
  - Is physical therapy needed for mobility issues?
  - What support or durable medical equipment does the patient need upon discharge from the hospital to support wound healing?
- Educate patients and caregivers on pressure injury prevention interventions.

Conclusion

Wound management and prevention of complications in the surgical setting encompasses many intrinsic and extrinsic factors and involves interdisciplinary collaboration and communication among health care staff. Raising awareness of wound care is of vital importance because surgical patients with wound complications are at risk of prolonged hospitalizations and further complications, putting a burden on both patients and health care facilities. Nurses have a unique opportunity to provide interventions in wound care, and providers often rely on their clinical judgment to know what to order for patients. Nurses also are in an ideal position to aid with the prevention and management of complications because they spend the most clinical time with patients in the acute care setting.

References

1. Gillespie BM, Walker RM, McInnes E, et al. Preoperative and postoperative recommendations to surgical wound care interventions: a systematic meta-review of Cochrane reviews. *Int J Nurs Stud.* 2020;102:103486. doi:10.1016/j.ijnurstu.2019.103486.
2. Copanitsanou P, Santy-Tomlinson J. The nurses' role in the diagnosis and surveillance of orthopaedic surgical site infections. *Int J Orthop Trauma Nurs.* 2021;41:100818. doi:10.1016/j.ijotn.2020.100818.
3. Salcido R. Healing by intention. *Adv Skin Wound Care.* 2017;30(6):246–247. doi:10.1097/01. ASW.0000516787.46060.b2.
4. Chhabra S, Chhabra N, Kaur A, et al. Wound healing concepts in clinical practice of OMFS. *J Maxillofac Oral Surg.* 2017;16(4):403–423. doi:10.1007/s12663-016-0880-z.
5. Rosenbaum AJ, Banerjee S, Rezak KM, et al. Advances in wound management. *J Am Acad Orthop Surg.* 2018;26(23):833–843. doi:10.5435/JAAOS-D-17-00024.
6. Wallace HA, Basehore BM, Zito PM. *Wound Healing Phases.* StatPearls Publishing; 2023.
7. Fencl J, Wood F, Gupta S, et al. Avoiding surgical site infections in neurosurgical procedures. *OR Nurse.* 2015;9(3):28–38.
8. Agency for Healthcare Research and Quality. Surgical site infections. The Patient Safety Network. September 7, 2019. https://psnet.ahrq.gov/primer/surgical-site-infections. Accessed September 30, 2022.
9. Goldberg B, Elazar A, Glatt A, et al. Perioperative interventions to reduce surgical site infections: a review. *AORN J.* 2021;114(6):587–596. doi:10.1002/aorn.13564.
10. Nasser R, Kosty JA, Shah S, et al. Risk factors and prevention of surgical site infections following spinal procedures. *Global Spine J.* 2018;8(4):S44–S48. doi:10.1002/aorn.12710.
11. Rosen RD, Manna B. *Wound Dehiscence.* StatPearls Publishing; 2022.
12. Fumarola S, Allaway R, Callaghan R, et al. Overlooked and underestimated: medical adhesive-related skin injuries. *J Wound Care.* 2020;29(3c):S1–S24. doi:10.12968/jowc.2020.29.Sup3c.S1.
13. Farris MK, Petty M, Hamilton J, et al. Medical adhesive-related skin injury prevalence among adult acute care patients: a single-center observational study. *J Wound Ostomy Continence Nurs.* 2015;42(6):589–598. doi:10.1097/WON.0000000000000179.
14. Cole M, Smith I, Vlad SC, et al. The effect of a skin barrier film on the incidence of dressing-related skin blisters after spine surgery. *AORN J.* 2020;112(1):39–48. doi:10.1002/aorn.13074.

15. McCaughan D, Sheard L, Cullum N, et al. Nurses' and surgeons' views and experiences of surgical wounds healing by secondary intention: a qualitative study. *J Clin Nurs.* 2020;29(13-14):2557–2571. doi:10.1111/jocn.15279.
16. Dhivya S, Padma VV, Santhini E. Wound dressings—a review. *Biomedicine (Taipei).* 2015;5(4):22. doi:10.7603/s40681-015-0022-9.
17. Oropeza K. What's the buzz about medical-grade honey? *Nursing.* 2014;44(7):59. doi:10.1097/01. NURSE.0000450793.03226.
18. Zaver V, Kankanalu Z. *Negative Pressure Wound Therapy.* StatPearls Publishing; 2022.
19. Faust E, Opoku-Agyeman JL, Behnam AB. Use of negative-pressure wound therapy with instillation and dwell time: an overview. *Plast Reconstr Surg.* 2021;147(1S-1):S16–S26. doi:10.1097/PRS.0000000000007607.
20. Silverman RP, Apostolides J, Chatterjee A, et al. The use of closed incision negative pressure therapy for incision and surrounding soft tissue management: expert panel consensus recommendations. *Int Wound J.* 2022;19(3):643–655. doi:10.1111/iwj.13662.
21. Wodash AJ. Wet-to-dry dressings do not provide moist wound healing. *J Am Coll Clin Wound Spec.* 2013;4(3):63–66. doi:10.1016/j.jccw.2013.08.001.
22. Edsberg LE, Black JM, Goldberg M, et al. Revised national pressure ulcer advisory panel pressure injury staging system: revised pressure injury staging system. *J Wound Ostomy Continence Nurs.* 2016;43(6):585–597. doi:10.1097/WON.0000000000000281.
23. Al Aboud A, Manna B. *Wound Pressure Injury Management.* StatPearls Publishing; 2022.
24. Alshahrani B, Sim J, Middleton R. Nursing interventions for pressure injury prevention among critically ill patients: a systematic review. *J Clin Nurs.* 2021;30(15-16):2151–2168. doi:10.1111/jocn.15709.
25. Kimsey DB. A change in focus: shifting from treatment to prevention of perioperative pressure injuries. *AORN J.* 2019;110(4):379–393. doi:10.1002/aorn.12806.

Questions

1. Susan, a 56-year-old female, is in the intensive care unit (ICU) after a craniotomy to remove a pituitary tumor. She is postop day 3. Her craniotomy incision is healing well. The wound edges are approximated, without drainage or erythema. Susan has been having significant pain at the operative site and reports lying on her back is the only position that provides any relief. Susan also reports having a poor appetite and eating ~25% of her meals. In addition, she has been refusing physical therapy. Per the patient's nurse, she has been refusing to reposition in bed and to sit in a chair. The only time she will leave her bed is to use the bedside commode, and she requires assistance from nursing staff to get to and from the commode. Currently what is your greatest concern with this patient?
    a. The patient's incision may not heal appropriately.
    b. The patient may become weaker since she is refusing physical therapy.
    c. The patient is at very high risk for developing a pressure injury.
    d. Discharge and placement will be a concern because the physical therapist cannot evaluate the patient.

2. Jill, a 28-year-old female, undergoes an anterior lumbar spine surgical approach. Upon inspection of the surgical incision site you find that the wound has dehisced. The wound is a full-thickness open wound, with healthy granular tissue and ~2 cm deep. There is a large amount of serosanguinous drainage, no odor, and no erythema to periwound. The patient reports she is eating well and denies having pain. What topical dressing will you recommend for this patient's dehisced surgical wound?
    a. Leave the wound open, without a dressing, because letting some air hit the wound will help it heal.
    b. Pack with a hydrofiber or calcium alginate dressing.
    c. Use a hydrocolloid dressing.
    d. Pack with a wet-to-dry gauze dressing.

3. Lyla, a 50-year-old female, is preparing to undergo posterior spine surgery for tumor debulking. Her past medical history includes breast cancer, treated with chemotherapy, radiation, and a right mastectomy. She regularly drinks alcohol, smokes a pack of cigarettes daily, and utilizes medical marijuana for pain relief. What is *not* a suggestion you should you make to Lyla to reduce the chances of her developing a surgical wound infection?
   a. Use a razor daily to ensure the area remains hair-free for surgery.
   b. Increase your intake of protein and water.
   c. Stop smoking.
   d. Apply a moisturizer regularly to the area if the skin appears dry or cracked.

4. Henry is precepting Jackson, a new nurse on the neurosurgical ICU. Jackson learns that most of the patients on the unit have decreased mobility from devastating brain and spinal cord injuries. What should Henry teach Jackson to do to help prevent the formation of pressure injuries in these patients?
   a. Inspect wounds and vulnerable skin areas regularly and recommend topical dressings to the provider to order.
   b. Keep bony prominences padded using foam dressing and check the skin underneath regularly.
   c. Advocate for high-protein oral or tube feeding nutrition, and blood glucose control using Accu-Checks or insulin drip.
   d. All the above

5. Cleo, a 34-year-old female, was recently hospitalized after a motor vehicle accident. She suffered a cervical spine injury and is now quadriplegic, ventilator dependent, and requires tube feed nutrition. During the initial stages of her hospitalization, she was depressed and refused turns, mobilization out of bed, and switching to a low air loss mattress. Once she became compliant with care, the nurses discovered an unstageable sacral pressure injury. The wound was initially covered by a dark area of eschar, and she underwent a bedside debridement. The wound care nurse now describes her sacrum as full-thickness tissue loss and notes undermining and tunneling. What stage is the wound?
   a. Remains classified as unstageable despite debridement
   b. Stage 1
   c. Stage 2
   d. Stage 3

Answers

1. c

2. b

3. a

4. d

5. d

CHAPTER 29

Nursing Management of Postoperative Fever

Shelly Gupta, MD

Introduction

Postoperative fever is defined as a temperature of >100.4°F on two consecutive postoperative days (POD) or >102°F on any single POD.[1] The timing of fever, along with the patient's underlying medical conditions, can help determine the most likely etiology of the fever and differentiate an infectious from noninfectious source. However, there may be more than one cause of fever, and an infectious and noninfectious source can exist simultaneously.[1] A physiologic fever may occur in the early postoperative period—up to 3 days postoperatively—and can be attributed to an inflammatory response triggered by tissue damage and exposure to foreign materials during surgery.[2,3] As the patient approaches POD 4, infectious causes for fever are more likely than noninfectious causes. Possible causes at this time can range from a urinary tract infection (UTI), pneumonia, or surgical site infection (SSI) to noninfectious causes that include drug fever, inflammatory reactions, and deep vein thrombosis (DVT). The patient's history, details regarding the development of fever and any associated symptoms, and a thorough physical examination are vital to correctly ascertaining the etiology of a postoperative fever. Identifying the causes for fever and implementing appropriate treatment in a timely manner can decrease morbidity and mortality.

Basics

Evaluation of postoperative fever starts with understanding the systemic inflammatory response syndrome (SIRS) criteria. The criteria establish a framework to remind clinicians when to be wary of infections and possible sepsis during but not limited to the postoperative period. Nevertheless, it is important to distinguish between SIRS (an exaggerated inflammatory defense response) and sepsis (the body's inflammatory response to infection requiring urgent treatment and antibiotics) when evaluating patients, as the two are not synonymous. The SIRS criteria consist of vital sign measurements and basic laboratory testing.

SIRS Criteria Parameters

- Temperature >100.4°F or <96.8°F
- Heart rate >90 beats per minute
- Respiratory rate >20 breaths per minute; or an arterial pCO2 <32 mmHg
- White blood cell counts <4 × 10/L or >12 × 10/L; or the presence of >10% bands
  - To meet SIRS criteria, two of the four parameters above must be present, which may be common postoperatively but does not always indicate that there is an infection.
  - To diagnose sepsis, two of the SIRS criteria need to be present in addition to a suspected source of infection.
  - To diagnose severe sepsis, there must be two of the SIRS criteria and a source of infection, PLUS evidence of organ dysfunction.

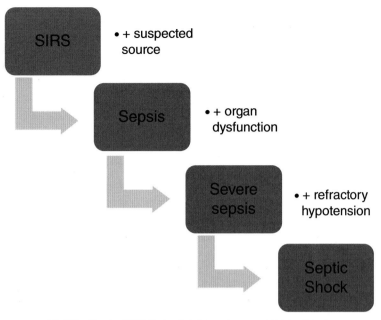

Fig. 29.1   Sepsis. *SIRS*, Systemic inflammatory response syndrome.

- To diagnose septic shock, a patient must meet SIRS criteria, have a source of infection and organ dysfunction, AND have hypotension refractory to fluid resuscitation (Fig. 29.1).

Signs of Organ Dysfunction
- Systolic blood pressure (BP) <90 mmHg or mean arterial pressure <65 mmHg
- Drop in BP >40 mmHg (especially important in patients with baseline hypertension)
- Lactate >2 mmol/L
- Urine output <0.5 mg/kg/hour for 2 consecutive hours
- Drop in Glasgow Coma Scale or abbreviated mental test score

TIMING

The timing of postoperative fever is an important factor in diagnosing its etiology. Fever after surgery is differentiated by the duration of time that has elapsed since the day of surgery (Fig. 29.2).

Subclassification of Fever by the Timing of Onset
- Immediate: usually occurring immediately after surgery, within the first few hours to POD 1
- Acute: occurring within the first week postop
- Subacute: onset between week 1 and 4 postop
- Delayed: >4 weeks postop

Immediate Postoperative Fever

Immediate fever can happen in the operating room or hours after surgery, up to 24 hours postoperatively. These fevers are usually from noninfectious causes and are mostly inflammatory and self-limited. Potential causes of immediate postoperative fever include surgically induced inflammation, immune-mediated reactions, malignant hyperthermia, preexisting infection, or fulminant SSI.

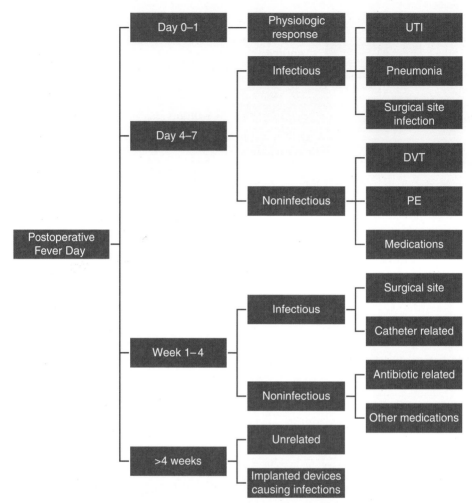

Fig. 29.2 Timing of postoperative fever. *DVT,* Deep vein thrombosis; *PE,* pulmonary embolism; *UTI,* urinary tract infection.

Inflammation can develop postoperatively as a consequence of surgical stress, which triggers the production of inflammatory markers and a febrile response.[4] Patients can also have a reaction to medications or blood products administered during or after surgery. These immune reactions may be accompanied by hypotension and a rash; when the offending agent is stopped, the reaction usually resolves. Malignant hyperthermia can occur intraoperatively within 30 minutes of administering anesthesia and is the result of an inherited disorder affecting the metabolism of general anesthesia. It can also occur after the cessation of anesthesia.[4]

Sometimes surgery is needed for a preexisting infection (e.g., wound washout for an infected surgical wound); in these cases, the patient should continue treatment for the initial infection postoperatively. Fulminant SSI is rare, but the two common bacteria that can be culprits are *Clostridium perfringens* and *group A Streptococcus,* which can lead to erythema and wound drainage.[4]

Acute Postoperative Fever

Acute postoperative fever is defined as a fever that occurs within the first week after surgery. It can be further classified as early, which occurs in the first 3 days postop, and late, which occurs after POD 3. The causes of acute postoperative fever include infections such as UTI, pneumonia, upper respiratory infection, SSI, wound infections, and catheter-associated infections. Noninfectious causes include pulmonary embolism (PE), venous embolism, thrombophlebitis, acute gout, myocardial infarction, acute pancreatitis, thyroid storm, adrenal insufficiency, alcohol withdrawal, and others.

Subacute Postoperative Fever

Subacute postoperative fever is defined as a fever occurring 1–4 weeks postoperatively.[1,5] In this time frame the most common infectious cause of fever is a SSI.[6,7] The most common noninfectious cause is medication and could be due to antimicrobials.[5,8]

Delayed Postoperative Fever

Delayed fever is defined as a fever occurring >4 weeks after surgery. In most cases this fever is unrelated to the initial surgery.[5] There are some exceptions, such as implanted devices and orthopedic prostheses, which can harbor an infection associated with the original procedure.[5,8]

Clinical Evaluation

Evaluating the cause of a postoperative fever starts with taking a history and doing a physical exam. This can help narrow the differential diagnosis and guide the diagnostic workup. Important questions to consider are the timing of the fever postprocedurally, and whether there was also fever present before the procedure. The clinician must take into consideration any medications given during the procedure or in the postoperative period that could also contribute to fever.

- Clinicians should inquire about pain, sputum production, vomiting or diarrhea, urinary symptoms, drainage from surgical site, catheters, and any new rashes.
- Nurses should complete a thorough physical examination, closely monitor the surgical site, and report any clinical changes to the provider.

Once the potential causes of fever have been identified, clinicians should proceed with a diagnostic workup that is appropriately customized to the patient's presentation, thereby minimizing waste of resources and maximizing the probability of correctly diagnosing the source.

- In a fever that occurs after POD 3, laboratory testing may include a basic metabolic panel, complete blood count (to check for an increase in the white blood cell count), urinalysis and urine culture, sputum cultures, and blood cultures (two sets from separate sites).
- Diagnostic imaging might include a chest radiograph, lower extremity duplex ultrasound, computed tomographic (CT) scan, or ultrasound/CT scan of the surgical area.

Treatment

The treatment of postoperative fever is dictated by its cause. If the diagnostic workup reveals an infection, then antibiotic therapy targeted to the culprit organism should be utilized. It is imperative for nurses to obtain cultures first, before starting antibiotics, and to use clean techniques when obtaining samples to minimize risk of bacterial contaminants.

If infection is strongly suspected, then clinicians may order broad-spectrum antibiotics even while cultures are pending and the workup remains in process, thereafter narrowing the antibiotic regimen once the organism and sensitivities are determined.[6] Timely administration of broad-spectrum antibiotics can help prevent further clinical deterioration of the patient. It is important to determine if the source of fever is an abscess, necrotizing infection, or an indwelling catheter. In

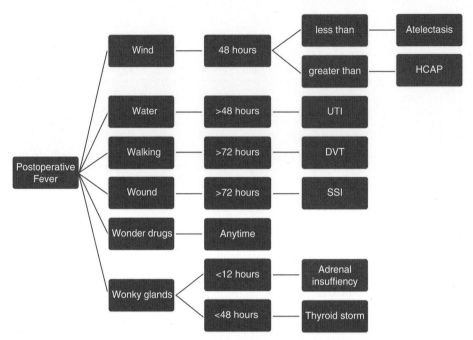

Fig. 29.3   Rule of W. *DVT*, deep vein thrombosis; *HCAP*, healthcare-associated pneumonia; *SSI*, surgical site infection; *UTI*, urinary tract infection.

these instances, source control must be achieved by surgically draining the abscess, removing the necrotizing tissue, or removing the catheter.[6]

Rule of W

The rule of W is a mnemonic that outlines the most common causes of postoperative fever in the order in which they occur[7]:

- Wind (atelectasis or pneumonia)
- Water (UTI)
- Wound (wound infection)
- Walking (venous thromboembolism)
- Wonder drug (drug fever)

This mnemonic has existed since the 1980s, and since then it has undergone numerous adaptations, including the addition of *waves* for myocardial infarction, *withdrawal* for alcohol or drug withdrawal, and *what did we do* for treatments given intraoperatively (e.g., medications, blood product transfusions, catheters placed). Endocrine disorders, such as adrenal insufficiency and thyroid storm, have also been proposed to be added as *wonky glands*[8] (Fig. 29.3).

WIND

Atelectasis is commonly seen postoperatively due to patients spending most of their time sitting or lying in bed, which leads to incomplete expansion of the lungs.[9] Sedation and pain can cause poor inspiratory effort, which contributes to decreased clearance of pulmonary secretions.[9] Atelectasis can also cause an inflammatory response.[9] In older studies, atelectasis was considered to be the leading cause of postoperative fever, but newer studies show no association between postoperative fever and the degree of atelectasis.[10] The incidence of atelectasis peaks during the first 48 hours after surgery, and after the first 48 hours rates of healthcare-associated pneumonia start to rise.[8,9]

Signs and symptoms of atelectasis include decreased breath sounds, crackles, tachypnea, dyspnea, cough, hypoxemia, and infiltrates seen on chest radiography.[9] Treatment for atelectasis includes incentive spirometry, early mobilization, chest physiotherapy, and bronchodilators.[9] Nurses are often in the best position to initiate these preventative measures, and these modalities can often prevent healthcare-associated pneumonia.[8]

A diagnosis of healthcare-associated pneumonia is considered when symptoms first appear after 48 hours in the hospital. Signs and symptoms of pneumonia can include fever, increased white blood cell count, purulence in sputum, and increase in oxygenation requirement.[11] Commonly ordered diagnostic tests include chest radiography, sputum cultures, blood cultures, and assays that specifically detect organisms such as *Legionella, Mycoplasma,* or *Chlamydophillia pneumoniae.*[11]

WATER

UTIs are the most common infections seen in the hospital.[11] Surgical patients have a higher rate of UTIs because of urinary catheter placement that typically occurs during surgery.[8] The signs and symptoms of a UTI include fever, suprapubic or flank pain, costovertebral tenderness, burning with urination (dysuria), increased urinary frequency, and urinary urgency.[8] UTIs are more common in females, older patients, diabetic patients, and patients with a history of previous UTIs.[12] The most significant risk factor for developing a catheter-associated UTI is prolonged use of the urinary catheter. Nurses should advocate for removal of urinary catheters as early as possible and provide proper catheter care to minimize the risk of infection.[13]

If a UTI is suspected, providers will order a urinalysis and culture to determine the organism and treat accordingly. The most common organisms that cause catheter-related UTIs are *Escherichia coli, Enterococcus* spp., *Candida* spp., *Pseudomonas aeruginosa,* and *Klebsiella* spp.[13] If the urinalysis is positive or the patient is symptomatic, empiric antibiotics may be started to treat a UTI while awaiting the culture results and the organism's antibiotic sensitivity profile. Once sensitivity results are finalized, antibiotics can be changed to treat the offending organism accordingly.

WOUND

SSI is an infection involving the skin and subcutaneous tissue at or near the surgical site. SSIs generally occur within 30 days of surgery or within 90 days if prosthetic materials are present.[14] Signs and symptoms of SSIs include erythema, warmth, tenderness, and purulent drainage from the incision site, which can start as early as 5–10 days after surgery.[15] Nurses should assess wounds frequently and monitor for such changes. Risk factors for SSI include a history of diabetes, older age, malnutrition, immunosuppression, smoking, obesity, and previous history of infections.[16]

Nurses can collect cultures of purulent drainage to help determine the organism and guide treatment, making certain to avoid culturing the skin itself, which is naturally colonized with bacterial flora.[8] If the patient has hemodynamic instability, high fevers, or leukocytosis, then further imaging (e.g., CT scan or magnetic resonance imaging [MRI]) may need to be obtained to look for a deeper soft tissue infection.[8] The most common pathogens that cause SSIs are *Streptococcus, Staphylococcus,* and *Enterococcus.*[17] Patients with SSIs may require surgery or interventional drainage to treat the infection and to obtain deep sterile cultures to ensure proper treatment. Empiric treatment can be started after cultures are obtained and should be narrowed once the organism and its antibiotic sensitivities are identified.

WALKING

Patients are often sedentary postoperatively, whether due to pain, deconditioning, or mobility impairment from surgery itself.[8] Postoperative immobility increases the probability of developing a

DVT; in fact, ~20% of all DVTs happen in the postoperative period.[18] Most patients with a DVT are asymptomatic, but some may have swelling in the affected extremity, accompanied by erythema, warmth to touch, and tenderness.[19] Inflammation of the deep vein system can cause fever.[20] DVTs can be diagnosed by ultrasound, and treatment includes anticoagulation when clinically safe from a surgical perspective. Patients undergoing surgeries for trauma, lower extremity orthopedic surgery, spinal surgery, and abdominal-pelvic surgery are at a higher risk of developing DVT.[21] Other risk factors for DVTs include cancer, previous DVT or PE, and clotting disorders. DVTs are more commonly seen during POD 3–5, but in high-risk patients they may be seen even sooner after surgery.[8] Nurses should educate patients on the importance of pharmacologic and mechanical DVT prophylaxis, encourage early postoperative ambulation, and report any concerns to the interprofessional team.

The risk factors for developing a PE are the same as those for developing an acute DVT. Clinically, symptoms of PE include decreased blood oxygen saturation, increased respiratory rate, and tachycardia. A PE can cause sudden death in the postoperative patient, so it is important to identify and treat PEs as soon as possible.[8] PEs can be detected by either a CT pulmonary angiogram or ventilation-perfusion scan. The preferred treatment for DVT and PE is therapeutic anticoagulation when deemed to be safe from a surgical standpoint.

WONDER DRUGS

The most common cause of noninfectious postoperative fever is medication induced. This fever can happen any time during the postoperative period, including immediately after or days later, and sometimes occurs in conjunction with a rash.[8] Interestingly, antimicrobials and heparin are the most common medications known to cause postoperative fever.[22] Furthermore, certain medications can cause febrile reactions, such as serotonin syndrome, malignant hyperthermia, or neuroleptic malignant syndrome. Frequently implicated medications include selective serotonin reuptake inhibitors, anesthetics, and antiemetic medications such as metoclopramide and promethazine.[8] If a drug reaction is suspected, nurses should stop or hold the offending agent and notify providers for further guidance.

Conclusion

A postoperative fever can occur at different times and for different reasons. In the hospital, nurses play a key role in the early recognition and evaluation of fever. Furthermore, nurses play an important role in educating patients and their families on what to do to prevent infection and fever outside of the hospital and what concerning signs and symptoms to monitor for. Familiarizing oneself with the most common causes of postoperative fever (especially the rule of W), diagnostic tests, and typical treatments can help prevent complications from surgery and promote optimal healing both in and outside the hospital setting.

References

1. Abdelmaseeh TA, Azmat CE, Oliver TI. *Postoperative Fever*. StatPearls Publishing; 2022.
2. Ghosh S, Charity RM, Haidar SG, et al. Pyrexia following total knee replacement. *Knee*. 2006;13(4):324–327. doi:10.1016/j.knee.2006.05.001.
3. Kennedy JG, Rodgers WB, Zurakowski D, et al. Pyrexia after total knee replacement. a cause for concern? *Am J Orthop (Belle Mead NJ)*. 1997;26(8):549–552 554.
4. Fry D. Surgical infection. In: O'Leary J, ed. *The Physiologic Basis of Surgery*. 3rd ed. Lippincott Williams & Wilkins; 2002:218–257.
5. Weed H, Baddour LM, Ho VP. Postoperative fever. UpToDate. 2011/2022;19. https://www.uptodate.com/contents/fever-in-the-surgical-patient . Accessed June 7, 2023.

6. Narayan M, Medinilla SP. Fever in the postoperative patient. *Emerg Med Clin North Am.* 2013;31(4):1045–1058. doi:10.1016/j.emc.2013.07.011.

7. Hyder JA, Wakeam E, Arora V, et al. Investigating the "rule of W," a mnemonic for teaching on postoperative complications. *J Surg Educ.* 2015;72(3):430–437. doi:10.1016/j.jsurg.2014.11.004.

8. Maday KR, Hurt JB, Harrelson P, et al. Evaluating postoperative fever. *JAAPA.* 2016;29(10):23–28. doi:10.1097/01.JAA.0000496951.72463.de.

9. Brooks-Brunn JA. Postoperative atelectasis and pneumonia. *Heart Lung.* 1995;24(2):94–115.

10. Mavros MN, Velmahos GC, Falagas ME. Atelectasis as a cause of postoperative fever: where is the clinical evidence? *Chest.* 2011;140(2):418–424. doi:10.1378/chest.11-0127.

11. Calandra T, Cohen J. International Sepsis Forum Definition of Infection in the ICU Consensus Conference. The international sepsis forum consensus conference on definitions of infection in the intensive care unit. *Crit Care Med.* 2005;33(7):1538–1548. doi:10.1097/01.ccm.0000168253.91200.83.

12. Wald HL, Ma A, Bratzler DW, et al. Indwelling urinary catheter use in the postoperative period: analysis of the national surgical infection prevention project data. *Arch Surg.* 2008;143(6):551–557. doi:10.1001/archsurg.143.6.551.

13. Centers for Disease Control and Prevention. Healthcare-associated infections (HAIs). Catheter-associated urinary tract infections (CAUTI). October 16, 2015. www.cdc.gov/hai/ca_uti/uti.html. Accessed June 7, 2023.

14. Centers for Disease Control and Prevention. Surgical site infection (SSI) event. www.cdc.gov/nhsn/PDFs/pscManual/9pscSSIcurrent.pdf. Accessed July 15, 2016.

15. Barie PS. Surgical site infections: epidemiology and prevention. *Surg Infect (Larchmt).* 2002;3(1):S9–S21. doi:10.1089/sur.2002.3.s1-9.

16. Mangram AJ, Horan TC, Pearson ML, et al. Guideline for prevention of surgical site infection, 1999. Centers for Disease Control and Prevention (CDC) hospital infection control practices advisory committee. *Am J Infect Control.* 1999;27(2):97–132 quiz 133-4; discussion 96.

17. Hidron AI, Edwards JR, Patel J, et al. NHSN annual update: antimicrobial-resistant pathogens associated with healthcare-associated infections: annual summary of data reported to the national healthcare safety network at the Centers for Disease Control and Prevention, 2006-2007. *Infect Control Hosp Epidemiol.* 2008;29(11):996–1011. doi:10.1086/591861.

18. Anderson Jr FA, Zayaruzny M, Heit JA, et al. Estimated annual numbers of US acute-care hospital patients at risk for venous thromboembolism. *Am J Hematol.* 2007;82(9):777–782. doi:10.1002/ajh.20983.

19. Geerts WH, Pineo GF, Heit JA, et al. Prevention of venous thromboembolism: the seventh ACCP conference on antithrombotic and thrombolytic therapy. *Chest.* 2004;126(3):S338–S400. doi:10.1378/chest.126.3_suppl.338S.

20. Nucifora G, Badano L, Hysko F, et al. Pulmonary embolism and fever: when should right-sided infective endocarditis be considered? *Circulation.* 2007;115(6):e173–e176. doi:10.1161/CIRCULATIONAHA.106.674358.

21. Geerts WH, Bergqvist D, Pineo GF, et al. Prevention of venous thromboembolism: American College of Chest Physicians evidence-based clinical practice guidelines (8th edition). *Chest.* 2008;133(6):S381–S453. doi:10.1378/chest.08-0656.

22. Mackowiak PA. Drug fever: mechanisms, maxims and misconceptions. *Am J Med Sci.* 1987;294(4):275–286. doi:10.1097/00000441-198710000-00011.

Questions

1. A 65-year-old female is admitted to the hospital for fevers and dizziness. She complains of cough and sputum production. Vitals on admission are 103°F, heart rate 122 bpm, respiratory rate 28 breaths per minute, BP 78/46 mm Hg, and 90% oxygenation saturation on 2 L oxygen. Lab work reveals a leukocytosis of 25 and a lactate level >2 mmol/L. A chest radiograph reveals infiltrates in the left lobe of the lung concerning for multifocal pneumonia. Due to her low BP she is resuscitated with intravenous (IV) fluid boluses three times. Despite appropriate fluid resuscitation, her BP remains 82/50 mm Hg. In what stage of sepsis criteria is the patient?

   a. SIRS
   b. Sepsis
   c. Severe sepsis
   d. Septic shock

2. A 52-year-old male presents to the emergency room with worsening back pain and fevers at home. On further review, he had an elective lumbar surgery 3 weeks ago. His vitals on presentation are significant for a fever of 102°F, heart rate 110 bpm, respiratory rate 12 breaths per minute, 98% oxygen saturation on room air, and BP 95/60 mm Hg. On examination of the patient's back, you notice purulent drainage coming from his incision site. Lab work was significant for a white blood cell count of 21. What is the best first step in management?
   a. Obtain culture from drainage.
   b. Obtain CT scan.
   c. Start antibiotics.
   d. Call surgery to take to the operating room.

3. A 42-year-old male with a history of IV drug use and untreated hepatitis C is admitted for worsening paralysis of his upper and lower extremities. On imaging he is found to have a cervical epidural abscess for which he undergoes surgical intervention. Postoperatively the patient does well, and cultures obtained from the abscess are positive for *Staphylococcus aureus*. The patient is started on cefazolin and discharged from the hospital. Two weeks later, the patient returns to the hospital with worsening neck pain, fevers, and slight drainage from the surgical site. What is the most likely cause of his fevers?
   a. UTI
   b. DVT
   c. Pneumonia
   d. SSI

4. A 48-year-old male with a past medical history of DVT undergoes a lumbar decompression. In the postoperative period the patient is immobile for the first few days due to pain. On POD 4, you notice swelling of his right lower extremity, but there is no swelling in his left lower extremity. Which test is the best choice for diagnosing a DVT in this patient?
   a. D-Dimer
   b. Ultrasound of lower extremity
   c. CT angiogram of right lower extremity
   d. MRI of right lower extremity

5. A 75-year-old female with a past medical history of chronic back pain and hypertension undergoes an elective thoracic discectomy. During surgery a urinary catheter is placed. The catheter is not removed until POD 5 due to failed trial of voids. Two days after the catheter is removed, the patient starts to have fevers, urinary urgency, and suprapubic tenderness. You are suspicious that she has a UTI. What should you do next?
   a. Start antibiotics immediately.
   b. Obtain a urinalysis and culture.
   c. Put urinary catheter back in.
   d. Consult infectious disease team.

Answers

1. d

2. a

3. d

4. b

5. b

Complex Issues in Pain Management and Substance Abuse

CHAPTER 30

Pain Management Using Multimodal Analgesia in the Neurosurgical Spine Patient

Newton Mei, MD

Introduction

Nurses play a vital role in a patient's pain management in the hospital setting. Nurses are front-line providers who are often the first to assess, and often reassess, a patient's pain. They provide direct patient care by administering medications and nonpharmacologic modalities to ameliorate a patient's pain. They are the patient's advocates, voicing to the interprofessional team when the patient's pain is inadequately controlled and notifying the team of adverse effects associated with the medication regimen. Therefore nurses need to be well versed in the fundamentals of pain management, especially in the care of neurosurgical patients who often have complex pain needs and significant perioperative pain.

Patients with spine disease, especially those who are admitted acutely to the hospital, often have complex pain needs. Their pain experience is shaped by the various biopsychosocial factors in their lives.[1,2] Neurosurgical patients may be on long-term pain medications for chronic pain caused by debilitating spine disease or underlying cancer. Some patients with spine infections may have underlying substance use disorders that predispose them to a heightened pain response (known as hyperalgesia) or to underlying opioid tolerance and dependence.[3] Mood disorders, such as depression or anxiety, may also affect how patients perceive painful stimuli and may affect how they cope with pain.[4] Lastly, patients' lack of social support or baseline malnourishment may prolong their recovery and exacerbate their pain experience.[2] Therefore treating pain is often challenging and requires a comprehensive multidisciplinary patient-centered approach.

Nursing Role and Assessment

A comprehensive and systematic approach should be taken to assess a patient's pain. For all providers, including nurses, it is important to obtain a thorough history from the patient. If a patient is a poor historian or unable to provide the history, obtaining collateral history from the patient's family members and other health care providers (such as primary care providers or providers from nursing homes or transferring facilities) can be helpful to better understand and characterize the patient's pain.[5]

To establish a baseline characterization of a patient's pain it is important to know the pain's location, onset, precipitating factors, ameliorating factors, exacerbating factors, quality, radiation, severity, timing, duration, and associated symptoms (Fig. 30.1).[6] It is also important to ask how the pain is affecting the patient's activities of daily living and functional status. Pain assessments can be conducted using validated tools:

- The Visual Analogue Scale and Numeric Rating Scale may be used to provide an objective rating of the pain severity.

Pain Assessment History	
Onset	*When did the pain start?*
Location	*Where is the pain located? Can you show me where the pain is?*
Precipitating Factors	*What triggers or brings on the pain?*
Ameliorating Factors	*What makes the pain better?*
Exacerbating Factors	*What makes the pain worse?*
Quality	*How would you describe the pain? Is the pain sharp, dull, achy, burning...?*
Radiation	*Does the pain move anywhere else in the body?*
Severity	*On a scale from 0-10 (10 being the worst imaginable pain), how would you rate your pain?*
Time	*How long have you had this pain? Is it getting worse, staying the same or getting better?*
Duration	*Does the pain come and go or is it constant? How long does each pain episode last?*
Associated Factors	*What other symptoms do you have with the pain? (Nausea, weakness, rash, swelling, etc)*
Past Medical History	*Any liver disease, kidney disease, neurologic disease, chronic pain syndromes, cancer?*
Past Surgical History	*What surgeries have you had? Any recent surgeries or procedures?*
Social History	*Any alcohol use? Any substance or drug use? Assess for support network*
Medications	*Review and confirm patient medications, paying close attention to pain medications. Review state patient drug monitoring program if available*
Allergies	*Update patient allergies and associated reactions*
Functional Status	*Assess the patient's baseline functional status/Activities of Daily Living (ADL) and how has the pain affected them*

Fig. 30.1 Pain assessment history.

- The McGill Pain Questionnaire is a validated and more comprehensive assessment of the severity and quality of a patient's pain.[7,8]
- The Roland Morris Low Back Pain and Disability and the Brief Pain Inventory can help with assessing a patient's ability to ambulate, work, and enjoy life.[9-11]

Once the initial assessment of the patient's pain is completed, the nurse can use this established baseline to monitor for any improvement with ongoing interventions and medications. Any worsening of the patient's pain control may suggest new or progressive pathology and should be investigated further with the interprofessional team.

After performing the initial pain evaluation, the next step is to elucidate the patient's biopsychosocial factors that may influence the pain management regimen. It is important to identify the patient's comorbid medical problems. For example, underlying liver or kidney disease may preclude the use of certain pain medications or, at minimum, alter their dosing. Underlying psychiatric illness, opioid use disorder, or other psychosocial barriers may be an indication to consult specialists from other disciplines such as social work, nutrition, physical therapy, occupational therapy, psychiatry, pain medicine, anesthesiology, or palliative care to provide a well-rounded approach and optimal pain relief for the patient.[6]

As part of the initial history taking, nurses can also assist by obtaining an up-to-date list of the patient's medications and any allergies or intolerances to medications. A patient's pharmacy or primary care provider is a great resource for getting an accurate medication list, including the most recently prescribed doses. Many states have implemented patient drug-monitoring programs (PDMP) that facilitate confirmation of dosing/frequency of prescribed controlled medications.[12] Reviewing this information helps providers formulate an appropriate pain control regimen for the patient. Knowing which pain medications the patient has used in the past offers guidance to providers when deciding how to adjust medication doses to effectively manage acute pain.

After the intake history, the physical exam is a critical component in the pain evaluation. The nurse should evaluate the area where the patient localizes pain, paying close attention to signs of inflammation (redness, swelling, induration, heat) and infection (purulence, drainage, wound breakdown, malodor).[13,14] Vital sign abnormalities such as tachycardia or elevated blood pressure can also signify pain or discomfort—these data points are especially important to keep in mind when caring for nonverbal neurosurgical patients. Nurses should be certain to evaluate and document all wounds, surgical sites, and lines (i.e., peripheral IVs, central lines, catheters, drains), as these all are potential sources of pain.[5] In the neurosurgical patient it is particularly important to document a baseline neurologic exam because pain can lead to weakness, decreased sensation, and impaired mobility.

Multimodal Analgesia Pain Management

Opioids are well known for their efficacy in the treatment of pain and were the cornerstone of pain management for many years. They bind to the opioid receptors in the brain to achieve their analgesic effect. However, opioids also come with a myriad of adverse side effects. Common side effects include nausea, vomiting, sedation, pruritus, constipation, ileus, urinary retention, hypotension, and respiratory depression.[7,15] Chronic opioid use can lead to tolerance and physiologic dependence, hyperalgesia, central sensitization, and hypothalamus-pituitary-adrenal (HPA) axis suppression leading to sexual dysfunction (Fig. 30.2).[16-18] Patients who have used opioids chronically require a longer time to achieve adequate pain relief in the perioperative setting.[19] Because of the side effects and addictive potential of opioids amid the growing opioid epidemic, research has shifted clinical practice to the concept of multimodal analgesia (MMA).

MMA has been studied and developed with the goal of optimizing a patient's perioperative pain control while minimizing opioid use.[7,20] The fundamental theory of MMA is that different categories of both nonpharmacologic and pharmacologic treatments achieve pain relief by using distinct pathways in the body. Using these modalities in combination can lead to a synergistic and additive analgesic effect for the patient. Pain management utilizing MMA also enables providers to prescribe lower doses of each pharmacologic agent, thereby decreasing the risk of side effects from each medication.[21,22]

- Nonpharmacologic modalities include patient education, setting appropriate expectations of postoperative pain, mindfulness, massage therapy, acupuncture, aromatherapy, cognitive behavioral therapy, ice packs, heating pads, and repositioning.[23] Some of these

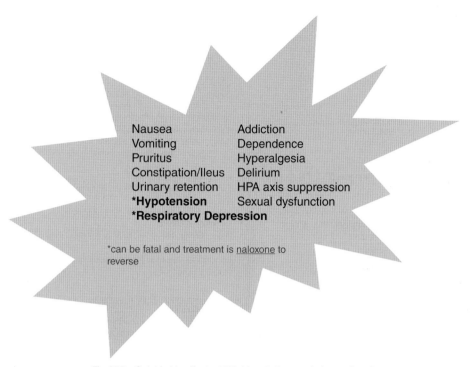

Nausea	Addiction
Vomiting	Dependence
Pruritus	Hyperalgesia
Constipation/Ileus	Delirium
Urinary retention	HPA axis suppression
*Hypotension	Sexual dysfunction
*Respiratory Depression	

*can be fatal and treatment is <u>naloxone</u> to reverse

Fig. 30.2 Opioid side effects. *HPA,* Hypothalamus-pituitary-adrenal.

nonpharmacologic modalities are nursing driven in the inpatient setting; others are currently only available in the outpatient setting.

- Pharmacologic modalities are medications that have proven their efficacy in the treatment of pain. They are usually prescribed based on evidence from studies that demonstrate their efficacy for a particular surgery or patient population.

Providers should customize the MMA pharmacologic regimen according to each patient's allergies, age, interactions with current medications, and medical comorbidities. When crafting an individualized MMA regimen, it can be helpful to use a checklist approach (Fig. 30.3).[24] Nurses should be familiar with the medications that might be incorporated in MMA regimens in the inpatient setting. With this knowledge, nurses can advocate proactively for their patients. After reviewing the MMA medication checklist (see Fig. 30.3), nurses can suggest the addition of different analgesic agents to optimize pain control or recommend discontinuation of the ones that may be affecting the patient adversely. Nurses are valuable members of the interprofessional team who are uniquely positioned to prevent unwanted outcomes, such as uncontrolled pain, patient dissatisfaction, patients leaving against medical advice, prolonged hospitalizations, and increased health care costs.[7,15,16]

Pharmacologic Options in Multimodal Analgesia

GABAPENTINOIDS

Gabapentinoids are medications that bind to the alpha-2–delta-1 subunit of N-type voltage-gated calcium channels in the presynaptic neurons and modulate the release of excitatory neurotransmitters within pain pathways.[7,15,25] Gabapentin and pregabalin are examples of commonly prescribed

Pharmacologic options (common route of administration)	Watch out for:
Gabapentinoids (PO) • Gabapentin • Pregabalin	• Kidney disease (doses will have to be adjusted • Elderly patients • Side effects: Sedation, delirium, confusion
SNRI (PO) • Venlafaxine • Duloxetine	• Side effects: high blood pressure, hyponatremia, GI upset, sweating, tachycardia, dry mouth, sedation, constipation, nausea, serotonin syndrome
Acetaminophen (PO, PR, IV)	• Can mask fevers • Cirrhosis, severe liver disease, significant alcohol use
NSAIDS (topical, PO, IV) • Celecoxib • Ketorolac • Ibuprofen • Diclofenac • Naproxen	• Can mask fevers • Side effects: GI upset, kidney injury, cardiac injury, bleeding • Long term use may lead to poor spinal surgery outcomes
Muscle Relaxants (PO) • Diazepam • Cyclobenzaprine • Baclofen • Metaxalone • Tizanidine • Methocarbamol	• Elderly patients • Side effects: sedation, delirium, confusion, addictive potential with diazepam
Dexamethasone (PO, IV)	• Elderly patients • Side effects: hyperglycemia, high brood pressure, osteoporosis, immunosuppression, high blood pressure, psychosis, confusion, poor wound healing
Ketamine (intranasal, IV)	• Elderly patients • Side effects: sedation, hallucination, nightmares, dizziness, blurry vision, nausea, vomiting
Lidocaine (subQ, patch, IV)	• Heating pads over lidocaine patches can increase systemic absorption • Side effects: sedation, perioral numbness, tinnitus, confusion, seizures, metallic taste, cardiac abnormalities
Opioids (PO, IV, patch) • Morphine • Hydromorphone • Hydrocodone • Fentanyl • Tramadol • Oxycodone • Codeine	• See Fig. 30-2

Fig. 30.3 Pharmacologic checklist for multimodal analgesia.

gabapentinoids. Clinically they have commonly been used in the treatment of conditions with neuropathic pain, such as diabetic neuropathy and postherpetic neuralgia.[15,26-29] Neuropathic pain is often described as a burning, pins-and-needles, ice, cold, or shooting pain.[30] In the spine literature, gabapentinoids have been shown to be effective in decreasing perioperative pain, decreasing perioperative opioid use, and improving patients' long-term functionality.[31] In light of their benefits, gabapentinoids should be incorporated in MMA for patients undergoing spine surgery.[15,32-34] Furthermore, studies have shown additional benefits, including decreased nausea/vomiting; decreased myalgias, pruritis, and fasciculations; improved sleep; reduced anxiety; and increased pain relief from spinal anesthesia and nerve blocks.[32,35,36]

Common side effects of gabapentinoids are sedation, dizziness, and confusion. There is a higher risk of respiratory depression when used in conjunction with opioids and benzodiazepines.[15,21] Elderly patients are more susceptible to the side effects of gabapentinoids. It is important to note that gabapentinoids are metabolized by the kidneys, so special attention should be paid to patients with kidney disease because doses of gabapentinoids will have to be adjusted.[37]

SELECTIVE NOREPINEPHRINE REUPTAKE INHIBITORS

Selective norepinephrine reuptake inhibitors (SNRIs) are approved for the treatment of mood disorders and have shown efficacy in the treatment of neuropathic pain.[38] SNRIs function by blocking the reuptake of serotonin and norepinephrine in neurons. The benefit of adding SNRIs to a patient's MMA regimen is to treat any underlying mood disorder that may be exacerbating a patient's pain and to treat underlying neuropathy from spinal disease and spine surgery. Considering that SNRIs have serotonergic properties, nurses should monitor for serotonin syndrome. This is a potentially serious side effect, and the risk is increased when the patient is taking other serotonergic medications. Symptoms of serotonin syndrome include high fevers, tachycardia, increased muscular tone, clonus, and change in mental status.[39] Common SNRIs include venlafaxine and duloxetine.

- Venlafaxine at doses >150 mg/day has shown benefits in relieving neuropathic pain.[40] Side effects associated with venlafaxine include cardiac conduction abnormalities, hypertension, hyponatremia, gastrointestinal (GI) upset, sweating, tachycardia, and dry mouth.[40]
- Duloxetine has also demonstrated modest efficacy in the treatment of neuropathic pain in cases of diabetic neuropathy. Side effects associated with duloxetine include somnolence, constipation, and nausea.[4]

ACETAMINOPHEN

Acetaminophen functions by inhibiting prostaglandin formation and activating the serotonergic pathways.[25,27] It is available in oral, rectal, and intravenous (IV) formulations. Acetaminophen has excellent perioperative analgesic properties and minimal side effects. Studies demonstrate improved perioperative pain control with acetaminophen usage in patients undergoing orthopedic surgeries.[27,41,42] Given its low side effect profile, acetaminophen is often included in MMA.

Despite its benefits for pain control, providers should be mindful that acetaminophen is an antipyretic and can mask fevers. This is important when a patient is being monitored for an infection. During periods of close fever monitoring, acetaminophen may be held or switched to be administered only as needed (PRN). Furthermore, acetaminophen is metabolized in the liver and should be used cautiously in patients with underlying liver disease, cirrhosis, or severe alcohol use. In the inpatient setting, a patient's liver function should be monitored while taking high doses of acetaminophen. The maximum dose of acetaminophen is 4 g in a 24-hour period for patients without cirrhosis or severe liver disease. For patients who have cirrhosis, a reduced dose of 2 g over a 24-hour period is recommended.[15,43]

NONSTEROIDAL ANTIINFLAMMATORY DRUGS

Nonsteroidal antiinflammatory drugs (NSAIDs) are a class of cyclooxygenase (COX) inhibitors that block the synthesis of proinflammatory prostaglandins.[25] Common NSAIDs include ibuprofen, ketorolac, naproxen, and celecoxib. Studies have shown that NSAIDs result in improved postoperative pain control and decreased use of morphine[44]; however, these medications can affect multiple tissues and organs in the body, including platelets, kidneys, GI tract, liver, and heart. Side effects of NSAIDs include cardiac injury, kidney injury, GI ulceration, and bleeding.[7,24] Additionally, studies have shown an association between NSAID use and an increased risk for nonunion, failure of fusion, and pseudoarthrosis.[25,45] NSAID use can also lead to platelet dysfunction and increase the risk of bleeding. As a result, spine surgeons are often hesitant to use NSAIDs for pain control in patients; however, recent spine literature has shown that these concerns can be mitigated with regular dosing and short-term use of NSAIDs.[46]

Recently, celecoxib has gained favor as a valuable component of MMA regimens. Celecoxib is the only selective COX-2 inhibitor available in the United States. It has minimal effects on COX-1 blockade, which allows preservation of platelet function and the GI tract's mucosa, thus lowering the risk of dyspepsia and stomach ulcers compared to nonselective NSAIDs.[7]

MUSCLE RELAXANTS

Despite the lack of clear evidence to demonstrate a significant analgesic benefit with the use of muscle relaxants in spine patients, they are often incorporated into the MMA regimen. Muscle relaxants are divided into two classes: antispasmodics and antispasticity agents.

- Antispasmodics are used to treat muscle spasms and include medications such as diazepam, cyclobenzaprine, and carisoprodol.
- Antispasticity medications, such as baclofen, are more commonly used in patients with spinal cord injury, stroke, and multiple sclerosis.

Muscle relaxants can lead to oversedation and delirium. Elderly patients are particularly vulnerable to these side effects. Patients should be counseled to take these medications when going to sleep and to avoid performing tasks that require focus and concentration when on these medications.[7]

DEXAMETHASONE

Dexamethasone is a steroid and potent antiinflammatory medication. It is often used in neurosurgical patients to decrease edema and inflammation in the brain or spinal cord. It is also very effective in treating bone pain. A review of the surgical literature suggests that dexamethasone can decrease postoperative pain across multiple types of surgeries, including spine surgery.[20,47] Nonetheless, dexamethasone's numerous side effects often outweigh its benefits for routine postoperative pain management. Common side effects of steroids include hyperglycemia, osteoporosis, poor wound healing, immunosuppression, hypertension, and psychosis.[20]

OPIOIDS

Opioids are effective pain medications and should be incorporated in MMA regimens for the treatment of acute postoperative pain. There is a wide variety of opioids that come in different formulations. Providers should review with the patient which opioids they have used in the past, whether certain formulations were more effective than others, and if there were any notable side effects. Opioids commonly used perioperatively in spine patients include tramadol and oxycodone.

- Tramadol is a weak mu-opioid agonist and inhibits serotonin and norepinephrine reuptake. Studies show a lower risk for addiction, constipation, and cardiovascular side effects in patients on tramadol.[21]
  - Tramadol can lower the seizure threshold and lead to serotonin syndrome when combined with other serotonergic medications.[21,48]
- Oxycodone is also favored in spine patients because it has been shown to cross the blood-brain barrier effectively. When compared to morphine, it has fewer side effects of nausea, hallucination, and pruritus.[49,50]

Patients who have been on chronic pain medications or have a history of opioid use disorder may be placed on IV opioid patient-controlled analgesia (PCA) pumps. With PCAs, the patient can press a button to self-administer a preset dose of an IV opioid. Each self-administered dose is followed by a lockout period during which the patient must wait before another dose can be administered. An important safety feature of PCAs is that pressing the button during a lockout period will not deliver a dose to the patient. PCA usage allows for the quantification of the patient's opioid requirement over a defined period. This then aids in the calculation of an effective dose for the transition to oral formulations. Since PCAs require the patient to press a button to activate the pump, nurses must ensure that the patient has the appropriate mental status, finger dexterity, and strength to use the PCA properly. Nurses should provide education to ensure that patients are using the PCA correctly and should monitor how often a patient is using the device.

- Patients who press their button frequently may need an increase in PCA dosage or the addition of other MMA medications. The frequency of which patients hit their button is also recorded within the pump and can be utilized to evaluate for undertreated pain.
- Patients who are not using their PCA often may be ready to transition to oral pain medications.

Acute Pain Management Service Medications

Certain medications that are commonly used in MMA protocols for spine patients fall under the purview of anesthesiologists or pain management specialists. These medications are often added for patients who would otherwise require excessively high doses of opioids, including those who have opioid tolerance due to chronic use.

KETAMINE INFUSION

Ketamine is an antagonist that binds to the N-methyl-D-aspartate receptor and blocks the formation of inflammatory cytokines.[51] Spine literature has shown significant pain relief and decreased opioid utilization in patients who are placed on ketamine infusions. Ketamine also decreases peripheral and central nerve sensitization and can modulate opioid receptors in patients with chronic opioid use, allowing for quick downward titration of a patient's opioid regimen.[7,20,52] Side effects of ketamine include sedation, hallucinations, nightmares, dizziness, blurry vision, nausea, and vomiting.[25,27] To combat these side effects, clonidine patches, antiemetics, and benzodiazepines are often ordered in conjunction with ketamine.

LIDOCAINE INFUSION

Lidocaine is commonly used as a local anesthetic via subcutaneous injection for bedside procedures. Lidocaine patches are also frequently prescribed both in the inpatient and outpatient setting to provide local topical pain relief. Recent studies have demonstrated the utility of lidocaine infusions for the treatment of postoperative pain after spine surgery. Lidocaine infusions also fall under the purview of pain specialist teams.[54] Lidocaine infusions have been used to treat fibromyalgia, complex regional pain syndrome, postherpetic neuralgia, diabetic neuropathy, cancer pain, and spinal cord injury pain.[53] With spine surgery, lidocaine infusions are effective at alleviating postoperative pain 6–48 hours after surgery, decreasing opioid use postoperatively, and reducing hospital length of stay.[54] Side effects include oversedation, perioral numbness, ringing in the ears, confusion, seizure, and a metallic taste. Cardiac complications include bradycardia and conduction abnormalities, so electrocardiograms are often checked before and after initiation of a lidocaine infusion.[55]

Conclusion

Patients with spinal disease have complex pain needs. MMA is used to optimize a patient's perioperative pain control and minimize the need for opioids. Nurses should be comfortable conducting a systematic and comprehensive pain assessment and exam, and they should be familiar with the nonpharmacologic and pharmacologic modalities available at their institution. Through understanding the common medications that comprise an MMA regimen and their potential side effects, nurses can advocate for the addition or discontinuation of certain medications according to their patients' needs. Being well versed in MMA management can improve a patient's satisfaction, outcome, and postoperative recovery.

References

1. Adams LM, Turk DC. Central sensitization and the biopsychosocial approach to understanding pain. *J Appl Biobehav Res*. 2018;23(2):e12125.
2. Meints S, Edwards R. Evaluating psychosocial contributions to chronic pain outcomes. *Prog Neuro-Psychopharmacol Biol Psych*. 2018;87:168–182.
3. Lee Y-C, Chen P-P. A review of SSRIs and SNRIs in neuropathic pain. *Exp Opin Pharmacother*. 2010;11(17):2813–2825.
4. Bayoumi AB, Ikizgul O, Karaali CN, et al. Antidepressants in spine surgery: a systematic review to determine benefits and risks. *Asian Spine J*. 2019;13(6):1036.
5. Herr K, Coyne PJ, Key T, et al. Pain assessment in the nonverbal patient: position statement with clinical practice recommendations. *Pain Manage Nurs*. 2006;7(2):44–52.
6. Fink RM, Gates RA, Montgomery R. Pain assessment *Oxford Textbook of Palliative Nursing*: Oxford University Press; 2010:137–160.
7. Devin CJ, McGirt MJ. Best evidence in multimodal pain management in spine surgery and means of assessing postoperative pain and functional outcomes. *J Clin Neurosci*. 2015;22(6):930–938.
8. Melzack R. The McGill pain questionnaire: major properties and scoring methods. *Pain*. 1975;1(3):277–299.
9. Keller S, Bann CM, Dodd SL, et al. Validity of the brief pain inventory for use in documenting the outcomes of patients with noncancer pain. *Clin J Pain*. 2004;20(5):309–318.
10. Cleeland C, Ryan K. Pain assessment: global use of the brief pain inventory. *Ann Acad Med Singap*. 1994;23(2):129–138.
11. Roland M, Fairbank J. The Roland–Morris disability questionnaire and the Oswestry disability questionnaire. *Spine*. 2000;25(24):3115–3124.
12. Lin H-C, Wang Z, Boyd C, et al. Associations between statewide prescription drug monitoring program (PDMP) requirement and physician patterns of prescribing opioid analgesics for patients with noncancer chronic pain. *Add Behav*. 2018;76:348–354.
13. Antonelli M, Kushner I. It's time to redefine inflammation. *FASEB J*. 2017;31(5):1787–1791.
14. Gardner SE, Frantz RA, Doebbeling BN. The validity of the clinical signs and symptoms used to identify localized chronic wound infection. *Wound Repair Regen*. 2001;9(3):178–186.
15. Mei N, Sharan AD. Perioperative optimization of pain control in patients undergoing spinal surgery using multimodal analgesia. In: Daniel RM, Harrop CM, eds. *Medical Management of Neurosurgical Patients*: Oxford University Press; 2019:213–232.

16. Dunn LK, Durieux ME, Nemergut EC. Non-opioid analgesics: novel approaches to perioperative analgesia for major spine surgery. *Best Prac Res Clin Anaesthesiol.* 2016;30(1):79–89.

17. Garimella V, Cellini C. Postoperative pain control. *Clin Colon Rectal Surg.* 2013;26(03):191–196.

18. Chou R, Turner JA, Devine EB, et al. The effectiveness and risks of long-term opioid therapy for chronic pain: a systematic review for a National Institutes of Health Pathways to Prevention Workshop. *Ann Int Med.* 2015;162(4):276–286.

19. Chapman CR, Davis J, Donaldson GW, et al. Postoperative pain trajectories in chronic pain patients undergoing surgery: the effects of chronic opioid pharmacotherapy on acute pain. *J Pain.* 2011;12(12):1240–1246.

20. Nielsen RV. Adjuvant analgesics for spine surgery. *Danish Med J.* 2018;65(3).

21. Wick EC, Grant MC, Wu CL. Postoperative multimodal analgesia pain management with nonopioid analgesics and techniques: a review. *JAMA Surg.* 2017;152(7):691–697.

22. De Jong R, Shysh AJ. Development of a multimodal analgesia protocol for perioperative acute pain management for lower limb amputation. *Pain Res Manag.* 2018.

23. O'Conner S, Heck C, Peltier C. Complementary and integrative therapies for pain management. In: Czarnecki ML, Turner HN, eds. *Core Curriculum for Pain Management Nursing.* 3rd ed.: Elsevier; 2018:505–532.

24. Schwenk ES, Mariano ER. Designing the ideal perioperative pain management plan starts with multimodal analgesia. *Korean J Anesthesiol.* 2018;71(5):345–352.

25. Kurd MF, Kreitz T, Schroeder G, et al. The role of multimodal analgesia in spine surgery. *J Am Acad Ortho Surg.* 2017;25(4):260–268.

26. Chincholkar M. Gabapentinoids: pharmacokinetics, pharmacodynamics and considerations for clinical practice. *Br J Pain.* 2020;14(2):104–114.

27. Pitchon DN, Dayan AC, Schwenk ES, et al. Updates on multimodal analgesia for orthopedic surgery. *Anesthesiol Clin.* 2018;36(3):361–373.

28. Rullán M, Bulilete O, Leiva A, et al. Efficacy of gabapentin for prevention of postherpetic neuralgia: study protocol for a randomized controlled clinical trial. *Trials.* 2017;18(1):1–9.

29. Snyder MJ, Gibbs LM, Lindsay TJ. Treating painful diabetic peripheral neuropathy: an update. *Am Fam Phys.* 2016;94(3):227–234.

30. Kehlet H, Jensen TS, Woolf CJ. Persistent postsurgical pain: risk factors and prevention. *Lancet.* 2006;367(9522):1618–1625.

31. Khurana G, Jindal P, Sharma JP, et al. Postoperative pain and long-term functional outcome after administration of gabapentin and pregabalin in patients undergoing spinal surgery. *Spine.* 2014;39(6):e363–e368.

32. Liu B, Liu R, Wang L. A meta-analysis of the preoperative use of gabapentinoids for the treatment of acute postoperative pain following spinal surgery. *Medicine.* 2017;96(37).

33. Yu L, Ran B, Li M, et al. Gabapentin and pregabalin in the management of postoperative pain after lumbar spinal surgery: a systematic review and meta-analysis. *Spine.* 2013;38(22):1947–1952.

34. Han C, Kuang M-j, Jian-xiong M, et al. The efficacy of preoperative gabapentin in spinal surgery: a meta-analysis of randomized controlled trials. *Pain Phys.* 2017;20(7):649.

35. Shimony N, Amit U, Minz B, et al. Perioperative pregabalin for reducing pain, analgesic consumption, and anxiety and enhancing sleep quality in elective neurosurgical patients: a prospective, randomized, double-blind, and controlled clinical study. *J Neurosurg.* 2016;125(6):1513–1522.

36. Park M, Jeon Y. Preoperative pregabalin prolongs duration of spinal anesthesia and reduces early postoperative pain: a double-blind, randomized clinical CONSORT study. *Medicine.* 2016;95(36).

37. Toth C. Pregabalin: latest safety evidence and clinical implications for the management of neuropathic pain. *Ther Adv Drug Safe.* 2014;5(1):38–56.

38. Aiyer R, Barkin RL, Bhatia A. Treatment of neuropathic pain with venlafaxine: a systematic review. *Pain Med.* 2017;18(10):1999–2012.

39. Wang RZ, Vashistha V, Kaur S, et al. Serotonin syndrome: preventing, recognizing, and treating it. *Cleveland Clin J Med.* 2016;83(11):810–817.

40. Sansone RA, Sansone LA. Pain, pain, go away: antidepressants and pain management. *Psychiatry (Edgmont).* 2008;5(12):16.

41. Sinatra RS, Jahr JS, Reynolds L, et al. Intravenous acetaminophen for pain after major orthopedic surgery: an expanded analysis. *Pain Prac.* 2012;12(5):357–365.

42. Sinatra RS, Torres J, Bustos AM. Pain management after major orthopaedic surgery: current strategies and new concepts. *JAAOS*. 2002;10(2):117–129.

43. Chandok N, Watt KD. Pain management in the cirrhotic patient: the clinical challenge. *Mayo Clin Proc*. 2010;85(5):451–458.

44. Jirarattanaphochai K, Jung S. Nonsteroidal antiinflammatory drugs for postoperative pain management after lumbar spine surgery: a meta-analysis of randomized controlled trials. *J Neurosurg Spine*. 2008;9(1):22–31.

45. Glassman SD, Rose SM, Dimar JR, et al. The effect of postoperative nonsteroidal anti-inflammatory drug administration on spinal fusion. *Spine*. 1998;23(7):834–838.

46. Sivaganesan A, Chotai S, White-Dzuro G. The effect of NSAIDs on spinal fusion: a cross-disciplinary review of biochemical, animal, and human studies. *Eur Spine J*. 2017;26(11):2719–2728.

47. De Oliveira GS, Almeida MD, Benzon HT, et al. Perioperative single dose systemic dexamethasone for postoperative pain: a meta-analysis of randomized controlled trials. *J Am Soc Anesthesiol*. 2011;115(3):575–588.

48. Beakley BD, Kaye AM, Kaye AD. Tramadol, pharmacology, side effects, and serotonin syndrome: a review. *Pain Phys*. 2015;18(4):395–400.

49. Cheung CW, Wong SSC, Qiu Q, et al. Oral oxycodone for acute postoperative pain: a review of clinical trials. *Pain Phys*. 2017;20(2S):SE33.

50. Boström E, Hammarlund-Udenaes M, Simonsson US. Blood–brain barrier transport helps to explain discrepancies in in vivo potency between oxycodone and morphine. *J Am Soc Anesthesiol*. 2008;108(3):495–505.

51. Kaye AD, Cornett EM, Helander E, et al. An update on nonopioids: intravenous or oral analgesics for perioperative pain management. *Anesthesiol Clin*. 2017;35(2):e55–e71.

52. Nielsen RV, Fomsgaard JS, Siegel H, et al. Intraoperative ketamine reduces immediate postoperative opioid consumption after spinal fusion surgery in chronic pain patients with opioid dependency: a randomized, blinded trial. *Pain*. 2017;158(3):463–470.

53. Tully J, Jung JW, Patel A, et al. Utilization of intravenous lidocaine infusion for the treatment of refractory chronic pain. *Anes Pain Med*. 2020;10(6):e112290.

54. Sun Y, Li T, Wang N, et al. Perioperative systemic lidocaine for postoperative analgesia and recovery after abdominal surgery: a meta-analysis of randomized controlled trials. *Dis Colon Rectum*. 2012;55(11):1183–1194.

55. Estebe J-P. Intravenous lidocaine. *Best Prac Res Clin Anaesthesiol*. 2017;31(4):513–521.

Questions

A 62-year-old male with a history of obstructive sleep apnea, morbid obesity, high blood pressure, chronic kidney disease, myocardial infarction in 1994, and type 2 diabetes presents to the emergency room with severe back pain that radiates down both legs, with numbness and tingling in the feet bilaterally. He has no known drug allergies. He provides you with a medication list: oxycodone 10 mg every 6 hours PRN for severe pain, lisinopril, atorvastatin, and insulin glargine 30 units every morning.

1. To better assess the patient's pain, what additional questions would you ask?
   a. When did the pain start?
   b. Are there any precipitating factors?
   c. Does the pain affect the patient's work and sleep?
   d. Both a and b
   e. All of the above

2. The patient's wife comes in and notes that her husband actually is taking 40 mg of oxycodone every 4 hours and that the medication list he provided on admission is incorrect. What should your next step be? (Select all that apply.)
   a. Call the team and request that the oxycodone be changed to 40 mg every 4 hours.
   b. Review PDMP or call the patient's pharmacy to confirm the oxycodone dose and frequency.
   c. Ignore the patient's wife because 40 mg of oxycodone is too high of a dose to be prescribed in an inpatient setting.
   d. Recommend a hydromorphone PCA, since the patient is on such a high dose of opioids at home.
   e. Recommend that morphine be tried instead.

3. The patient is on postoperative day (POD) 1 after spine surgery and complains of 10/10 pain. His labs from the morning are notable for a creatinine of 3.1 mg/dL, increased from his baseline of 1.4 mg/dL. Which of the following should you *not* add to the patient's MMA regimen at this time?
a. Acetaminophen
b. Lidocaine patch
c. Celecoxib
d. Ketamine
e. Ice packs

4. On POD 4, the patient appears to be more lethargic than usual. Which of the following medications could be contributing to the patient's sedation?
a. Pregabalin
b. Tizanidine (muscle relaxant)
c. Acetaminophen
d. Both a and b
e. All of the above

5. The patient has not had a bowel movement in 5 days, and you believe it is a side effect from one of his pain medications. What are some other side effects that this class of pain medications can cause?
a. Dilated pupils
b. Respiratory depression
c. Suppressed HPA axis
d. Both a and b
e. Both b and c

Answers

1. e

2. b, d

3. c

4. d

5. e

CHAPTER 31

Nursing Management of the Patient With Opioid Use Disorder

Allison M. Lang, MSN, CRNP, AGACNP-BC ■ Johanna Beck, MD

Introduction

The opioid epidemic has created many challenges in the inpatient health care setting. The *Diagnostic and Statistical Manual of Mental Disorders*, Fifth Edition, defines opioid use disorder as "a problematic pattern of opioid use leading to problems or distress."[1] For a formal diagnosis, the patient must exhibit two of the following within a 12-month period:

1. Taking larger amounts or taking drugs over a longer period than intended
2. Persistent desire or unsuccessful efforts to cut down or control opioid use
3. Spending a great deal of time obtaining or using the opioid, or recovering from its effects
4. Craving, or a strong desire or urge to use opioids
5. Problems fulfilling obligations at work, school, or home
6. Continued opioid use despite recurring social or interpersonal problems
7. Giving up or reducing activities because of opioid use
8. Using opioids in physically hazardous situations
9. Continued opioid use despite ongoing physical or psychological problems likely to have been caused or worsened by opioids
10. Tolerance (i.e., need for increased amounts or diminished effect with continued use of the same amount)
11. Experiencing withdrawal (opioid withdrawal syndrome) or taking opioids (or a closely related substance) to relieve or avoid withdrawal symptoms[1]

Patients with opioid use disorder generally require extensive psychotherapy in conjunction with pharmacotherapy to maintain abstinence. Neurosurgical patients with opioid use disorder pose unique challenges in perioperative pain management due to the physiologic changes resulting from the chronicity of their opioid use, coupled with possible paradoxic hyperalgesia or increased pain perception. These patients likely require higher doses of opioid pain medications during the acute postoperative period in combination with other nonopioid pain medications. To better understand how to effectively treat postoperative pain in this patient population, it is important to understand the pharmacologic treatment options available.[2]

Agonists, Partial Agonists, and Antagonists

- An agonist is a chemical substance that binds to and activates a physiologic receptor to produce a full response.
- A partial agonist similarly activates a physiologic receptor but with lower efficacy and a suboptimal response even if occupying the total number of receptors.
- An antagonist blocks or inactivates the receptor from producing a response.
- The affinity of the drug determines how effective the drug will be at binding to and competing with other drugs at the receptor.[3,4]

- There are three opioid receptor types: mu, delta, and kappa
  - The mu-opioid receptor is predominantly affected by opioid agonists, partial agonists, and antagonists.
  - The mu receptor is responsible for the sensations of pain relief, physical dependence, mood changes, and respiratory effects experienced by patients using opioids.

Commonly Used Medications in the Patient With Opioid Use Disorder

OPIOID AGONISTS

Commonly used opioid agonists in the postoperative neurosurgery patient include hydromorphone, morphine sulfate, and oxycodone. These highly potent medications are typically chosen to treat postoperative pain in most neurosurgical patients especially those with opioid use disorder. These are considered to have a higher affinity profile among other opioid agonists. They bind tightly to the mu-opioid receptor to produce an analgesic response in the brain.[5,6] However, there is increasing evidence that administering higher and higher doses of opioids not only increases the risk of adverse effects, such as respiratory depression, but also can actually produce an opposite effect known as opioid-induced hyperalgesia.[2]

- Methadone is a commonly used opioid agonist used to treat opioid use disorder. It is often used in the inpatient setting to both control cravings and treat pain. Although methadone fully binds to the mu-opioid receptor (similarly to other opioid agonists), it does so slowly, and it does not produce the euphoric effect that other opioid agonists would in the opioid-dependent patient.[3] Many patients with opioid use disorder follow with a methadone clinic in the outpatient setting to help control their cravings for illicit substances and prevent relapse.
  - In the outpatient setting, patients receiving methadone therapy will need to present to a methadone clinic daily to receive their dose. Their dose will be titrated as indicated by trained physicians and advanced practice providers.
  - It is important to collaborate care with the patient's home methadone clinic to coordinate accurate dosing both in the hospital and on discharge.
    - These patients should always be continued on their outpatient doses of methadone while inpatient, unless clinically contraindicated.
  - During the acute postoperative pain period, some patients may benefit from having their methadone dose split into twice daily or three times daily dosing to help control the acute pain, while concurrently managing addictive cravings.
    - These split doses need to be consolidated into once-daily dosing upon discharge to be continued at an outpatient methadone clinic.
  - In the methadone-naive patient, baseline and daily electrocardiogram monitoring should be obtained to monitor the QTc interval both prior to initiating and while titrating this QTc prolonging medication.[7]
    - Prolonged QT interval can lead to a deadly cardiac arrhythmia known as torsades de pointes.

OPIOID PARTIAL AGONIST

The most known opioid partial agonist is buprenorphine (Subutex) sublingual. Buprenorphine has been proven in various studies to be an effective illicit opioid use deterrent in patients and an alternative to methadone.[7] This medication has a high affinity but a low efficacy at the mu-opioid receptor and produces only a partial effect. However, because of its affinity for the mu-opioid receptor, buprenorphine can displace already present opioid agonists on the receptor, which may then precipitate sudden opioid withdrawal in the patient. For this reason, it is often recommended that prior to initiating buprenorphine treatment, patients with known opioid use disorder should (1) wait ≥4 hours after their last opioid use and (2) wait until they are beginning to experience mild symptoms of opioid withdrawal. This ensures an adequate opioid washout period, reducing the chance of precipitated withdrawal. Opioid withdrawal symptoms can be monitored using standardized scoring systems, such as the Clinical Opiate Withdrawal Scale (COWS) score.

- Buprenorphine also comes in a formulation that is paired with naloxone (Suboxone) sublingual, an opioid receptor antagonist. The naloxone component is used primarily to prevent misuse if the patient injects the drug intravenously (IV) or intramuscularly (IM) instead of taking the medication sublingually.
  - Naloxone has very little effect if the patient takes it appropriately via the sublingual route.
  - If the medication is injected IV or IM, the naloxone will be absorbed effectively and will prevent buprenorphine from binding to the opioid receptors and taking effect.

NALOXONE

Naloxone (Narcan) is an opioid receptor antagonist that competes at the opioid receptor site to displace full or partial agonists and prevent/reverse the opioid agonists' effects on the patient. In the inpatient setting, naloxone is commonly used in suspected opioid overdose situations, such as when a patient is nonresponsive after recent opioid medication administration or has developed concerning symptoms, such as a diminished respiratory drive.[3,4]

OPIOID-INDUCED HYPERALGESIA

This paradoxic phenomenon is described as an overly nociceptive sensitive state caused by prolonged exposure to opioids. The prolonged use of opioids results in peripheral and central nervous system changes that eventually lead to the sensitization of the pain pathways in the affected patient. Patients experiencing opioid-induced hyperalgesia become more sensitized to painful stimuli despite adequate treatment with opioid analgesics.

- Patients experiencing this condition will often express continued uncontrolled pain despite escalation in pain regimen.
- Management of these patients will ideally include the tapering off of opioids and use of a multimodal analgesia regimen for pain control (Table 31.1, Fig. 31.1).[8]

COWS Score Monitoring

To successfully initiate medication therapy, the nurse's assessment of the patient's current withdrawal status is imperative. COWS scoring is a universal tool used by nursing to assess the severity of withdrawal

TABLE 31.1 ■ Commonly Used Medications to Treat Opioid Use Disorder and Their Dosages

Commonly Used Drugs	Initiation Dosages	Dose Ranges
Buprenorphine	2–8 mg sublingual tablets x 1 day, then 8–16 mg daily x 1–2 days	4–24 mg/day
Buprenorphine/naloxone	2/0.5 mg–4/1 mg sublingual x 1, may increase by 2/0.5 mg–4/1 mg every 2 hours up to 8/2 mg on first day	2/0.5 mg–24/6 mg sublingual
Methadone	Initiate at 10–30 mg (tablet or liquid) by prescriber's assessment; max 40 mg on day 1	May up titrate by 10 mg/day. Common maintenance doses range 60–120 mg

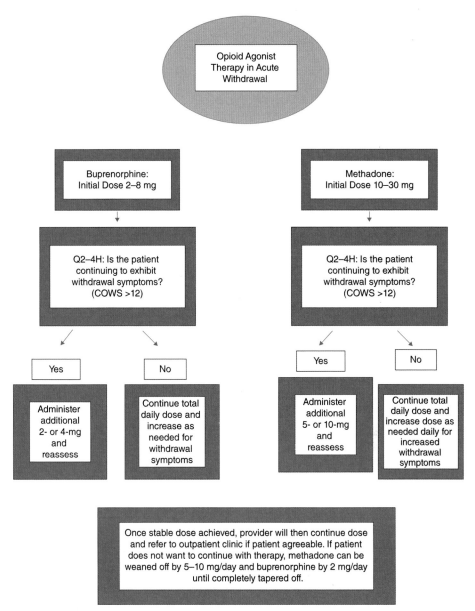

Fig. 31.1 Algorithm illustrating how buprenorphine and methadone are prescribed in an acutely withdrawing patient.

in a patient with opioid use disorder. The COWS score incorporates common physiologic symptoms and signs that may be present in a patient undergoing opioid withdrawal. It is a critical assessment made by nursing at specifically ordered intervals to help assess the patient's current withdrawal status. It helps the provider know how to best treat the patient and when to initiate treatment with partial agonist therapy. Nursing should use clinical judgment when assigning the score. After assigning the patient a COWS score, the nurse should communicate the score to the provider to help facilitate treatment in a timely fashion.[9] Fig. 31.2 shows COWS scoring used in many medical facilities worldwide.

Patient's Name:_____   Date and Time____/____/____:_____

Reason for this assessment:_____

Resting Pulse Rate: _____beats/minute *Measured after patient is sitting or lying for one minute* 0 pulse rate 80 or below 1 pulse rate 81–100 2 pulse rate 101–120 4 pulse rate greater than 120	**GI Upset:** *over last 1/2 hour* 0 no GI symptoms 1 stomach cramps 2 nausea or loose stool 3 vomiting or diarrhea 5 multiple episodes of diarrhea or vomiting
Sweating: *over past 1/2 hour not accounted for by* *room temperature or patient activity.* 0 no report of chills or flushing 1 subjective report of chills or flushing 2 flushed or observable moistness on face 3 beads of sweat on brow or face 4 sweat streaming off face	**Tremor** *observation of outstretched hands* 0 no tremor 1 tremor can be felt, but not observed 2 slight tremor observable 4 gross tremor or muscle twitching
Restlessness *Observation during assessment* 0 able to sit still 1 reports difficulty sitting still, but is able to do so 3 frequent shifting or extraneous movements of legs/arms 5 unable to sit still for more than a few seconds	**Yawning** *Observation during assessment* 0 no yawning 1 yawning once or twice during assessment 2 yawning three or more times during assessment 4 yawning several times/minute
Pupil size 0 pupils pinned or normal size for room light 1 pupils possibly larger than normal for room light 2 pupils moderately dilated 5 pupils so dilated that only the rim of the iris is visible	**Anxiety or Irritability** 0 none 1 patient reports increasing irritability or anxiousness 2 patient obviously irritable or anxious 4 patient so irritable or anxious that participation in the assessment is difficult

Bone or Joint aches *If patient was having pain*
previously, only the additional component attributed
to opiates withdrawal is scored
0 not present
1 mild diffuse discomfort
2 patient reports severe diffuse aching of joints/muscles
4 patient is rubbing joints or muscles and is unable to sit
    still because of discomfort
	Gooseflesh skin
	0 skin is smooth
	3 piloerrection of skin can be felt or hairs standing up
	    on arms
	5 prominent piloerrection

Runny nose or tearing *Not accounted for by cold* *symptoms or allergies* 0 not present 1 nasal stuffiness or unusually moist eyes 2 nose running or tearing 4 nose constantly running or tears streaming down cheeks	Total Score_____ The total score is the sum of all 11 items Initials of person completing assessment: _____

Score: 5-12 = mild; 13-24 = moderate; 25-36 = moderately severe; more than 36 = severe withdrawal

Fig. 31.2 Clinical Opiate Withdrawal Scale (COWS). (From Wesson DR, Ling W. The clinical opiate withdrawal scale (COWS). *J Psychoactive Drugs.* 2003;35[2]:253–259.)

Nursing Considerations

The nursing care of patients with opioid use disorder may be challenging at times and requires a greater understanding of the underlying mental health disorders that coincide with substance use. Many patients with opioid use disorder are concurrently diagnosed with mental health disorders, such as bipolar disorder, schizophrenia, posttraumatic stress disorder, and other mood disorders. Their care requires skillful interviewing techniques, along with compassion and patience while building rapport. The literature shows that a majority of nurses generally harbor a negative perception of these patients for a variety of reasons. Many nurses are mistrustful of patients with substance use disorder because such patients will frequently utilize manipulative behaviors to satisfy their addiction cravings. Nurses have also expressed safety concerns because these patients may become agitated if their withdrawal symptoms and other underlying mental health disorders are not adequately treated, causing them to become frustrated with care.[10]

While caring for this patient population, it is important for the nurse to be aware of the surroundings. Deescalation training is imperative for all nursing staff involved in the care of this patient population. Nurses are often the first to respond to potentially dangerous situations with these patients, and they should utilize their resources within their health care institution, such as having security present early, when a patient begins to exhibit unsafe or violent behavior. Patients with opioid use disorder may attempt to have visitors deliver illicit substances while they are inpatient or alternatively may have hidden illicit substances on their person or in their belongings for use while hospitalized. Frequent monitoring of these patients for any behavior changes can help prevent adverse events from occurring.

- If nurses suspect recent substance use while in the hospital, they should contact the medical team immediately for patient evaluation, potential reversal of the substance, and drug screen. Security should perform a room search; if an illicit substance is found, the patient should have visitors restricted for the duration of the stay to ensure patient safety.
- Ultimately, ensuring patient safety and stability (such as making sure a patient is adequately protecting their airway, breathing, circulation [ABCs]) takes precedence over drug screening and searching.

Conclusion

Patients with opioid use disorder can be very challenging in many aspects of their care. However, it is important to note that they should be treated with dignity and respect. Having a better understanding of addiction and the treatments available will help the nurse care for these patients with compassion and expertise.[11]

References

1. American Psychiatric Association. Opioid-related disorders. In: *Diagnostic and Statistical Manual of Mental Disorders*, 5th ed. Author; 2013.
2. Angst MS, Clark JD. Opioid-induced hyperalgesia: a qualitative systematic review. *Anesthesiology.* 2006;104(3):570–587.
3. Helm S, Trescot AM, Colson J, et al. Opioid antagonists, partial agonists, and agonists/antagonists: the role of office-based detoxification. *Pain Phys.* 2008;11(2):225–235.
4. National Institute on Drug Abuse. Medications to treat opioid use disorder research report 2018.
5. Berg KA, Clarke WP. Making sense of pharmacology: inverse agonism and functional selectivity. *Int J Neuropsychopharmacol.* 2018;21(10):962–977.
6. Tallarida RJ, Cowan A. The affinity of morphine for its pharmacologic receptor in vivo. *J Pharmacol Exp Ther.* 1982;222(1):198–201.
7. Nielsen S, Larance B, Degenhardt L, et al. Opioid agonist treatment for pharmaceutical opioid dependent people. *Cochrane Database Syst Rev.* 2016;(5):CD011117.
8. Lee M, Silverman SM, Hansen H, et al. A comprehensive review of opioid-induced hyperalgesia. *Pain Phys.* 2011;14(2):145–161.
9. Wesson DR, Ling W. The clinical opiate withdrawal scale (COWS). *J Psychoactive Drugs.* 2003;35(2):253–259.
10. Donroe JH, Holt SR, Tetrault JM. Caring for patients with opioid use disorder in the hospital. *CMAJ.* 2016;188(17-18):1232–1239.
11. Neville K, Roan N. Challenges in nursing practice: nurses' perceptions in caring for hospitalized medical-surgical patients with substance abuse/dependence. *J Nurs Adm.* 2014;44(6):339–346.

Questions

Joel is a 42-year-old male with past medical history of opioid use disorder who presented with a 4-day history of fevers and chills, along with worsening lower back pain. He states that he uses heroin IV daily, and he last used the day of admission. On admission, his temperature was 103°F. Infectious workup was notable for magnetic resonance imaging spine with an epidural abscess at the L5 level and blood cultures positive for methicillin-resistant *Staphylococcus aureus* bacteremia. The patient was admitted and received a lumbar decompression and fusion with washout with neurosurgery. Due to the intensity of his pain, acute pain services were consulted; they started Joel on a hydromorphone patient-controlled analgesia to help control his pain during his perioperative course. The patient is now medically stable for discharge and has expressed interest in beginning treatment with buprenorphine-naloxone (Suboxone) for his opioid use disorder while he receives continued antibiotic treatment at a rehabilitation facility.

1. When initiating buprenorphine therapy, it is most important to first:
   a. Give the first dose to the patient immediately to keep him calm.
   b. Give the patient a dose of naloxone prior to initiating treatment.
   c. Wait at least 4 hours after last dose of opioid until the patient begins to exhibit withdrawal symptoms.
   d. Educate the patient on the alternative IV and IM routes of administration.

2. The nurse caring for this patient has had negative experiences in the past with other patients with opiate use disorder. The patient calls the nurse and states he is in 10/10 pain and asks if she can notify the provider to see if he can have anything additional for pain control. The nurse ignores the request and tells the patient that he can't have anything else. She continues to ignore his requests throughout the day. What is wrong with the nurse's response to this situation?
   a. The nurse is not setting clear boundaries with the patient.
   b. The nurse is not treating the patient with dignity due to own unconscious bias.
   c. This will cause the patient to become distrustful of staff and frustrated with care.
   d. Both b and c.

3. The patient calls the nurse to ask for an additional dose of hydromorphone. The nurse informs the patient that he is not due for his dose for another hour. The patient becomes visibly upset and quickly escalates, yelling at the nurse. What should the nurse do next?
   a. Exit the room and call security for assistance.
   b. Tell the patient he needs to "just calm down."
   c. Yell back at the patient and tell him he won't get any more pain medication if he continues to act like this.
   d. Request the patient be transferred to another unit in the hospital.

4. The patient calls the nurse to the room to bring him a can of soda. While in the room, the nurse notices the patient exhibiting strange behavior, and the two visitors in the room leave abruptly. The nurse is suspicious that the patient may have had illicit substances delivered to him. What are the next steps the nurse should take?
   a. Ignore it and hope nothing bad happens to the patient.
   b. Notify the provider to examine the patient as well as security to perform a room search.
   c. Scold the patient and tell him that using drugs in the hospital is only going to make his situation worse.
   d. Confront the visitors to ask them directly.

5. The nurse goes to assess the patient on hourly rounds and finds him to be very lethargic but arousable to light touch. He is breathing at a rate of 12 respirations per hour and his oxygen saturation is 92% on room air. How should the nurse respond initially?
   a. Wait a few hours and see if he will wake up more on his own.
   b. Pinch him repeatedly until he is more arousable.
   c. Continue frequent monitoring, notify the provider, and ensure naloxone is available if needed.
   d. Request the provider initiate methadone or Suboxone at this time.

Answers

1. c

2. d

3. a

4. b

5. c

CHAPTER 32

Social Work Management of the Patient With Opioid Use Disorder

Khadija Israel, MSW, LMSW ■ Laura Esquivel Martinez, PhD Candidate, LMSW

Introduction

As opioid-related care continues to increase the burden on the health care system,[1-5] it has become evident that addressing the opioid epidemic within the acute setting requires a multidisciplinary approach. In the acute care setting, patients with opioid use disorder (OUD) often have multifaceted structural, social, and clinical barriers that complicate care.[6] Though medical contributions to recovery have been linked to increased treatment engagement[7-9] and drug-free days postdischarge,[10] these outcomes are often short lived without ultimately addressing the psychosocial and systemic components that often complicate inpatient care.[11-13] Sustained recovery for this population may be improved with the administration of holistic care.[14,15] Therefore clinicians must utilize other resources at their disposal when administering opioid-related care, including the consultation of social workers.

The role of the inpatient social worker is often overlooked by hospital staff, who tend to relegate the position to case managers.[16,17] Often social workers are not consulted until nearing discharge, when highly disenfranchised and vulnerable populations (the unhoused, people with mental illness, adults with special needs, etc.) are transitioned back into the community. At this point, social workers are commonly used to conduct a social-environmental assessment to facilitate transitioning these populations into resource-limited communities.[18] However, the entire taxonomy of social work roles, skills, and competencies are quite vast and can be utilized throughout a patient's hospital stay to aid with the following[19]:

1. Rapid assessment of patient's misuse to identify risk level
2. Providing an interdisciplinary perspective within collaborative efforts
3. Enacting the role of a bridge between the patient/family and the medical team
4. Providing services and care to enhance patient's overall well-being
5. Providing access points to community resources while ensuring a postdischarge continuum of care
6. Ensuring quality care through enacting patient-centered, evidence-informed practice
7. Promoting accountability within the care team
8. Translating social work's unique contributions across other professions

Adequate dissemination of the scope of these roles to the medical, nursing, and other supplemental staff is critical to ensure that social workers are appropriately consulted and utilized. Providing effective treatment to neurosurgical patients with OUD requires the creative implementation of these distinctive skill sets and responsibilities.

Neurosurgical patients often present with ample medical complications from chronic opioid use that are exacerbated by low social support and limited/no access to essential postdischarge resources. In addition, the stigma attached to providing care and treatment options to these patients often results in an elevated incidence of self-directed discharge (also known as discharge against medical advice), which ultimately exacerbates the burden on the health care system.[20,21] To better understand how to treat this patient population effectively, it is essential to understand the unique contributions social workers can provide to the interdisciplinary team.

Screening and Assessment

Care for patients with OUD needs to be administered through a syndemic framework, which focuses on the relationship between disease and social condition. Adequate screening for risky use/OUD is an essential tool to assist in pain management navigation and the early introduction of secondary pharmacologic and nonpharmacologic interventions.[22] Often adverse interactions of health inequities caused by poverty, stigma, and structural deficits work in synergy with infections from misuse, reinforcing and exacerbating comorbidities.[23] Integrating social work management into the screening process ensures that the psychosocial, environmental, and systemic factors are appropriately addressed.

The current evidence-based screening program endorsed by the Substance Abuse and Mental Health Services Administration (SAMHSA) is Screening, Brief Intervention, and Referral to Treatment (SBIRT). SBIRT is a comprehensive three-component model that uses validated tools and clinical judgment to provide brief intervention and referral to treatment.[24] Unfortunately, implementation studies of this model have found that medical and nursing staff, plagued by the push for shortened hospital stays, view the screening for this model as "one more thing to do" in their already overburdened role.[25,26] As a result, utilizing social workers to oversee this role and screening process provides interdisciplinary collaboration with the space, expertise, and skillset to implement this model effectively and efficiently.

In the acute care setting, typical patient-staff interactions may be only a few minutes long. The SBIRT tool is quick to administer and easy to score/interpret, which allows for a successful intervention to occur in a short duration.[27] The SBIRT tool is used to identify cases of substance abuse in the initial stages (prior to developing abuse or dependence diagnoses) or those that may have otherwise gone unnoticed in an acute care setting (when the primary reason for admission is often not related to substance use).[27] In fact, results from the SBIRT can be used to help providers predict, plan for, and treat withdrawal symptoms in acute care settings, while helping to facilitate access to treatment for patients postdischarge.[27] The three components of the SBIRT are:

- Screening: This component is used to screen patients for drug or alcohol use behaviors and serves as the gateway for further intervention.[27]
  - Uses/validates screening tool to ask about substance use in nonjudgmental and consistent ways[24]
  - Common screening tools include:
    - Alcohol Use Disorders Identification Test (AUDIT)
    - Drug Abuse Screening Test (DAST)
    - CAGE (Cutting down, annoyance, guilty, eye opener)
- Brief intervention: This component is used to target people exhibiting mild to severe symptom levels and address substance use.[24]
  - Commonly uses motivation interviewing (MI) to help patients recognize the reality associated with harmful substance use and resolve ambivalence about making changes in their lives.[24]
  - MI is particularly appropriate for patients who are ambivalent regarding changing their substance use behaviors.[24]
- Referral to treatment: This component is used to refer appropriate individuals to treatment.
  - It can include either a recommendation to seek treatment after hospital discharge or a referral to a specific outpatient treatment facility upon discharge (Fig. 32.1).[24]

Brief Screening - Ask	In the past 12 months, have you used drugs other than those required for medical reasons?	Positive screen (yes) should yield a social work consult
(+) Positive on Brief Screen		**(−) Negative on Brief Screen**

(+) Positive on Brief Screen

Assess

Use a brief assessment instrument (see table below) to determine level of risk severity based on DSM criteria for substance abuse and dependence

	DAST-10ᵃ (adult drug use)	CRAFFT (adolescent alcohol & drug use)
Hazardous use (risky use)	Score 3-5	Score of 2 or more positive items indicates need for further assessment
Harmful use (use plus consequences)	Score 6-8	
Possible dependence (compulsive use)	Score 9-10	

Patients with Hazardous/Harmful Use

Willing to Work on Change

- Discuss health risks of opioid use emphasizing health problems related to use, possible interactions with medications.
- Provide clear, supportive feedback: "At this level of consumption, you are at increased risk for health problems and injuries."
- Determine the patient's willingness to make a change attempt.
- Assist patient with setting goals through motivational interviewing.
- Administer brief therapy for patients with substantial level of use or with difficulty changing use pattern.
- Referral to appropriate post-discharge treatment.

(−) Negative on Brief Screen

Administer Reinforcement

Reinforce positive decisions.
Rescreen at each readmission.

Patients with Hazardous/Harmful Use

Patient Not Willing to Work on Change

- Communicate your concern and willingness to help.
- Increase knowledge around safer substance use
- Introduction to community support (Peer support specialists)
- Provide access to Fentanyl test strips, Naloxone and overdose education kits
- Provide access to safe smoking supplies and sterile syringes and other injection equipment to prevent and control the spread of infectious diseases

Fig. 32.1 Screening, Brief Intervention, and Referral to Treatment flow chart. Rapid screening determines the appropriate level of treatment by assessing the severity of substance use. (From University of Missouri-Kansas City Screening, Brief Intervention, and Referral to Treatment for Substance Use. Clinician tools. https://www.sbirt.care/tools.aspx.)

Interventions

For patients with OUD the need to employ psychosocial interventions in tandem with medical interventions is well documented within the literature.[28] Brief interventions within the medical setting have been shown to influence postdischarge health outcomes positively and, due to this effectiveness, have been incorporated into many acute care programs.[10,11,26,29] Social workers, when appropriately consulted, are uniquely and aptly suited to perform these brief intervention services.[30,31] Types of brief therapeutic interventions include motivational interviewing and motivational enhancement therapy. These are considered nonjudgmental, patient-centered approaches; their utilization, in conjunction with a social worker's psychosocial training, promotes the efficacy of implementation. In the acute care setting these interventions are used most effectively to[32]:

- Encompass motivation-driven dialogue
- Empower patients by increasing their awareness of substance use and its consequences
- Provide feedback
- Motivate patients toward behavioral change, if feasible and desired

Social work interventions have been shown to play a pivotal role in addressing the opioid epidemic and the ever-changing syndemic that accompanies it. Recent studies have also outlined emerging effective social work interventions that address the comprehensive symptomology of patients with OUD. Clinical trials of Motivational Orientated Recovery Enhancement, a mindfulness-based integrative social work intervention, reported significant reductions in chronic pain symptoms, opioid dosing, and psychological distress after a 9-month follow-up.[33,34]

In addition, patients with OUD present as a heterogeneous population with varying levels of misuse severity, social support, resources, traumas, and self-efficacy. Social workers can address each patient's unique needs by providing a wide range of tailored interventions, including short therapeutic consultations, information, self-help materials, and harm reduction education. These tools can benefit the interdisciplinary team because they contest the unwritten rule of abstinence, which is implicit within acute medical care.

In patients with low interest in abstinence or treatment, social work management is conducted through a harm reduction lens. The use of harm reduction strategies has been substantiated within the literature,[35] and example resources include:

- Ensuring that patients are provided with drug use education
- Outlining access to sterile syringe distribution
- Providing access to supervised consumption facilities (where people can use preobtained drugs under the supervision of medical staff)
- Providing patients with access to naloxone kits

The implementation of harm reduction strategies has been associated with reducing the adverse risk of substance misuse, assuaging iatrogenic suffering and stigma, and encouraging candid and transparent discussions between patients and health care providers.[21] Furthermore, a harm reduction perspective creates an environment that can:

1. Target risks while simultaneously outlining the root cause
2. Tailor preadministered medical/social intervention to reduce potential risks
3. Acknowledge any positive change made within patients' lives to facilitate positive reinforcement
4. Recognize dignity and compassion are primarily cultivated when staff accept patients as they are
5. Protect the patient's rights to quality care regardless of use[35]

In the medical field, social stigma has been known to undermine disease prevention efforts and wellness enhancement.[36] Nurturing an atmosphere with these tenets fosters a sense of acceptance, compassion, and autonomy within patients. This promotes self-efficacy and circumvents internalized stigma created by negative patient and staff interactions. Creating an environment that minimizes stigma and promotes self-efficacy is crucial due to self-efficacy's association with treatment engagement and reduction of opiate misuse during OUD treatment.[37]

It is also important to recognize that treatment plans for patients with OUD work best when they are considered in the context of the patient's stage of change. The harm reduction model and the transtheoretical model of change are well paired in understanding individuals' goals to stop or reduce using opioids.

- These models indicate that when a person considers a behavior change, the individual may move in a different stage before making the desired change
  - Stages range from precontemplation to relapse, and are nonlinear.
- Utilizing a social worker to explore harm alongside the stage of change can help individuals and professionals support specific behavior goals.

Referral

Referral to treatment is the most prominent role of social work management. Social workers act as the liaison between the acute care team, outpatient health services, mental health services, and community resources during the postdischarge transition process.[19] Consequently, this discipline is tasked with navigating a complex, oversaturated, fragmented system of care to ensure that patients acquire adequate postdischarge treatment.[38,39] A social worker's role in acquiring postdischarge care is crucial because care is administered through an ecologic lens. This lens ensures that a patient's unmet social needs are addressed in conjunction with addiction services.

Current research indicates that utilizing comprehensive health care–based interventions that address patients' unmet social needs positively impacts health outcomes.[40] Effective integration of social work management throughout the transitional process allows multiple points of contact to address the patient's determinants of health. Overall, this can be leveraged to mitigate recurrent hospital utilization and adverse consequences of opioid misuse.

In settings where shortages of health care personnel are particularly pronounced, addiction medicine consultation may be more effective and efficient for treating the population of opioid-using patients. Addiction medicine consultation services utilize an interprofessional team to provide consultation and addiction expertise. The team may consist of nurse practitioners, social workers, physician assistants, psychologists, and peers (recovery-trained peers).[41] Addiction consultation services have become the emerging standard of care. They allow for seamless integration of medical and social work management to address the unique needs of patients with OUD without burdening already overburdened health care staff. Five fundamental core services are offered by addiction medicine consultation[41]:

1. Assessments of mental health and OUD
2. Psychotherapeutic intervention
   a. This may include brief intervention, brief cognitive-behavioral therapy, brief dialectical-behavioral therapy, and motivational interviewing.
   b. The type of psychological techniques will ultimately depend on disciplines represented on the team.
3. Medical management of opioid use through pharmacotherapy-related clinical activities
4. Medical management of pain
5. Linkage of care via referral to treatment, utilization of care pathways, and/or bridge clinics

Conclusion

Adequate care for neurosurgical patients with OUD requires a greater understanding of psychosocial interactions that impact and influence treatment needs. In fact, medical management, though effective, is often incomplete and optimized when nonpharmacologic interventions are administered during admission. Social workers are specifically trained, and the role is specifically tailored, to provide evidence-based interventions to patients. They can be an indispensable option for overworked nursing staff with high patient loads.

Furthermore, the utilization of social workers can deescalate the tension and stigma often salient throughout medical care administration due to negative patient-staff interactions. Inadequate management of withdrawal symptoms and other underlying mental health disorders can create a hostile environment that stifles self-efficacy and acts as a barrier to recovery. Social workers have the knowledge and skillset to navigate this environment and empower patients to facilitate change. This can create a more effective healing environment for patients and medical staff.

References

1. Zadoretzky C, McKnight C, Bramson H, et al. The New York 911 Good Samaritan law and opioid overdose prevention among people who inject drugs. *World Med Health Policy*. 2017;9(3):318–340.
2. Naeger S, Mutter R, Ali MM, et al. Post-discharge treatment engagement among patients with an opioid-use disorder. *J Subst Abuse Treat*. 2016;69:64–71. doi:10.1016/j.jsat.2016.07.004.
3. Priest KC, Englander H, McCarty D. "Now hospital leaders are paying attention": a qualitative study of internal and external factors influencing addiction consult services. *J Subst Abuse Treat*. 2020;110:59–65. doi:10.1016/j.jsat.2019.12.003.
4. Priest KC, McCarty D. Making the business case for an addiction medicine consult service: a qualitative analysis. *BMC Health Serv Res*. 2019;19(1):822.
5. Wakeman SE, Rigotti NA, Herman GE, et al. The effectiveness of post-discharge navigation added to an inpatient addiction consultation for patients with substance use disorder; a randomized controlled trial. *Subst Abus*. 2021;42(4):646–653. doi:10.1080/08897077.2020.1809608.
6. Gryczynski J, Nordeck CD, Welsh C, et al. Preventing hospital readmission for patients with comorbid substance use disorder: a randomized trial. *Ann Intern Med*. 2021;174(7):899–909.
7. Liebschutz JM, Crooks D, Herman D, et al. Buprenorphine treatment for hospitalized, opioid-dependent patients: a randomized clinical trial. *JAMA Intern Med*. 2014;174(8):1369–1376.
8. Wakeman SE, Metlay JP, Chang Y, et al. Inpatient addiction consultation for hospitalized patients increases post-discharge abstinence and reduces addiction severity. *J Gen Intern Med*. 2017;32(8):909–916. doi:10.1007/s11606-017-4077-z.
9. McNeely J, Troxel AB, Kunins HV, et al. Study protocol for a pragmatic trial of the consult for addiction treatment and care in hospitals (CATCH) model for engaging patients in opioid use disorder treatment. *Addict Sci Clin Pract*. 2019;14(1):5. doi:10.1186/s13722-019-0135-7.
10. Weinstein ZM, Wakeman SE, Nolan S. Inpatient addiction consult service: expertise for hospitalized patients with complex addiction problems. *Med Clin North Am*. 2018;102(4):587–601. doi:10.1016/j.mcna.2018.03.001.
11. Wilson JD, Altieri Dunn SC, Roy P, et al. Inpatient addiction medicine consultation service impact on post-discharge patient mortality: a propensity-matched analysis. *J Gen Intern Med*. 2022;37(10):2521–2525. doi:10.1007/s11606-021-07362-8.
12. Weinstein ZM, Cheng DM, D'Amico MJ, et al. Inpatient addiction consultation and post-discharge 30-day acute care utilization. *Drug Alcohol Depend*. 2020;213:108081.
13. Glass JE, Ilgen MA, Winters JJ, et al. Inpatient hospitalization in addiction treatment for patients with a history of suicide attempt: a case of support for treatment performance measures. *J Psychoactive Drugs*. 2010;42(3):315–325.
14. Vogel E, Ly K, Ramo DE, et al. Strategies to improve treatment utilization for substance use disorders: a systematic review of intervention studies. *Drug Alcohol Depend*. 2020:108065.
15. Murphy MK, Chabon B, Delgado A, et al. Development of a substance abuse consultation and referral service in an academic medical center: challenges, achievements and dissemination. *J Clin PsycholMed Settings*. 2009;16(1):77–86. doi:10.1007/s10880-009-9149-8.
16. Kitchen A, Brook J. Social work at the heart of the medical team. *Soc Work Health Care*. 2005;40(4):1–18. doi:10.1300/J010v40n04_01.
17. Cowles LA, Lefcowitz MJ. Interdisciplinary expectations of the medical social worker in the hospital setting. *Health SocWork*. 1992;17(1):57–65.
18. Holliman D, Dziegielewski SF, Teare R. Differences and similarities between social work and nurse discharge planners. *Health Soc Work*. 2003;28(3):224–231.

19. Maramaldi P, Sobran A, Scheck L, et al. Interdisciplinary medical social work: a working taxonomy. *Soc Work Health Care*. 2014;53(6):532–551. doi:10.1080/00981389.2014.905817.

20. Simon R, Snow R, Wakeman S. Understanding why patients with substance use disorders leave the hospital against medical advice: a qualitative study. *Subst Abus*. 2020;41(4):519–525. doi:10.1080/08897077.2019.1671942.

21. Hyshka E, Morris H, Anderson-Baron J, et al. Patient perspectives on a harm reduction-oriented addiction medicine consultation team implemented in a large acute care hospital. *Drug Alcohol Depend*. 2019;204:107523. doi:10.1016/j.drugalcdep.2019.06.025.

22. Punches BE, Ali AA, Brown JL, et al. Opioid-related risk screening measures for the emergency care setting. *Adv Emerg Nurs J*. 2021;43(4):331–343. doi:10.1097/TME.0000000000000377.

23. Singer M, Bulled N, Ostrach B, et al. Syndemics and the biosocial conception of health. *Lancet*. 2017;389(10072):941–950.

24. Thoele K, Draucker CB, Newhouse R. Implementation of screening, brief intervention, and referral to treatment (SBIRT) by nurses on acute care units: a qualitative descriptive study. *Subst Abus*. 2021;42(4):662–671. doi:10.1080/08897077.2020.1823549.

25. Keen A, Thoele K, Newhouse R. Variation in SBIRT delivery among acute care facilities. *Nurs Outlook*. 2020;68(2):162–168. doi:10.1016/j.outlook.2019.09.001.

26. Keen A, Thoele K, Oruche U, et al. Perceptions of the barriers, facilitators, outcomes, and helpfulness of strategies to implement screening, brief intervention, and referral to treatment in acute care. *Implement Sci*. 2021;16(1):44. doi:10.1186/s13012-021-01116-0.

27. Mitchell SG, Gryczynski J, O'Grady KE, et al. SBIRT for adolescent drug and alcohol use: current status and future directions. *J Subst Abuse Treat*. 2013;44(5):463–472.

28. Lusk SL, Stipp A, Rumrill PD, et al. Opioid use disorders as an emerging disability. *J Vocation Rehab*. 2018;48(3):345–358. doi:10.3233/jvr-180943.

29. Weinstein ZM, Cheng DM, D'Amico MJ, et al. Inpatient addiction consultation and post-discharge 30-day acute care utilization. *Drug Alcohol Depend*. 2020;213:108081. doi:10.1016/j.drugalcdep.2020.108081.

30. Senreich E, Ogden LP, Greenberg JP. A postgraduation follow-up of social work students trained in "SBIRT": rates of usage and perceptions of effectiveness. *Social Work Health Care*. 2017;56(5):412–434. doi:10.1080/00981389.2017.1290010.

31. Martin MP, Woodside SG, Lee C, et al. SBIRT training: how do social work students compare to medical learners? *Soc Work Health Care*. 2021;60(10):631–641. doi:10.1080/00981389.2021.2001711.

32. Holt M, Reed M, Woodruff SI, et al. Adaptation of screening, brief intervention, referral to treatment to active duty military personnel in an emergency department: findings from a formative research study. *Mil Med*. 2017;182(7):e1801–e1807. doi:10.7205/MILMED-D-16-00333.

33. Garland EL, Hanley AW, Riquino MR, et al. Mindfulness-oriented recovery enhancement reduces opioid misuse risk via analgesic and positive psychological mechanisms: a randomized controlled trial. *J Consult Clin Psychol*. 2019;87(10):927–940.

34. Garland EL, Manusov EG, Froeliger B, et al. Mindfulness-oriented recovery enhancement for chronic pain and prescription opioid misuse: results from an early-stage randomized controlled trial. *J Consult Clin Psychol*. 2014;82(3):448–459.

35. Huhn AS, Gipson CD. Promoting harm reduction as a treatment outcome in substance use disorders. *Exp Clin Psychopharmacol*. 2021;29(3):217–218.

36. Clarke K, Harris D, Zweifler JA, et al. The significance of harm reduction as a social and health care intervention for injecting drug users: an exploratory study of a needle exchange program in Fresno, California. *Soc Work Public Health*. 2016;31(5):398–407.

37. Phillips KT, Rosenberg H. The development and evaluation of the harm reduction self-efficacy questionnaire. *Psychol Addict Behav*. 2008;22(1):36–46.

38. McKay JR. Impact of continuing care on recovery from substance use disorder. *Alcohol Res*. 2021;41(1):1.

39. McKay JR. Continuing care research: what we have learned and where we are going. *J Subst Abuse Treat*. 2009;36(2):131–145.

40. Gurewich D, Garg A, Kressin NR. Addressing social determinants of health within healthcare delivery systems: a framework to ground and inform health outcomes. *J Gen Intern Med*. 2020;35(5):1571–1575. doi:10.1007/s11606-020-05720-6.

41. Priest KC, McCarty D. The role of the hospital in the 21st century opioid overdose epidemic: the addiction medicine consult service. *J Addict Med*. 2019;13(2):104–112.

Questions

Millie is a 26-year-old female who was unresponsive upon admission. She has a past medical history of opioid misuse. The patient's friend was present and reported that when he found the patient, he administered intranasal naloxone, and emergency technicians administered another dose. When the patient awoke, she removed the oropharyngeal airway and was noted to be alert and oriented, with a respiratory rate of 16 breaths per minute, but had significant weakness in her legs. Oxygen was administered through a nasal cannula at a rate of 6 L/min. Upon evaluation, the patient was admitted for spinal osteomyelitis. When admitted, Millie started experiencing withdrawal symptoms, extreme pain, and was notably agitated. A social worker was consulted to administer the brief inpatient intervention and address postdischarge options for the management of misuse.

1. When caring for patients, social workers are only consulted:
   a. If the patient has a diagnosis of OUD
   b. If a patient is denied/refused OUD therapy postdischarge
   c. When there is any indication of opioid misuse and screening, intervention and management can be implemented
   d. To assist with finding supplemental income and housing for homeless patients

2. Millie consistently complains of "10/10 pain" and withdrawal symptoms, but the nurse suspects that the patient is utilizing manipulative behaviors to gain additional pain medication management. What is the appropriate response?
   a. Consult the provider about pain management and social work to address symptoms of misuse with brief inpatient nonpharmacologic intervention.
   b. Avoid consulting additional staff due to fear of behavior escalation.
   c. The nurse should bargain with Millie and administer additional pain medication *only* if she agrees to initiate Suboxone therapy.
   d. Continue to delay administering medications until the patient leaves against medical advice.

3. Millie calls the nurse to ask for an additional dose of hydromorphone. The nurse informs the patient that she is not due for his dose for another hour. She becomes visibly upset and quickly escalates, yelling at the nurse. What should the nurse do next?
   a. Validate the patient's feelings of discomfort and consult social work to provide nonpharmacologic management until his dose is due.
   b. Tell the patient she needs to "just calm down."
   c. Tell the patient she won't get any more pain medication if she continues to act belligerent.
   d. Apply restraints to the patient and place on 1:1.

4. A nurse enters the room and notices Millie exhibiting strange behaviors. The nurse becomes suspicious that she is continuing to use (drugs) within the facility. What are the next steps the nurse should take?
   a. Notify the provider for medical management and educate the patient on the counteracting effects of inpatient use.
   b. Follow option (a) and consult social work to discuss hospital protocols and avenues for harm reduction if the patient is not ready to be abstinent.
   c. Ignore the patient's request for any additional assistance and tell her that using drugs in the hospital has made her unworthy of care.
   d. Call administration to have the patient forced out of the hospital to make room for patients willing to comply with treatment.

5. Upon discharge, Millie should be provided with which of the following?
   a. Access to naloxone to avoid future overdose incidences
   b. Adequate case management services to ensure a safe discharge
   c. Follow-up appointment with an outpatient health care provider to ensure the continuation of care
   d. All the above

Answers

1. c

2. a

3. a

4. b

5. d

Posthospitalization Care

CHAPTER 33

Rehabilitation of the Neurosurgical Patient

Kelly Hufford, PT, DPT

Introduction

Physical therapists (PT) and occupational therapists (OT) play a vital role in the recovery after surgery by providing early and progressive patient-centered interventions, which can reduce hospital length of stay, decrease delirium, and improve functional independence.[1] A comprehensive therapy evaluation includes obtaining the patient's history, conducting a systems review, performing tests to identify and measure deficits, and assessing the patient's ability to perform functional tasks.[2] Therapists then generate a plan of care that includes an analysis of the medical information obtained, social history, and the patient's clinical findings upon presentation, in comparison to the baseline level of function. This plan includes specific types of skilled interventions, goals for the patient's progressive recovery, and recommendations regarding postacute resources for discharge planning.[3] PT and OT must collaborate closely with other health care professionals such as nurses, physicians, speech-language pathologists (SLP), case managers, and social workers to create an interdisciplinary plan of care and ensure a safe discharge process.

Patients may benefit from a therapy evaluation after neurosurgical procedures if they demonstrate a decline in functional mobility or the performance of an activity of daily living (ADL), suffer a change in mental status or a new cognitive impairment, or require skilled training to maximize independence in functional mobility and self-care tasks. PT and OT roles often overlap in the immediate postoperative period, and each will focus on increasing mobility, maximizing independence with daily tasks, educating on postoperative precautions and restrictions, and recommending assistive devices or adaptive equipment. Therapists may offer suggestions regarding environmental adaptations to assist with physical, perceptual, and cognitive functioning, as well as provide caregiver training to maximize safety in the home.[1]

Role of the Physical Therapist Versus Occupational Therapist

Physical therapists assess the quality and efficiency of movement to develop and facilitate interventions focused on restoring an individual's functional independence.[3] Important tasks regularly addressed by PT include bed mobility, transfers, gait training, wheelchair assessment and training, stair training, brace management, and recommendations for assistive devices. In the acute care setting, interventions may include strengthening, endurance training, neuromuscular reeducation, and balance activities. The use of weights and resistance bands is typically avoided, however, until the patient is cleared by the surgeon for these more strenuous activities. Therapists educate patients on upper and lower extremity exercises that can be performed while sitting or standing. Balance exercises may be performed while sitting or standing and are advanced by progressively decreasing the amount of support provided or by adding dynamic movements. For example, once a patient tolerates static standing with or without a device, the therapist may progress the activity to standing at the sink to perform a self-care task. Therapists might challenge the patient's balance during ambulation by removing the assistive device or incorporating head turns or obstacles. Before discharge to home, PT frequently make recommendations regarding the use of assistive devices, review mobility techniques, and provide training to caregivers to maximize the patient's safety and success while at home.

Occupational therapists review the patient's prehospitalization level of function, evaluate patient's current capacity for participation, assess cognitive status, estimate the likelihood of resuming previous roles, and develop individualized goals to optimize recovery. OT interventions focus on restoring the patient's ability to complete ADLs. Neurosurgical patients with postoperative limitations often benefit from self-care retraining using adaptive equipment and compensatory strategies, including brace management and custom splint fabrication. An OT cognitive evaluation of the patient contributes to the individualized treatment plan and includes an assessment of attention, memory, and executive function.[1] Older patients are more susceptible to hospital-acquired delirium after surgery and may present with fluctuating levels of consciousness, decreased attention, disorientation, delusions, or hallucinations. An OT consultation may be warranted if nursing staff is concerned about the patient's ability to follow commands, recall information or recent events, or if there are new vision impairments. An OT evaluation might include recommendations for increasing the patient's level of participation, implementing safety precautions, and training caregivers in preparation for discharge.

Discharge Recommendations

PT and OT collaborate with the interdisciplinary team to determine an appropriate discharge disposition for each patient. When making a recommendation for discharge, therapists consider the patient's current level of function and disability, the patient's wishes and needs, the current living situation (including home setup and availability of resources and support), and the patient's ability to participate in the postacute rehabilitation required to maximize recovery potential.[2] Table 33.1 includes a summary of common discharge dispositions and their corresponding resources, indications, and requirements.

Activity Measure for Post-Acute Care

The Activity Measure for Post-Acute Care (AM-PAC) is a validated tool that measures functional limitations in patients across different health care settings.[4,5] In the acute care setting, AM-PAC "6-Clicks" short forms are used to score the patient's performance of basic mobility and daily activities. The Basic Mobility Short Form addresses bed mobility, transfers, ambulation, and staircase management; the Daily Activity Short Form focuses on dressing, bathing, toileting, grooming, and eating. Both forms consist of six items, each of which is scored on a scale of 1 (unable, total assistance required) to 4 (no difficulty, no assistance required) according to the degree of assistance that the patient requires to complete the task. The total score for each form ranges from 6 to 24, with higher scores indicating a higher level of function.

Studies have shown that Basic Mobility and Daily Activity scores are predictive of the patient's discharge needs and most likely destination (e.g., home or rehab). Patients with Basic Mobility scores ≥17 have better odds of being discharged to home, whereas scores ≤16 indicate a need for increased support and possibly discharge to a postacute care facility. A Daily Activity score >19 also is predictive of discharge to home, and patients who score ≤19 are more likely to be discharged to a facility.[6]

Scoring of the forms is based on clinical judgment through direct observation of the patient's performance. It can be completed by PT or OT during each session or by trained nursing staff at

TABLE 33.1 ■ Common Discharge Recommendation Terms Used by Physical Therapy (PT) and Occupation Therapy (OT)

Home	
With or without assistance	Necessity and amount of assistance are dependent on the patient's level of function, ability to perform activities of daily living, use of an assistive device (which may impede the performance of household tasks), and understanding of and compliance with safety precautions.
Home PT/OT	Therapists perform in-home safety evaluations and recommend home modifications, assess carryover of learning, and progress patient's mobility to community level.
Outpatient PT/OT	Once cleared by the surgeon, patients can maximize their balance, fine- and gross-motor coordination, endurance, or strength.
Inpatient Rehabilitation Facility	
Acute level	• Must tolerate 3–4 hours of PT/OT/speech-language pathology (SLP) per day
	• Must have comprehensive rehab needs from multiple disciplines (PT/OT/SLP) and rehabilitation physicians (physical medicine and rehab [PM&R]/rehabilitation psychiatry)
	• Must have significant functional loss with medical complexity requiring daily physician involvement
	• Patients with short length of stay should have good potential for return home with consideration of family support and home setup
	• Typical diagnoses: spine injury or surgery with spinal cord involvement, new diagnosis or exacerbation of neuromuscular disorder resulting in change from baseline level of function, traumatic brain injury
	• Spinal cord injury (SCI) rehab: specialized for patients after trauma or tumor removal with SCI presentation requiring extensive durable medical equipment needs, transfers/mobility training, SCI education, and family training
	• Brain injury rehab unit (BIRU): for patients presenting with severe attention issues in need of significant cognitive therapy in addition to functional retraining
	• Low-stimulation BIRU: specialized program for patients after severe brain injury who are showing signs of emergence; goal of program to increase tracking, arousal, and command following to progress to BIRU program
Subacute level	• Must tolerate 2–3 hours of PT/OT/SLP per day
	• Must have rehab needs from at least two disciplines (PT/OT/SLP/PM&R)
	• Appropriate for patients with decreased activity tolerance that need less intense rehabilitation over a longer duration to achieve goals before returning home
Long-Term Acute Care Hospital (LTACH)	• Not a therapy recommendation
	• Patients may receive therapy services while at an LTACH, but primary focus is on maximizing medical stability through ventilator weaning, wound care, antibiotic administration, etc.

regular intervals. When completed by nursing staff, the AM-PAC score can serve as a guide for optimal inpatient therapy consultation. Patients with only minimal functional limitations (e.g., raw scores >18) may not require inpatient therapy consultation, but these cases should still be discussed with the interprofessional team to ensure collective agreement on the plan of care.[7] For example, patients who were independent preceding surgery typically can be mobilized by nursing staff without waiting for a therapy evaluation. Nursing-led mobilization of patients with higher

AM-PAC scores has the added benefit of expediting the patient's recovery, reducing hospital length of stay, and minimizing unnecessary therapy consultations, which allows the reallocation of therapy resources to patients with greater degrees of impairment.[7,8]

Brace Utilization After Spinal Surgery

The goal of bracing after spine surgery is to limit the mobility of the spine, reduce postoperative pain, improve rates of fusion, and prompt patients to avoid movements that may compromise their recovery. Despite the intended benefits of bracing, a systematic review concluded that there is low to moderate evidence suggesting no significant differences in disability, pain, quality of life, functional impairment, or radiographic outcomes between braced and nonbraced individuals after spine surgery.[9] Due to the limited evidence available, spine surgeons often rely on their clinical experience to determine their own postoperative bracing protocols. Table 33.2 summarizes various types of braces that may be utilized after spine surgery.

Patients and staff should follow the surgeon's instructions regarding brace requirements. After a traumatic spinal injury, patients may need to wear the brace at all times or don the brace in the supine position (using the log roll technique) until the spine is stabilized. Postoperatively, some patients may need to wear a rigid collar at all times; others may be allowed to wear a soft collar in bed, a rigid collar when out of bed, and a separate collar (such as the Philadelphia collar) for showering. In other cases, patients may have to wear a rigid cervical collar in bed but don more supportive bracing, such as a CTO brace, when getting out of bed. Patients who have undergone elective thoracic and/or lumbar surgery may be permitted to don the brace while sitting or standing. PT, OT, and nursing staff play a pivotal role in educating patients about proper bracing techniques.

Proper wear and care of the brace are important for patient comfort and adherence. Brace management should be reviewed frequently with patients and families to reinforce the correct use of the brace and their understanding of its purpose. Cervical collar padding should be replaced and cleaned as needed to prevent infection. Thoracic and lumbar orthoses should be worn over a thin shirt, rather than against the skin, to protect the surgical incision and prevent skin breakdown. If nursing staff suspect that the collar or brace does not fit properly, causes pain, or is missing components, they should alert the surgical team and orthotist to refit or replace the brace before the patient is discharged.

Precautions and Restrictions After Neurosurgery

Postoperative precautions and mobility restrictions promote healing and prevent complications. Patients should be informed that their mobility and completion of ADLs might require modified techniques during the postoperative period. Educating patients regarding their postoperative precautions and encouraging adherence to the plan of care are important interprofessional efforts and shared responsibility.

SPINAL PRECAUTIONS

After spine surgery, standard precautions and restrictions should be followed for 6–8 weeks or as instructed by the surgeon. If the surgeon recommends additional activity restrictions, these should also be implemented and reviewed with the patient in anticipation of discharge. Spinal precautions typically include:

- No bending, lifting, or twisting
  - Avoid excessive bending other than to perform mobility
  - Avoid lifting anything over 5 lb
  - Use the log roll technique to get in and out of bed

TABLE 33.2 ■ Braces Commonly Utilized After Neurosurgical Spine Surgery

Cervical Collars

Soft Collar	Rigid Collar[14]	Cervical-Thoracic Orthosis (CTO)[15]
• For pain control or to support the neck after injury or surgery	• Supports the neck and restricts head and neck movement; chin should rest on support and collar should be snug (e.g., Miami J, Aspen collar, Philadelphia collar)	• Rigid brace that restricts neck and upper back movement • Often similar to rigid cervical collars but connects to anterior and posterior thoracic sections, which wrap around the chest 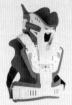

Back Braces[16]

Lumbar-Sacral Orthosis (LSO)	Thoracic-Lumbar-Sacral Orthosis (TLSO)	Custom-Molded Orthosis
• Provides lumbar support and prevents excessive bending, lifting, or twisting; brace should be positioned just above the hips, waist panels connected, and pull tabs utilized to create compression	• Provides support of lower and upper spine and prevents excessive bending, lifting, or twisting • Some TLSO designs resemble a backpack with shoulder straps connecting the rigid posterior piece with the waist strap • A TLSO with a rigid sternal piece provides anterior and posterior support to the wearer; sternal piece should be adjusted to sit ~1–2 inches below the sternal notch	• Molded plastic fabricated as either two pieces that fasten together on the sides (clam-shell style) or one large wraparound piece • May be LSO or TLSO or modified as needed, such as TLSO with a leg extension or custom CTLSO • Due to the custom design, these braces may be more difficult for patients and caregivers to don and doff; contact the orthotist for issues with fit or areas of irritation, or a physical or occupational therapist to assist with positioning

Images from: Second row: Left/center, Courtesy Mayfield Clinic; right, courtesy Össur. Bottom row: Left/center top, Courtesy Aspen Medical Products; center bottom, courtesy Mayfield Clinic.

■ If ordered by the surgeon, wear a brace as instructed
■ Avoid sitting for prolonged periods of time by standing or ambulating every hour
■ No strenuous activity (such as raking, shoveling, vacuuming) or driving until cleared by the surgeon

CRANIAL PRECAUTIONS

The objectives of cranial precautions are to decrease swelling and avoid increasing intracranial pressure. These precautions are most relevant for patients who have undergone a craniotomy for tumor resection or hematoma evacuation, craniectomy, suboccipital craniectomy, arteriovenous malformation embolization, or treatment of an aneurysm (e.g., coiling, stenting, clipping). Activity precautions should be followed until the surgeon clears the patient to resume unrestricted activity. Cranial precautions include:

- Avoid excessive bending and keep the head above the level of the heart.
- Avoid pushing, pulling, or lifting objects weighing more than 5–10 lb.
- Avoid lying flat by using pillows to keep the head elevated.
- No strenuous activity (such as raking, shoveling, vacuuming) or driving until cleared by the surgeon.
- If a bone flap was removed (craniectomy), then a helmet might be necessary when out of bed (depending on the size of the craniectomy) unless instructed otherwise by the surgeon. After the bone flap is replaced or a cranioplasty is performed, patients no longer need to wear a helmet.

Mobility Considerations After Neurosurgery

BED MOBILITY AND POSITIONING

While in bed, patients should reposition frequently to prevent skin breakdown and pressure injuries. If patients are unable to reposition independently, caregivers should assist with turning every 2 hours. Proper positioning includes a semi-side-lying position with a pillow or wedge under the back to offload the sacrum. A pillow positioned between the patient's knees can alleviate pressure on the bony prominence and promote correct spinal alignment. Pillows should also be placed under the patient's calves to float the heels above the mattress, thereby minimizing the risk of developing pressure injuries. The head of the bed should be no higher than 30 degrees to avoid shearing forces, except for brief periods when patients are eating. Patients with decreased lower extremity strength or impaired mobility may also benefit from the application of a multipodus boot or pressure-relief ankle-foot orthosis (PRAFO) to assist with offloading and to avoid plantar flexion contractures. Firm PRAFO boots can be used if the patient is able to achieve neutral ankle positioning, and they should be worn for 2 hours at a time, alternating on/off throughout the day to prevent skin breakdown. Softer heel protection boots should be selected if the patient has a plantar flexion contracture or increased tone in the lower extremities. These can be worn in conjunction with intermittent pneumatic compression devices.

After spine surgery, patients should use the log roll technique for bed mobility to maintain neutral spine positioning. Flattening the head of the bed will help maintain spinal precautions during mobility.

- Supine to sitting on the edge of the bed: After flexing the knees, the patient should reach for the rail and push through the legs to roll onto the side. Both legs should be brought over the edge of the bed, then the patient can push with the arms into a seated position.
- Sitting to supine: From the seated position, the patient should lower onto the shoulder, reaching the opposite arm in front of the body toward the railing. Both legs should be lifted onto the bed to achieve a side-lying posture before rolling back into a supine position.
- Caregivers should support the patient's shoulders and hips for rolling, bringing the lower extremities over the edge of the bed, and righting the trunk. Caregivers should never pull on the patient's neck or arms (Fig. 33.1).

TRANSFERS

Patients may require physical assistance or cueing to perform transfers safely after neurosurgical procedures. If a patient actively participates in bed mobility and safely sits at the edge of the

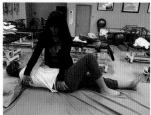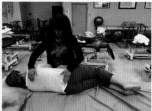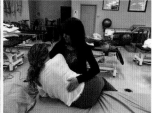

Fig. 33.1 Bed mobility technique. (From Vatwani A. Caregiver guide and instructions for safe bed mobility. *Arch Phys Med Rehabil.* 2017;98[9]1907–1910.)

bed with minimal or no assistance, an active transfer to the chair can be attempted. If a patient requires maximal assistance for bed mobility or is unable to maintain sitting balance, an overhead or mechanical lift is recommended for transfers out of bed.

- Sit-to-stand transfers: Patients should push up with the upper extremities from the seat or armrests while leaning forward and utilizing the lower extremities for upward force production. If utilizing a walker or other assistive device, the patient should keep at least one hand on the seat for support. If physical assistance is needed, caregivers should stand on either or both sides, facing the patient, and provide stabilization at the shoulder while assisting with one hand under the buttocks. Once standing, the patient can bring the other hand to the walker or to a caregiver's handheld assist.
- Stand-to-sit transfers: Before sitting down, the patient should feel the surface of the seat on the back of the legs. Patients should reach back with at least one hand for the surface before sitting. Holding onto the walker could lead to it tipping over, causing a loss of control and possibly a fall. If the patient is unable to perform the action safely, caregivers should help maintain control by slowly lowering the patient into the chair.
- Stand pivot transfers: If able to take small steps, a patient can transfer to a chair, commode, or other surface positioned close to the bed. Caregivers can provide stability by handheld assistance, supporting the waist, or utilizing an assistive device, and they should remain close to the patient. Depending on the patient's cognition and functional level, caregivers should offer verbal or tactile cueing to advance the lower extremities and take steps toward the next surface.

AMBULATION

Mobility is a vital component of recovery after all surgical procedures. Among patients who undergo an elective lumbar spine procedure, those who ambulate on the day of surgery have a decreased incidence of urinary retention, urinary tract infections, and ileus. Same-day ambulation is also associated with a decreased length of stay, increased likelihood of discharge to home, and decreased rate of readmission for patients after spinal fusions.[10,11] Patients who ambulated with an assistive device (e.g., cane or walker) preoperatively may feel more comfortable using the same device postoperatively. For patients who were ambulatory without assistance preoperatively or who appear uncomfortable managing a new assistive device postoperatively, PT should be consulted to assist in selecting the optimal device and providing training on its safe and appropriate use.

Due to a restricted range of neck motion, patients who need to wear a cervical collar may have a limited view of their environment. These patients should be instructed to scan their environment during ambulation. Upon returning home, patients and their families should be advised to remove obstacles from common routes, remove rugs to avoid tripping, and maintain close supervision when performing higher-level mobility, such as stair negotiation or ambulation in the community.

ACTIVITIES OF DAILY LIVING

After a neurosurgical procedure, patients may need to modify the techniques previously used to perform daily activities. OT can recommend alternative strategies and adaptive equipment to maximize patients' independence while following precautions.[12,13]

- Dressing: Loose clothing (button-down shirts, V-neck shirts, sweatpants) enhance the ease with which patients can get dressed. Patients should dress their lower body while seated, crossing one leg over the other or using an adaptive device to avoid bending. OT can train patients to dress with the assistance of a dressing stick, long-handled reacher, sock aid, or shoehorn.
- Toileting: After spine surgery, patients may experience difficulty with personal hygiene due to restrictions on bending and twisting or limitations imposed by braces. If a patient does not have assistance at home, OT can recommend tools and techniques to maximize independence.
- Bathing: Patients should perform lower body bathing in a seated position using a shower chair or bench to ensure safety and conserve energy. Spine patients may need to wear a different collar during showering.

SEATING

Postsurgical patients with impaired mobility may benefit from specialized support surfaces to promote skin protection. These surfaces should be considered for patients who have previously had or currently have a pressure injury (especially in the sacral region), bony prominences at high risk for skin breakdown, impaired nutrition, increased moisture on the skin, obesity, or impaired sensory perception. Pressure redistribution surfaces, such as a pressure-relieving air cushion (e.g., wheelchair with a Roho cushion), may be indicated. PT and OT can identify an appropriate seating and cushion combination for the patient based on the degree of injury, risk level, and the patient's body type and size.

Regardless of the type of surface, patients should perform weight shifts every 30–60 minutes while seated. Weight shift techniques include standing for several minutes, performing a seated pushup and holding for 5–10 seconds, anterior lean to offload the ischial tuberosities, or lateral lean held for at least 1 minute while ensuring that the ischial tuberosity is offloaded. If a patient has limited mobility and is unable to participate in weight shifts, then the patient may benefit from a wheelchair that enables caregivers and staff to perform tilt back weight shifts for 5 minutes every 30 minutes and regular skin assessments to monitor areas of concern. Nursing staff, patients, and families ought to discuss the specific details regarding weight shift techniques with PT or OT to be certain that they achieve proper offloading of areas at risk for pressure injury.

Considerations for Nursing

To prevent workplace injuries, nursing staff should utilize proper body mechanics while providing patient care. When assisting patients with mobility, hospital staff should:

- Maintain a center of gravity over the base of support and avoid reaching and leaning.
- Keep feet at shoulder width apart to maintain balance and base of support.
- When lifting, use a squat position with force production coming from the legs.
- Use a draw sheet under the patient to aid in repositioning in bed.
- Avoid bending over by elevating the height of the bed to the waist level of the shortest staff member when performing care or repositioning the patient.
- If tolerated, position the bed in Trendelenburg for gravity to assist when repositioning larger patients.
- If available, utilize a repositioning sling with overhead lift systems for rolling or repositioning bariatric patients in bed. High-back or split-leg slings can be used with the overhead lift system to transfer a patient from the bed to a chair or commode.

Patients undergoing neurosurgical procedures may have cognitive deficits that inhibit their ability to follow commands, process information, or initiate a response. When working with patients who have cognitive deficits, caregivers should provide simple, one- or two-step instructions, along with tactile cues or gestures as needed. Patients should be given ample time to process instructions and initiate mobility.

Conclusion

Mobility is a critical component of the postoperative recovery process. Nurses play a central role in patient mobilization by assisting patients out of the bed and into a chair, helping patients get to the bathroom, and ambulating patients in between therapy sessions. Collaboration between nursing and therapy staff can maximize patients' performance and recovery by coordinating therapy sessions with pain medication administration, communicating a shared plan of care to patients and their families, and preparing the patient for discharge from the hospital.

References

1. Roberts P, Robinson M, Furniss J, et al. Occupational therapy's value in provision of quality care to prevent readmissions. *Am J Occup Ther*. 2020;74(3):7403090010p1-7403090010p9.
2. Smith BA, Fields CJ, Fernandez N. Physical therapists make accurate and appropriate discharge recommendations for patients who are acutely ill. *Phys Ther*. 2010;90(5):693–703.
3. Masley PM, Havrilko CL, Mahnensmith MR, et al. Physical therapist practice in the acute care setting: a qualitative study. *Phys Ther*. 2011;91(6):906–919.
4. Jette DU, Stilphen M, Ranganathan VK, et al. Validity of the AM-PAC "6-clicks" inpatient daily activity and basic mobility short forms. *Phys Ther*. 2014;94(3):379–391.
5. Jette DU, Stilphen M, Ranganathan VK, et al. AM-PAC "6-clicks" functional assessment scores predict acute care hospital discharge destination. *Phys Ther*. 2014;94(9):1252–1261.
6. Warren M, Knecht J, Verheijde J, et al. Association of AM-PAC "6-clicks" basic mobility and daily activity scores with discharge destination. *Phys Ther*. 2021;101(4):pzab043.
7. Probasco JC, Lavezza A, Cassell A, et al. Choosing wisely together: physical and occupational therapy consultation for acute neurology inpatients. *Neurohospitalist*. 2018;8(2):53–59.
8. Martinez M, Cerasale M, Baig M, et al. Defining potential overutilization of physical therapy consults on hospital medicine services. *J Hosp Med*. 2021. https://shmpublications.onlinelibrary.wiley.com/doi/abs/10.12788/jhm.3673. Accessed October 18, 2021.
9. Zhu MP, Tetreault LA, Sorefan-Mangou F, et al. Efficacy, safety, and economics of bracing after spine surgery: a systematic review of the literature. *Spine J*. 2018;18(9):1513–1525.
10. Adogwa O, Elsamadicy AA, Fialkoff J, et al. Early ambulation decreases length of hospital stay, perioperative complications and improves functional outcomes in elderly patients undergoing surgery for correction of adult degenerative scoliosis. *Spine*. 2017;42(18):1420–1425.
11. Zakaria HM, Bazydlo M, Schultz L, et al. Ambulation on postoperative day #0 is associated with decreased morbidity and adverse events after elective lumbar spine surgery: analysis from the Michigan Spine Surgery Improvement Collaborative (MSSIC). *Neurosurgery*. 2020;87(2):320–328.
12. Bondoc S, Lashgari D, Hermann V, et al. Occupational therapy in acute care. American Occupational Therapy Association. Updated 2017. https://www.aota.org/about-occupational-therapy/professionals/rdp/acutecare.aspx. Accessed October 18, 2021.
13. University of Washington Medical Center Health Online. Activities of daily living after a craniotomy: for your healing and safety. Updated April 2019. https://healthonline.washington.edu/sites/default/files/record_pdfs/Activities-Daily-Living-After-Craniotomy.pdf. Accessed October 18, 2021.
14. Mayfield Brain & Spine. Braces for your neck. Updated April 2020. https://mayfieldclinic.com/pe-braces-neck.htm. Accessed October 18, 2021.
15. Mayfield Brain & Spine. Braces for your cervical-thoracic spine. Revised April 2020. https://mayfieldclinic.com/pe-ct-braces.htm. Accessed October 18, 2021.
16. Mayfield Brain & Spine. Braces for your back. Revised April 2020. https://mayfieldclinic.com/pe-back-braces.htm. Accessed October 18, 2021.

Questions

Janet is an 82-year-old female with a past medical history of hypertension, diabetes, left hip replacement, and chronic low back pain caused by spinal stenosis. She has maintained her independence, walking without an assistive device, until recently. Due to the pain, her mobility has become more limited, she has had two recent falls, and she now relies on her family to perform household tasks. Conservative treatments, including physical therapy, epidural injections, and various pain medications, have had minimal effect on her pain. Janet wants to regain her independence and return to participating in community activities, so she has been admitted for a posterior lumbar decompression and fusion from L3–L5. Postoperatively she is instructed to wear an LSO brace when out of bed.

1. After surgery, Janet is hesitant to get out of bed. Which of the following are benefits of postoperative mobility? (there may be more than one correct answer)
   a. Decreased incidence of ileus
   b. Increased length of stay
   c. Increased likelihood of discharge to home
   d. Decreased need for spine-stability bracing

2. When helping Janet to get out of bed, what is the best technique to use?
   a. Allow her to swing her legs off the bed and pull on the rail to sit upright.
   b. Utilize the log roll technique to maintain a neutral spine.
   c. Pull on her arm to help her come to a seated position.
   d. Use the overhead lift regardless of mobility to reduce risk of falls.

3. Janet requires a minimal level of assistance for bed mobility and moderate assistance to stand from the edge of the bed and take a few steps to the chair. She is unable to ambulate further or attempt stair negotiation. What is the AM-PAC Basic Mobility Short Form score?
   a. 8
   b. 12
   c. 14
   d. 20

4. Janet is motivated to walk to the bathroom, but you are concerned about her balance, strength, and activity tolerance. What is the best option for safely toileting this patient?
   a. Walk her to the bathroom with handheld assistance.
   b. Make her use the bedpan until PT/OT can evaluate her.
   c. Assist her with utilizing the bedside commode until her mobility improves.
   d. Request Foley catheter placement.

5. Janet lives alone in a two-story house with no bathroom on the first floor. She must negotiate a full flight of steps to reach her bathroom with the tub. Based on the information from the previous questions and the patient's home setup, what is the most appropriate discharge option for this patient?
   a. Inpatient rehab (subacute)
   b. Home with intermittent assistance from family who stop by once a day to help with meals
   c. Home with outpatient PT
   d. Remain inpatient until her home can undergo appropriate renovations

Answers

1. a, c
2. b
3. b
4. c
5. a

Note: Page numbers followed by '*f*' indicate figures, and '*t*' indicate tables.